THE CAMBRIDGE ILLUSTRATED HISTORY OF
Medicine

THE CAMBRIDGE ILLUSTRATED HISTORY OF

Medicine

EDITED BY ROY PORTER

CAMBRIDGE
UNIVERSITY PRESS

Published by the Press Syndicate of the University of Cambridge
The Pitt Building, Trumpington Street, Cambridge CB2 1RP
40 West 20th Street, New York, NY 10011-4211, USA
10 Stamford Road, Oakleigh, Melbourne 3166, Australia

First published 1996

Project editor: Sarah Bunney
Picture research: Sara Waterson
Layout: Andrew Shoolbred
Indexer: Barbara Hird
Cartography by European Map Graphics Ltd, Finchampstead

Origination by HiLo Offset, Colchester

Printed in Great Britain at the University Press, Cambridge

A catalogue record for this book is available from the
British Library

Library of Congress cataloguing in publication data
The Cambridge illustrated history of medicine / edited by
Roy Porter.
p. cm. – (Cambridge illustrated history)
ISBN 0-521-44211-7
1. Medicine – History. I. Porter, Roy, 1946– . II. Series.
R131.C232 1996
610'.9--dc20
95-38000
CIP

ISBN 0 521 44211 7 hardback

Half-title: A woodcut from Paracelsus's *Opus Chyrurgicum* (1565)
shows physicians and nurses attending a patient

Title-page: The old sick ward of St John's Hospital, Bruges,
by Johannes Beerblock, 1778

Contents

Introduction

Never have people in the West lived so long, or been so healthy, and never have medical achievements been so great. Yet, paradoxically, rarely has medicine drawn such intense doubts and disapproval as today. No-one could deny that the medical breakthroughs of the past 50 years – the culmination of a long tradition of scientific medicine – have saved more lives than those of any era since the dawn of medicine. So blasé have we become about medical progress, that it is worth taking stock of just some of the tremendous innovations taken for granted today yet unavailable a century or two ago. These advances are discussed and explained at length in the chapters that follow. By way of introduction, here is a brief summary of the most dramatic changes that have occurred during the second half of the twentieth century.

At the outbreak of the Second World War, penicillin was still at the laboratory stage and remained rationed for several years. Before the advent of such antibiotic 'magic bullets', pneumonia, meningitis, and similar infections were still frequently fatal. Tuberculosis – dubbed the 'white plague' to contrast it with the Black Death (and because sufferers had a characteristic pallor) – was long the single most important cause of death in the developed world. But that was given the *coup de grâce* by the introduction of the BCG vaccine and streptomycin in the 1940s. The 1950s extended the 'first pharmacological revolution' on to a broad front. The new biological drugs beat the bacteria, improved the control of deficiency diseases, and produced effective medications (such as the psychotropic drug chlorpromazine) for mental illnesses. The first vaccines against polio arrived at the same time.

Other drug breakthroughs, notably steroids such as cortisone, made it feasible to capitalize on the growing understanding of the immune system. By tackling the rejection problem, the development of immunosupressants opened up vast new fields for plastic and transplant surgery. Cardiology also blossomed. One milestone was the first surgical intervention in 1944 for 'blue babies' born with congenital heart disease; thereafter, paediatric cardiology forged ahead. Open-heart surgery dates from the 1950s; bypass operations, another leap forward, began in 1967.

By that time, surgery was beginning to resemble space travel, and it was also capturing the public's imagination; it seemed to know no bounds. Organ replacement was developed, first with kidneys. Transplants became banner headlines in 1967 when Christiaan Barnard sewed a woman's heart into Louis Washkansky, who lived for 18 days. By the mid-1980s, hundreds of heart transplants were being conducted each year in the USA alone, with two-thirds of the recipients surviving for 5 years or more. During the past 50 years, surgery has not just grown: its nature has been transformed. Early in the twentieth century, its essence lay in

Opposite: A woman's body revealed by false-colour magnetic resonance imagery (MRI). MRI is one of several recent scanning techniques developed within high-tech medicine in the past few decades. Specifically useful for the detection of abnormalities in the soft tissues of the body, its images are reconstructed by computers. Renaissance anatomy developed techniques for exploring the dead body; the invention of X-rays a century ago provided a vision of the hard parts of the living body; and now, today, the body's entire structure is becoming visible.

extirpation: locate the lesion and cut it out (often effective but rather crude). Now, its philosophy has become far more sophisticated: that of continuous repair and (perhaps endless) replaceability.

Alongside these practical leaps forward in intervention, science has been contributing to healing. Such technological breakthroughs as electron microscopes, endoscopes, computerized axial tomography (CAT), positron emission tomography (PET), magnetic resonance imaging (MRI), lasers, tracers, and ultrasound have created a revolution in medicine's diagnostic capacities. Lasers brought microsurgery. Iron lungs, kidney-dialysis machines, heart-lung machines, and pacemakers have all taken their place in medicine's armoury. Meanwhile, research in basic science has transformed our understanding of the body and its battles with disease. In particular, genetics and molecular biology developed rapidly after Francis Crick and James Watson's discovery of the double-helical structure of DNA and the cracking of the genetic code in 1953. Genetic screening and engineering have been making great headway. At the same time, brain chemistry

The 1940s brought the first surgical intervention for congenital heart disease, the so-called blue-baby syndrome, which heralded the beginnings of modern cardiac surgery. First undertaken at Johns Hopkins Hospital in Baltimore on 29 November 1944, the operation was pioneered by Helen Taussig, an American paediatrician who went on to become the first woman to be appointed a full professor at Johns Hopkins University. Taussig worked on congenital heart disease in association with the cardiac surgeon Alfred Blalock. She was actively involved in the diagnosis and aftercare of the patients on whom Blalock operated. Here she is (on the right of the photograph) with one of her patients in about 1945. The black box is a hearing aid (Taussig was partially deaf at the time).

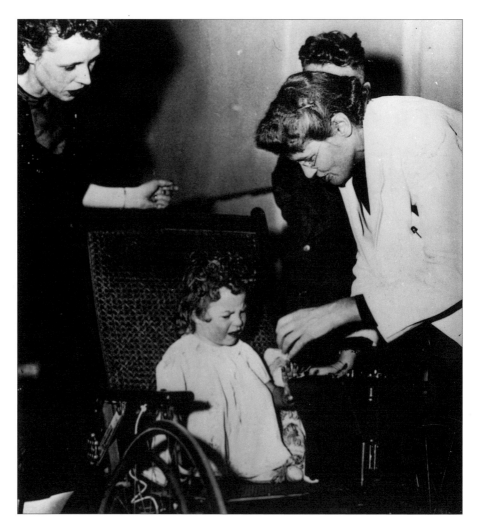

opened new horizons for medicine: research on endorphins has been laying bare and mastering the secrets of pain; synthetic manipulation of neurotransmitters such as L-dopa has provided treatments for Parkinson's disease and other disorders of the central nervous system. So long a Cinderella, clinical science – the application of scientific methods to the actual experience of sickness – has come into its own, thanks partly to the randomized clinical trial, developed from the mid-1940s.

Such advances in science and therapeutics have not blossomed in a desert. They have arisen from the vast endowment of medicine as a social utility (discussed in Chapter 9). In the UK, the creation of the National Health Service (NHS) in 1948 remains a red-letter day, but nations worldwide have been devoting ever larger public and private resources to medicine. In the USA and several European Union nations, more than 10 per cent of gross national product now goes on health. The World Health Organization (WHO) continues to expand. Its programmes of disease prevention and eradication, especially in developing countries, have had some striking successes, notably the global eradication of smallpox in 1977.

To put developments in a nutshell, two facts give powerful (if conflicting) evidence of the growing significance of medicine. First, the doubling of world population in the past 50 years (from around 2,500 million in 1950 to an estimated 6,250 million by the year 2000), no small percentage of which has been caused by new medical interventions and preventions. Second, the introduction of the contraceptive pill, which, in theory at least, paved the way for a safe and simple means to control that population. These developments are well known, but familiarity does not detract from the achievement. Many revolutions have occurred in human history – the introduction of agriculture, the growth of cities, printing, the great scientific advances in the seventeenth century, and the industrial revolutions. But not until the last half of the twentieth century has there been a medical revolution with dramatic therapeutic implications, if we take as our yardstick the dependable ability to vanquish life-threatening disease on a vast scale. The healthiness and longevity of the rich world, and the populousness of the poor world, alike attest this.

A major aim of this volume is to set those changes in medicine in their historical context. We trace the long tradition that arose out of Ancient Greece, which first set medicine on a rational and scientific foundation. We examine the transformations stimulated by the Renaissance and the Scientific Revolution, which presented medicine with the triumphs of physics and chemistry. And we consider

A page from a manuscript of William Harvey's called *De Musculis* (1619), now in the British Museum. Medicine advanced from traditional practice to scientific research once Renaissance anatomists, such as Harvey, began the systematic dissection of the human body and laid bare for the first time its various systems. Observation and experiments in the seventeenth century put medicine on a new footing.

the remarkable contribution of nineteenth-century medical science, with its advances in public health, cell biology, bacteriology, parasitology, antiseptis, and anaesthetic surgery. Major advances were made early in the twentieth century: X-rays, immunology, the understanding of hormones and vitamins, chemotherapy, even psychoanalysis.

As the following chapters show, a historical understanding of medicine is far more than a cavalcade of triumphs. It involves the attempt to explain the more distant and indirect antecedents of modern changes, to show why one path was taken and not another, to examine the interconnections of the theoretical and practical aspects of medicine, science, and healing, and doctor and patient; to analyse the relations between the broad trends and leading individuals; and, not least, to lay bare the thinking – often to our minds bizarre and unscientific – that lay behind the physiological and therapeutic systems of the past.

But *The Cambridge Illustrated History of Medicine* also attempts to go beyond simply telling the story of the rise of medicine and its interplay with science, society, and the public. It aims, through historical analysis, to put medicine under the microscope, and to raise questions about the great forces that have fuelled medical change over the centuries and continue to do so. Who has controlled medicine? Has it been shaped by supply or by demand, by money and market forces? How adequately has it met the needs of the sick? How responsive has it been to the wishes of the medical profession? What has been the role of the state in financing and directing healing?

The volume thus poses questions about medicine's social and political roles. For if healing has, obviously, been medicine's task, has it also had hidden programmes, which, as some critics have alleged, may have an unsavoury side? The

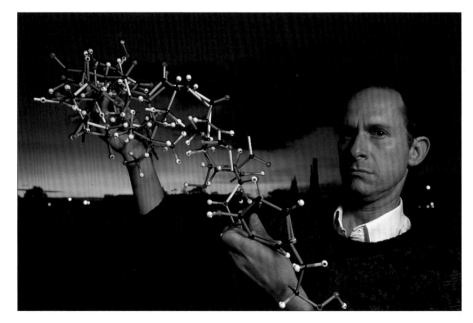

Colombian scientist Manuel Patarroyo with a model of his new chemical vaccine against malaria, a disease that affects more than 300 million people and kills around 2 million people each year, most of them children in tropical Africa. In 1995, Patarroyo gave the World Health Organization the rights to develop, distribute, and sell the vaccine – known as SPf66. Field trials in Africa have yielded contradictory results. But an effective vaccine is urgently needed because drug-resistant strains of the malaria parasite are spreading.

involvement of German doctors and scientists with the Nazi final solution, from unethical and deadly human experimentation to the supervision of the gas chambers at Auschwitz and elsewhere, needs to remembered alongside the selfless dedication of innumerable other physicians and health professionals. Partly by way of recoil from the atrocities of the Second World War, doctors have been conspicuous in humanitarian movements during the past 50 years, including campaigns for nuclear disarmanent and against torture.

Questioning the roles of medicine is important, not for any cynical reasons but because if we are to understand the directions medicine is taking now – its priorities, funding, and regulation – it is crucial that we have a historical perspective on how it has come to be. That is why it is helpful to return to the paradoxical state of medicine today.

In spite of all the tremendous advances, an atmosphere of disquiet and doubt now prevades medicine. The flag-waving optimism of the 1960s has disappeared. Euphoria bubbled up over penicillin, over the coming of heart transplants, and over the first test-tube baby, Louise Brown, in 1978. Now, fears are growing over the strange powers that medicine might assume as genetic engineering and biotechnology expand. At the same time, as health costs get out of hand, prospects loom of real medical cutbacks in major Western societies. Will the development of scientific medicine make it unaffordable to many people? Will it

Medicine has reduced infant mortality and increased life expectancy in the past 100 years but this has led to a steady rise in the world's population. Excessive numbers increase poverty and worsen disease. The World Health Organization estimated in 1995 that a fifth of all the people in the world live in extreme poverty, almost a third of the world's children are undernourished, and that half the global population does not have access to essential drugs. But international relief campaigns directed at the developing world have repeatedly faltered before the 'population' problem.

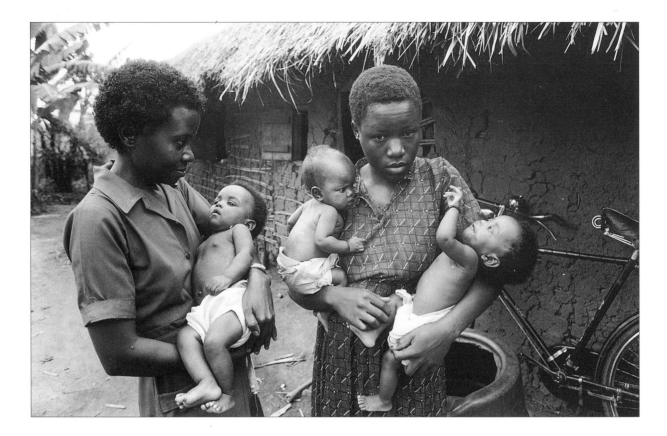

Triplets with suspected AIDS in Uganda. Their father died of the disease. Growing awareness in the 1980s of the vast scale of infection with the human immunodeficiency virus in Africa led to different responses in the West. There were calls to strengthen medical help to the Third World. Fears also arose about further terrible diseases that might be transmitted from tropical environments to Western nations, in which infectious diseases were believed to have been 'conquered'. Media hysteria about epidemics of new and deadly viral infections, such as Ebola and Marburg disease, continue to enflame the latter reaction.

succumb to an inverse square law – growing costs and complexity entailing diminishing utility?

Now that the big battles have been won, medicine is more open to criticism. Setbacks, major and minor, naturally do not help. For example, thalidomide proved disastrous; iatrogenic (doctor-caused) illness has grown; research on cancer, schizophrenia, multiple sclerosis, Alzheimer's, and other degenerative diseases creeps forwards at a snail's-pace; and doubts remain about the medical basis of psychiatry. In Britain, the NHS has been turned into a political football and faces disintegration or possible dismantling; in the USA, insurance and litigation scandals dog the profession. In rich countries, the needy still get a poor medical deal. In the developing world, for lack of international will, malaria and other tropical diseases remain rampant, while diphtheria and tuberculosis, once thought to have been routed, are resurgent in the former USSR and other industrialized nations. Not least, the pandemic of AIDS (acquired immunodeficiency syndrome) destroyed any naive faith that disease itself has been conquered.

Medicine is arguably going through a serious crisis, one that is in large part the price of progress and unrealistically high expectations that have been whipped up by the media and indeed by the medical profession itself. Medicine may appear to be losing its way, or rather having to redefine what its goals are. In 1949, in an article in the *British Medical Journal*, the distinguished physician Lord Horder posed the question: 'Whither Medicine?', and returned the answer direct: 'Why, whither else but straight ahead'.[1] Today, who even knows where 'straight ahead' lies?

For centuries, the medical enterprise was too paltry to attract radical critiques of itself. It had its mockers, yet those who could invariably called the doctor when sick. As Edward Shorter suggests in Chapter 4, in what might paradoxically be called the good-old-bad-old-days, things were simple: people did not have high expectations of medicine, and when the Old Doc typically achieved rather little, his patients did not blame him too much. Medicine was a profession, but it carried no great prestige and had rather little power. In the twentieth century, by contrast, medicine has claimed greater authority, and has become immensely costly. Once medicine grew mighty, it drew critics. And once it proved effective, the scourge of pestilence was forgotten, and the physician became exposed to being viewed primarily as a figure of authority, the tool of patriarchy, or the servant of the state.

In one other key respect, medicine has become the prisoner of its own success. Having finally conquered many grave diseases and provided relief for suffering, its goals have ceased to be so clear and its mandate has become muddled. What are its aims? Where is it to stop? Is its prime duty to keep people alive as long as possible, whatever the circumstances? Is its charge to make people lead healthy lives? Or is it but a service industry, to fulfil whatever fantasies its clients may frame for their bodies – for instance, a facelift or cosmetic remodelling?

In the particular case, many of these quandaries can be resolved reasonably satisfactorily with the aid of common decency, good will, and a sensible ethics committee. But in the wider world, who can decree for the directions medicine may now be taking? Now that (in the rich world at least) medicine has accomplished most of its basic targets as understood by Hippocrates, William Harvey, or Lord Horder, who decides its new missions?

In this situation, public alarm is bound to grow over the high-tech 'can do, will do' approach apparently embraced by scientific medicine at the cutting edge – medicine led by an elite that sometimes seems primarily interested in extending its technical prowess, with scant regard for ends and values, or even the individual sufferer. Where patients are seen as 'problems' and reduced to biopsies and lab tests, no wonder sections of the public vote with their feet, and opt for styles of holistic medicine that present themselves as more humane.

What may be more disquieting than the switch to alternative treatments is the public's fixation on medicine. Ironically, the healthier Western society becomes, the more medicine it craves; indeed, it comes to regard maximum access to medicine as a political right and a private duty. Especially in the USA, where a free market operates, intense pressures are created – by, for example, the medical profession, medi-businesses, the media, and compliant (or susceptible) individuals – to expand the diagnosis of treatable illnesses. Scares about new diseases and conditions arise. People are bamboozled into more and more lab tests, often of dubious reliability. Thanks to 'diagnostic creep', ever more disorders are revealed, or, as many would say, concocted. Extensive and expensive treatments are then urged. In the USA, the physician who choses not to treat leaves himself exposed to accusations of malpractice. Anxieties and interventions spiral upwards. Practitioners, lawyers, and pharmaceutical companies do well, even if patients don't get well; and medicine is increasingly blown off course.

To understand the roots of the trouble, particularly in the USA but elsewhere too, we need to examine these elements in the light of historical change. The problem is endemic to a system in which an expanding medical establishment, faced with a healthier population of its own creation, is driven to medicating normal life events (such as the menopause), to converting risks into diseases, and to treating trivial complaints with fancy procedures. Doctors and 'consumers' alike are becoming locked within a fantasy that unites the creation of anxiety with gung-ho 'can-do, must-do' technological perfectibilism: everyone has something wrong with them, everyone can be cured. Medical success may be creating a Frankenstein's monster, what has been called by Ivan Illich, a critic of modern medicine, the 'medicalization of life'. To air these predicaments is not antimedical spleen – a churlish reprisal against medicine for its victories – but simply a realization of medical power that is growing not exactly without responsibility but with dissolving goals. Even though this may be in medicine's finest hour, it might also be the dawn of its dilemmas.

For centuries medicine was impotent and hence unproblematic. From the Greeks to the First World War, its job was simple: to struggle with lethal diseases and gross disabilities, to ensure live births, and to manage pain. It performed these uncontroversial tasks mostly with meagre success. Today, with mission accomplished, medicine's triumphs are dissolving in disorientation. The task facing medicine in the twenty-first century will be to redefine its limits even as it extends its capacities.

The triumphs and trials of modern medicine can be understood only in a historical framework. That understanding must be based on proper scholarship. All too often oversimplified and caricatured visions of the rise of medicine are reproduced in books and newspapers. For example, the late and extremely distinguished American physician, Lewis Thomas, wrote that

> The history of medicine has never been a particularly attractive subject in medical education and one reason for this is that it is so unbelievably deplorable ... bleeding, purging, cupping and the administration of infusions of every known plant, solutions of every known metal, every conceivable diet including total fasting, most of them based on the weirdest imaginings about the cause of disease, concocted out of nothing but thin air – this was the heritage of medicine until a little over a century ago.[2]

One understands the emotions behind Professor Thomas's statements. His view, however, amounts to extremely bad history: almost every statement contained in the quotation above will be shown, somewhere in this volume, to be untrue. If we reduce the history of medicine to a travesty, through gross oversimplification, how can we expect to achieve more than a superficial grasp of trends at work now? One of the main aims of this volume is to create the sense that medicine has been constantly remaking itself, demolishing old dogmas, building on the past, forging new perspectives, and redefining its goals. In one respect, of course, medicine has always been about the same thing: healing the sick. But what that has entailed – imaginatively, organizationally, scientifically, humanely – has forever been (as this volume shows) in a state of transformation.

A few further words of explanation are due. This volume does not attempt to be a universal history of medicine worldwide, and some topics – such as primary care, surgery, and psychiatry – are covered in more detail than, for example, tropical medicine, dentistry, medical jurisprudence, and complementary therapies. The book is essentially a history of the roots, rise, and present state of the major specialities of Western medicine, or, as it might be called, scientific medicine. Very little is said about the medical systems to be found in the hundreds of tribal societies the world over; nor are there chapters on Chinese medicine, Islamic medicine, the Ayurvedic medicine of India, and the many medical systems that have flourished in Asia. The omission of those traditions is not a comment on their historical importance or value. To have done such subjects justice – and to have included more detail on other subjects – would have doubled the length of the work. These topics have been sacrificed for coherence and concentration. We have chosen instead to examine in detail the historical roots of Western scientific medicine, which, to a greater or lesser degree, is now becoming the dominant system of the world. Why this is so is one of the questions we address in this volume.

As the story told here shows, we are today living through momentous times for medicine but ones also full of doubt. During the past two centuries, and especially in recent decades, medicine has grown ever more powerful and successful. Yet there is deep personal anxiety and public debate about many of the directions in which medicine may be heading. The paradox involved (better health and longer life, but greater medical anxieties) may be understood, if not resolved, by the historical perspectives that this volume offers.

Roy Porter

Kenneth F. Kiple

CHAPTER 1

The History of Disease

Humans have been fighting the diseases of 'civilization' since they began congregating in large numbers. There is written and pictorial evidence of this from Egypt and Mesopotamia around 1000 BC, India about 750 BC, Greece of the sixth century BC, and China about 100 BC. Yet, as the Canadian physician and historian William Osler commented, 'Civilization is but a filmy fringe on the history of man'. By this he meant that the past four or five millennia represent a tiny fraction of 1 per cent of the time since human ancestors first appeared on earth. There is, of course, no recorded history of the ailments of people before the emergence of civilizations and thus before the diseases that they spawned, but we can make informed guesses about them from skeletons and other archaeological remains.

BEFORE FARMING

For at least 4.5 million years, human ancestors (hominids) were hunters and gatherers. They lived in scattered groups of perhaps 50 to 100 individuals. The low numbers and low densities of the populations reduced the incidence of viral and bacterial infections so that people were not troubled by contagious diseases such as smallpox or measles, whose pathogens require large and dense populations for survival. Moreover, the lifestyle of hunter-gatherers spared them other illnesses. They were restless folk, often on the move, and thus not tied to a neighbourhood long enough to pollute water sources with human wastes that transmit disease, nor to pile up refuse that attracts disease-carrying insects. Finally, hunter-gatherers had no domesticated animals. Tamed animals helped to create civilizations with their meat, hides, milk, eggs, and bones but also transmitted many diseases.

Our hunting, fishing, and gathering ancestors did not escape diseases altogether but they were less exposed to them than are modern humans. There were two principal sources of disease in those far-off times, one of them wild animals. Infections (zoonoses) were acquired by eating or just being in contact with animals. The second threat of disease came from organisms that were present in pre-hominid ancestors and continued to evolve with humans. In this second category were numerous worms, lice, and bacteria such as *Salmonella* and *Treponema* (the agent of yaws and syphilis).

The zoonotic illnesses in the first category may have included trichinosis, sleeping sickness, tularaemia (rabbit fever), tetanus, schistosomiasis (bilharziasis), and leptospirosis (Weil's disease). Other possibilities are one or more of the various forms of typhus, malaria, and even yellow fever. Encounters with these infections would have been mostly incidental and individual and would seldom, if ever, have affected many members of a group, especially in view of the mobility of hunter-gatherers and their tendency to abandon areas when food became short.

An early human ancestor may have suffered from a chronic disease caused by an excess of vitamin A. The disease, hypervitaminosis A, affects bone structure and scientists claim to have identified the characteristic pathology in the fossilized bones of a hominid (probably *Homo erectus*) that lived near Lake Turkana in Kenya about 1.65 million years ago. A rival theory is that the hominid had the treponemal disease yaws. The preserved parts of its skeleton are shaded black on this diagram.

Such mobility also put hunter-gatherers within reach of a wide range of wild plant and animal food that presumably helped establish the kinds and quantities of the nutrients that humans need today. Studies of the few remaining hunter-gatherers of present times point to the consumption of a truly astounding variety of foodstuffs. If such variety was characteristic of hunter-gatherer diets of the past, it may partly explain anomalies of modern humans, such as the ability to develop scurvy if food contains insufficient vitamin C (ascorbic acid). Humans and only a few other animals cannot synthesize their own ascorbic acid. Because of the importance of vitamin C to metabolic processes (see page 46), it seems unlikely that an ability to synthesize it would have been lost in evolution, unless it had been rendered superfluous – unnecessary because ascorbic acid had been well supplied by the diet over hundreds of thousands of years.

If, however, early humans were blessed with nutritional plenty and a life relatively untroubled by disease, why is it that they remained hunter-gatherers for more than 99.5 per cent of the 2.5 million years that 'cultural' (that is, toolmaking) people have been on earth? Why did human populations not quickly mushroom in just a few thousand of those years to the point where people could no longer feed themselves with hunting and gathering strategies?

Such population crises may, in fact, have occurred countless times. Famine must often have intervened to bring population size back into line with the available food supply. Doubtless, too, many lives were lost in high-risk, high-return endeavours associated with scavenging and hunting of large animals. Doubtless many were lost in the higher-risk, higher-return business of killing fellow humans. Other checks on population growth may also have operated to permit hunting and gathering to continue for so long. Childbirth was risky and many

Forest clearance for crop-growing in northern Thailand. When farming began 11,000-10,000 years ago the act of breaking the sod for cultivation brought humans into new and intimate contact with many disease-causing organisms and the crops created new environments for small populations of parasites to grow into large ones. Agriculture also intensified the exploitation of natural resources. Environmental degradation has typically been the consequence.

infants probably died from natural causes. Infanticide may also have been practised. Indeed, viewed within the context of the restlessness of hunter-gatherers on
the one hand, and the fact that, when moving, they had to carry everything they
owned, on the other, it is difficult to believe that infanticide was not an important
factor in checking the growth of ancient populations.

In spite of these restraints, populations grew. If a hunter-gatherer band became
too large to function efficiently, it split into two. This kind of multiplication took
ancient humans into every corner of the Old World after 1.8–1.5 million years
ago. From their ancestral home in Africa, *Homo erectus* populations expanded into
the tropical regions of Asia and later into more temperate zones, continuing their
peripatetic existence. Even the first modern humans (*Homo sapiens*), with brains
the size of ours, continued as hunter-gatherers for some 100,000 years.

The advent of a sophisticated tool culture around 40,000 years ago led to effi-
ciencies in hunting and food preparation but there was no major change in the
nomadic lifestyle until 12,000–10,000 years ago at the end of the last ice age. This
presents us with another puzzle, especially for those who believe that replacing
hunting and gathering with the domestication of plants and animals was a major
improvement in the human condition.

American anthropologist Mark Cohen has argued that people were wise
enough to know when they were well off – they became farmers only because
increasing population pressure left them little choice. By at least 50,000 years ago,
humanity had spilled over from the Old World to Australasia and sometime before
12,500 years ago to the Americas as well. During the coldest parts of the ice age it
was possible to walk over to these new continents on land. When the ice caps
melted 12,000 to 10,000 years ago and the seas rose to seal off this kind of migration, there was simply no place to absorb surplus populations. Stone Age technology was strained to its utmost to support people in all the habitable parts of the
Old World, and in the words of an American historian, Alfred Crosby, humankind
was now faced with the choice of becoming 'either celibate or clever. Predictably,
the species chose the latter course': people settled down and took up producing
their own food.

FARMING AND DISEASE

Once set on that course, events moved with dizzying speed – at least when measured against the 5 to 6 million years that the human family has been around. As
Mark Cohen has remarked, around 10,000 years ago almost everybody lived
exclusively on wild food; by 2,000 years ago, most people were farmers. Such a
transition was indisputably the most important event ever engineered by
humankind.

Wild grasses were tamed and tinkered with until they became domesticated
varieties of wheat, rye, barley, and rice. Dogs were probably the first animals to be
domesticated (around 12,000 years ago) and over the next few thousand years

The dog was probably the first animal to be domesticated, first by late Ice Age hunters for use as retrievers and later by early farmers for used as herders and guarders of tamed livestock. With domesticated animals came many diseases. The earliest evidence for a close relationship between dogs and people comes from the burial of an elderly woman with her puppy (top right) at the Natufian site of Ain Mallaha in northern Israel (about 9600 BC).

they were followed by cattle, sheep, goats, pigs, horses, and fowl. The few square miles that a hunter-gatherer band might have quickly picked clean were thus transformed into a base that could support many more people indefinitely. The population expanded dramatically because those who surrendered their mobile lifestyle were no longer constrained in the number of offspring they might have. Rather, the more people there were, the more hands for the fields and security for the elderly. It was from this crucible of the agricultural revolution that people began learning to manipulate the planet – to rearrange its ecological systems, not to mention the genes of the plants and animals within those systems. They began the enterprise of undoing a self-regenerating nature without knowing what they were doing, an unthinking process that has continued to the present.

The agricultural revolution thus had ecological downsides, the depths of which we cannot yet fathom. One of these downsides embraces the many realms of parasites. By inventing agriculture, humans also cultivated disease. Pathogens of domesticated animals now found their way into human bodies and began adapting to them as well. According to William McNeill, an American historian, humans share some 65 diseases with dogs, 50 with cattle, 46 with sheep and goats, 42 with pigs, 35 with horses, and 26 with poultry. These animals joined with humans in fouling drinking water with their bodily wastes. Humans scattered those wastes on the cultivated land, which maximized the opportunities of parasitic worms and attracted disease-spreading insects.

Permanent dwellings attracted other domesticates, albeit self-appointed ones. Mice and rats learned to take shelter with humans, enjoy their warm surroundings, and eat the same food. After several thousand years of co-evolution the day has long passed when these small, furry animals could live without humans, to

As populations rose with the growth of civilizations, humans provided perfect environments for a range of living parasites, such as hair lice. This ancient louse revealed by scanning electron microscopy was found attached to the hair of an Eygptian mummy buried in the Early Dynastic Period (*c.* 3000 BC) at Abydos. Lice and ticks carry typhus and other so-called 'filth diseases' that are associated with dirty clothes and poor domestic hygiene.

which they have become adapted so well. All too often, however, these commensals have helped spread disease.

Permanent settlements attracted mosquitoes and other assorted blood-sucking insects, which now had many human bodies to feed on. Mosquito breeding sites were available in forest clearings and in stagnant water near dwellings. Faeces-feeding houseflies flourished in these new settlements and their 'dirty feet' on food intended for the human stomach insured a variety of self-perpetuating diarrhoeal diseases and bacillary dysentery. Fleas and lice colonized the outside of the human body, and amoebas, hookworms, and countless other parasitic worms moved into its interior. All would proliferate easily because people lived in close proximity.

In spite of such disease-producing squalor, human breeding ability insured that the festering villages became home for increasing numbers of people. Infant and child mortality rates doubtless increased but birth rates soared even higher, which meant more and more individuals living within spitting, coughing, and sneezing distance of one another to lay the groundwork for a myriad of airborne illnesses.

Farming itself also promotes disease. Irrigation farming in the early river valley civilizations, such as that of the Yellow River (Huang He) in China and the Nile, especially the flooding of lands for the cultivation of rice, had the desired effect of killing off competing plant species. But in the warm, shallow waters of the paddy fields lurked parasites able to penetrate the skin and enter the bloodstream of wading human rice farmers. Foremost among these is a blood fluke called *Schistosoma* that uses aquatic snails as an intermediate host through successive stages of development and produces the debilitating, and often deadly disease called schistosomiasis (or bilharziasis). Evidence of the presence of the disease has been found in Egypt in the kidneys of 3,000-year-old Egyptian mummies.

Slash-and-burn agriculture – a method of land clearance in which vegetation is cut, allowed to dry, and then burned before crop-planting – created niches in which relatively small populations of parasites could breed into very large ones. In Africa south of the Sahara, for example, it has been shown that this type of cultivation led to the proliferation of the mosquito *Anopheles gambiae* that spreads falciparum malaria, the most dangerous of malarial diseases.

Finally, just the act of breaking the sod for cultivation brought humans into new and intimate contact with numerous insects and worms, not to mention bacteria, viruses, protozoans, and the rickettsias (microorganisms intermediate between bacteria and viruses) carried by ticks, fleas, and lice.

Clearly, then, the establishment of permanent settlements from about 12,000 years ago and the cultivation of land around them did human health no good. But, even worse, disease came from the domestication of animals. Cattle contributed their poxes to the growing pool of pathogens; pigs, birds, and horses, their influenzas. Measles is probably the result of rinderpest, or canine distemper, oscillating back and forth between humans and cattle or dogs; smallpox is probably the product of a long evolutionary adaptation of cowpox to humans.

One says 'probably' because, although there is little doubt that humans acquired most of their diseases after they became farmers, one can only speculate about distant evolutionary changes. It was a process in which viruses and bacteria ricocheted back and forth between various domesticated animal species that had never before been in close contact and between those animals and their human owners. In this new pathogenic crucible, microorganisms incubated, combined, altered, perished, and prospered. Their prosperity was often a function of still more evolutionary trial and error, in which pathogens found their way to intermediary hosts, which serve as staging areas for later assaults on humans. Similarly,

The daily grind of work in an early farming community is revealed by damaged bones of skeletons recovered from a burial site at Abu Hureyra in northern Syria. Injuries to these two neck vertebrae, for example, were probably caused by the carrying of heavy loads on the head. Telltale signs of other injuries caused by demanding physical activity, such as grinding grain, are visible on other skeletal parts.

it probably took other microorganisms a long time to acquire vectors to shuttle them about from intermediary host to people as well as from person to person.

Some diseases such as smallpox and measles were so perfectly adapted to humans when they emerged from this crucible that they no longer needed their old host or hosts to complete their life cycle. They were also so contagious that they spread with remarkable ease from human to human. Indeed, the appearance of these 'new' diseases that require only human hosts – but many of them – is testimony to the population explosion that occurred after people gave up hunting and gathering. This happened in spite of the declining health of people. As small settlements grew into large ones they became even more squalid, and population pressure dictated the concentration of the diet on fewer and fewer foodstuffs (see page 45). In other words, people became nutritionally impoverished as disease became more ubiquitous, opening the door to a synergistic union of malnutrition and pathogens.

THE RISE OF NEW DISEASES

The roundworm (*Ascaris*), which was probably acquired from pigs, and the hookworm, both spread by faecal pollution of soil, would have joined in this assault on the human body. These worms live in the gut and compete with their human hosts for protein, causing anaemia. Deprived of nutrients important in combating disease, early farmers, especially their children, would have been less able to withstand the next wave of pathogens to invade them: and so the cycle continued.

Ironically, then, as humans switched their activities from living off nature to vigorously manipulating it, they were increasingly parasitized by microorganisms with a vigour of their own. The microorganisms had a clear advantage because they reproduce with lightning speed and can go through several thousand life cycles while humans are still working their way from infancy to reproductive age.

Humans were not totally defenceless in this apparently uneven struggle. Those that survived a disease were, at best, left with an ability to escape completely its next visitation or, at worst, with some immunity against its ravages. Humans hence began developing sophisticated immune systems to enable them to live with their invaders. Pathogens co-operated in this immunological development. Although the most susceptible humans they infected died out, so, too, did the most virulent pathogens, which killed themselves by killing their hosts. Thus invader and invaded reached a compromise: the host survived but passed on the pathogens to other hosts.

Immunities, developed by mothers against diseases they encountered, were delivered across the placenta, which provided the newborn with some defence against the inevitable invasion of germs. Some individuals are also protected genetically from disease. In the case of the dangerous falciparum malaria, for example, individuals with the sickle-cell trait, a deficit in energy metabolism called glucose-6-phosphate dehydrogenase (G6PD) deficiency, beta-thalassaemia,

Protection against malaria

Malaria is believed to have originated among African primates. In humans, it is caused by one of four species of protozoan parasites (genus *Plasmodium*) that are transmitted from one human host to another by the bite of a female mosquito (genus *Anopheles*). As the parasites enter the bloodstream to feed on red corpuscles (erythrocytes), bodily defences are summoned: white blood cells capture the parasites and digest them, and the spleen filters the debris out of the system.

Parasite preferences can help to limit the extent of an infection. *Plasmodium vivax*, for example, only parasitizes young erythrocytes whereas *P. malariae* goes after mature ones. Thus, *P. falciparum*, which invades both types of cell indiscriminately, is much more likely than the other malaria parasites to achieve a life-threatening level of parasitic activity.

Malaria immunities that hold down the parasite count can be innate or acquired. In the latter case, the body develops an ability to produce antibodies that prevent the proliferation of parasites. But this occurs only after a person has survived several attacks and somebody who has earned resistance does so only to one strain while remaining susceptible to others. As a result, natural selection in malarious regions has gradually supplemented acquired immunities by evolving innate resistance to the multiplication of parasites.

Most of these mechanisms were developed against falciparum malaria, which seems to be the newest as well as the deadliest of the malaria types. Vivax malaria is much older and more benign, but at one time it must have been considerably more lethal. This is because almost all people whose origins are in Africa south of the Sahara have acquired a genetic trait (an absence of the Duffy blood-group determinants FY^a and FY^b) that protects them against vivax malaria.

Duffy-negative red blood cells do not seem to be harmful, but possession of the sickle trait – the best known of the defences against *Plasmodium falciparum* – can be fatal. Sickle-shaped blood cells, which discourage the multiplication of parasites, save lives in areas where falciparum malaria occurs. But the odds are one in four that if both parents have the trait, then their child will be a victim of sickle-cell anaemia.

Other, less-costly mechanisms of protection include a deficiency in glucose-6-phosphate dehydrogenase (G6PD, a blood enzyme), and thalassaemia traits alone and in combination with the sickle trait. None of these is restricted to persons of African ancestry, but they occur most frequently among them because of their long association with malaria.

Such an association has also prompted suggestions that other blood anomalies among black people may confer resistance to malaria. Certainly, the recent linkage between malaria protection in West Africans and histocompatibility antigens on the surfaces of cells seems still more important evidence of the ability of humans to change in the face of endemic disease.

Red blood cells infected with the microscopic protozoan parasite *Plasmodium*.

A brass statuette of Juara, the Hindu goddess of malaria fever, with three heads, three legs, and six arms. The image was probably used as an icon to ward off attacks.

or several other blood anomalies have increased resistance to the disease. Genes for such traits have proliferated in malarious areas.

Where parasitic worms are widespread, people develop a tolerance for the worms – or, as it were, a partial immunity to them. Indeed, the rule seems to be that those who live in close proximity to a particular pathogen for long enough develop an ability to 'live' with the disease that the pathogen provokes.

Other diseases are, however, far more difficult to live with. These are the pathogens that first emerged when human numbers increased sufficiently to support them in their new form. Speculation about when and where these new plagues of humankind first manifested themselves is fascinating but is little more than quesswork, given the dearth of archaeological data and the frequently contradictory nature of what there is. It was certainly not much before 3000 BC. Around that time, cities with populations as large as 50,000 were springing up in Mesopotamia and Egypt. In the Indus Valley in the Indian subcontinent, too, large populations were also emerging. These had substantial cattle herds, from which several pathogens, including perhaps that of smallpox, spread to humans. Evidence to strengthen the suspicion that smallpox was present quite early in southern Asia lies in the existence of ancient Indian temples that appear to have been erected to worship a smallpox diety. In addition, smallpox inoculation seems to have been practised in India in ancient times.

Focusing a little nearer present times, William McNeill decided that the period beginning about 500 BC was when pathogens began to have an impact on the growth of civilizations in Asia and Europe. These were the microparasites that trigger smallpox, diphtheria, influenza, chickenpox, mumps, and numerous other illnesses. They pass quickly and directly from human to human and need no intermediary carrier. These new illnesses changed the course of human history. Populations in which a particular disease had arisen presumably developed some immunity against it, just as they had developed resistance to the older diseases in their immediate locale. But marauders, merchants, missionaries, and marching armies did not long permit civilizations to flourish in exotic isolation. Moving from one place to another, they also linked their pools of pathogens. Thus, one people's familiar disease became another people's plague.

The immediate consequence of an invasion by novel pathogens would have been a massive epidemic and a dramatic fall in population as the most susceptible individuals were eliminated. The survivors would have then begun the painful process of population recovery, only to be set upon by another new disease, and yet another. Populations that had grown large enough to host such illnesses would have suddenly become too small to do so. With almost everybody immune and few non-immune individuals being born, the illnesses themselves would have disappeared, only to return after the populations had grown large again and were full of people with low resistance.

While one group enjoyed an epidemiological respite, the new diseases attacked other populations that had grown large, often near the limits of their food supplies. In short, the new diseases became important in preventing human overpopulation while immunologically tempering those that survived them.

CITIES AS MAGNETS FOR DISEASE

By limiting population growth, such diseases also made possible the agricultural surpluses that sped the growth of cities. These in turn became magnets for pathogens as well as people. Until relatively recently, cities were generally so unhealthy that their populations could not replace themselves by reproduction. They maintained their numbers or grew in size only because of migration from the surrounding countryside. Many who were attracted to gregarious living perished from the gauntlet of disease that accompanied city life. But those that survived joined a growing immunological elite of urbanites – a teeming infectious multitude that was acutely dangerous to less immunologically developed neighbours. When such biologically dangerous peoples had the urge to expand their territories, their pathogens often spearheaded the effort.

Hence, wherever armies marched pathogens flourished. The Peloponnesian war (431–404 BC) was one of the earliest and best examples of this. Before the war we know from the Hippocratic treatises (see page 58) that, whereas the ancient Greeks suffered from malaria and probably tuberculosis, diphtheria, and influenza as well, they seemed to have been spared killer epidemic diseases such as smallpox. However, growing populations, especially that of Athens, helped to kindle the flames of imperial ambition. Those flames were abruptly extinguished during Athens's war with Sparta and the sudden advent of epidemic disease.

The famous description by the Greek historian Thucydides tells us much about this epidemic that reputedly began in Africa, spread to Persia, and reached Greece in 430 BC. He claimed that initially it killed 25 per cent of the Athenian forces; then lingered in southern Greece for the next 4 years, killing up to 25 per cent of the civilian population. On the basis of the symptoms described, plague, smallpox, measles, typhus, or even syphilis and ergotism have been proposed as likely candidates. Whatever the disease was it seems to have destroyed the Greek people's ability to host it by killing or immunizing them. Whereupon it disappeared, leaving in its wake the wreckage of Athenian dreams of hegemony, which has been called a 'turning point' in the history of Western civilization.

Disease occasioned other turning points. Roman conquest knitted together much of the known world and most of its deadly pathogens by successively embracing Macedonia and Greece (146 BC), Seleucid Asia (64 BC), and finally Egypt (30 BC). Disease began affecting the Empire and Rome from the second century AD onwards. The first widespread epidemic, the so-called Antonine plague, may have killed from a quarter to a third of the populations in infected areas between AD 165 and 180, whereas a second,

The rise of cities brought about the spread of infectious diseases. In the absence of effective medicines, religious healing thrived. Votive offerings such as this Graeco-Roman terracotta head of a sick man were made in the hope of a cure or in gratitude for relief.

which struck between 211 and 266, scourged both Rome and the countryside. In short, after AD 200 epidemics and barbarians joined in first battering and ultimately bringing down the Roman Empire. A shrinking world also resulted in wider and wider pools of diseases shared by more and more people in South Asia, the Middle East, and East Asia; that is, centres from which diseases rotated outwards to draw other Old World populations into their vortices. The example of Japan is a classic in this regard. Before AD 552, the Japanese seem to have escaped the epidemic diseases that had long scourged mainland populations. In that year, however, Buddhist missionaries from Korea visited the Japanese court, and shortly after many Japanese died from what may have been smallpox.

In 585 – after a new, non-immune generation had arisen in Japan – there was another outbreak of disease that seems clearly to have been smallpox or measles. Once again many died. Then a century seems to have elapsed without notable outbreaks of illness. The seventh century, however, was brought abruptly to an end with the beginning of Japan's 'age of plagues' (700–1050). During the eighth century, the country was rocked with thirty-four epidemics; in the ninth century, it suffered through thirty-five; in the tenth century, twenty-six; and in the eleventh century, twenty-four, sixteen of which had occurred by mid-century.

An approximate chronology of the Black death as it spread across Europe from Asia in the middle of the fourteenth century.

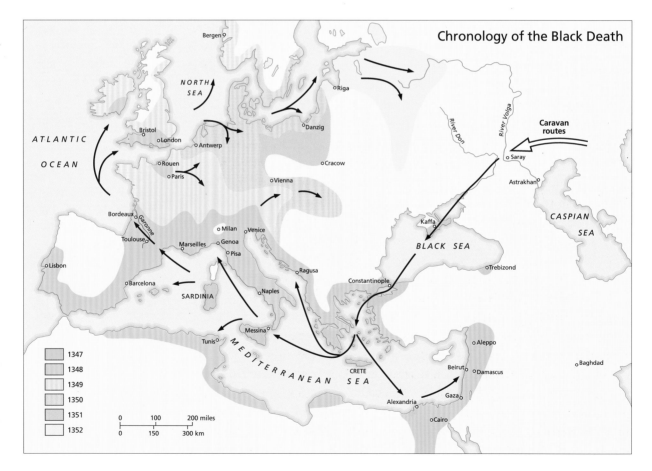

In the forefront of the diseases known to have triggered these epidemics were smallpox and measles, although influenza, mumps, and dysentery were also well represented. All continued to pound Japan during the period 1050–1260 but not with the same intensity, and the population finally began to grow after stagnating for centuries. Much of the reason for this renewed growth may be found in the fact that, by about 1250, smallpox and measles had come to be regarded as childhood diseases.

Viewed from the present day, such a transformation of plagues into childhood illnesses stands out as a large milestone in the epidemiological history of humankind. In the case of the Japanese, it meant that almost all of the adults had already suffered illnesses that they could not get again. But it also meant that they were producing enough non-immune children to hold onto the illnesses so that they dwelled generation after generation in the bodies of the young – and did not escape to return at a later date as devastating plagues. Epidemic diseases that became endemic diseases were not only substantially less disruptive of political, social, and economic life, they were also less wasteful of human life because many epidemic diseases tend to affect the young less severely than they do adults.

Yet, if larger populations had the effect of taming many of the epidemic diseases, such populations remained exposed to other serious infections. These were diseases against which its members were immunologically defenceless because they were diseases of animals, not usually of humans. One such illness is bubonic plague, which has assaulted humans with extreme ferocity whenever and wherever populations have accidentally been caught in a crossfire of disease transmission involving rats, fleas, and the plague bacillus.

As had happened so often in the past, a killer disease (in this case, plague) made its appearance when populations were enjoying a substantial period of growth, and in Europe the next few centuries witnessed demographic stagnation with populations reasserting themselves at different rates. After the Great Plague of London in 1665, for example, the disease withdrew from northwestern Europe but not the Mediterranean. Spain, which had suffered cruelly from epidemics in 1596–1602 and 1648–52, also endured another 9 years of plague from 1677 to 1685. The timing of these epidemics seems especially significant when one recalls the rise in English fortunes during this period and the decline of those of Spain.

In the fifteenth and sixteenth centuries, however, not even plague was able to stop the inhabitants of the Iberian Peninsula from engineering the beginning of the European expansion. The Portuguese followed up the capture of Ceuta in 1415 (the year their queen, Philippa, died of plague) with the voyages of trade and exploration that would ultimately take them into the Indian Ocean and on to the threshold of a huge East Indies empire. Meanwhile the Spaniards were also active in waters off the African coast as they conquered the Canary Islands. There, the native resistance of the Guanches, although initially stiff, crumbled in the face of diseases that eventually annihilated them. Sugar plantations were operated by

The cause of plague

The rodent disease that produces plague in humans is *Yersinia pestis* (once called *Pasturella pestis*). It reaches humans through frantic infected fleas searching for another living rat after their infected host has died, but willing to board a less-satisfactory host for a while.

After the flea bites its new host, the bacillus enters the lymphatic system and heads for the nearest lymph node, causing the characteristic swelling or 'bubo' in the groin, armpit, or neck, depending on the location of the bite. This form of the disease is called bubonic plague, which historically brought death to about 60 per cent of those infected.

The septicaemic form, which is almost always fatal, occurs when the insect injects the bacillus directly into the bloodstream of the victim, giving the lymph nodes no chance of containing it. The most deadly form of all, pneumonic plague, usually develops from bubonic plague. This, in addition to being invariably fatal without antibiotic treatment, needs no insect vector for transmission because it spreads directly and quickly from person to person on breath and in clothing. The cradle of the disease is believed to be along the edge of the Himalayas where China and India share a border – in part because the species of black rat (*Rattus rattus*) that has traditionally been implicated in carrying plague seems to have originated in those parts.

The first documented outbreak of plague was in the Roman Empire, which reportedly lost about a quarter of its population to this disease that had abruptly joined with other factors to topple it. Called the Plague of Justinian, the disease is credited with devastating Constantinople in AD 542 and spreading from there into Western Europe, after which it ricocheted around the Mediterranean for the following two centuries.

It was the second cycle of plague, however, that left its greatest imprint on the known world. In its early stage, the pandemic was sometimes known as the Black Death (see also page 78). Around 1300 it began a rampage in Asia that then swept westwards, cutting huge swathes in populations from the Middle East to North Africa and Europe. Between 1347 and 1350 Europe alone is said to have lost some 20 million people to the disease.

This pandemic, however, was just the first wave of a pestilence that continued to erupt until about 1800, when the second plague cycle mercifully came to an end.

Doubtless the complex circumstances that impelled plague on this deadly tour can be found in many monumental events of the period linking East and West – the expansion of Islam; the Crusades; the imperialism of the Ottoman Turks; and the Mogul conquests. Nonetheless, in its wake plague left some epidemiological mysteries that have not been resolved.

One has to do with its point of origin and another with the perigrinations of *Rattus rattus*, which moved from Asia into the Middle East and Europe. Perhaps the most fascinating mystery, however, revolves around the question of the failure of the plague to establish an endemic focus in Europe, meaning that epidemics in Europe always represented a reintroduction of the disease from the Middle East.

A final mystery lies in why the plague did, in fact, disappear, and why Europe was spared the third cycle of plague, which began in Asia about the middle of the eighteenth century and reached out as far as the Americas on one side of the world and Australia on the other.

Other questions about the plague have to do with its relationship to other diseases. Leprosy, for example, which had been present in Europe since at least the sixth century AD, abruptly receded in the face of the plague's initial onslaught in the middle of the fourteenth century. But tuberculosis simultaneously established a beachhead in the European disease ecology, which would expand for many centuries to come (see page 37).

The 'plague banner' of the Madonna della Misericordia, Chiesa del Gonfalone, Perugia (detail). The effects of the Black Death were cultural and religious no less than epidemiological. It induced a late medieval culture haunted by the figure of Death.

A sixteenth-century panoramic view of Lisbon. From the fifteeth century, Western Europe was poised on the brink of a dramatic expansion, which, in the next two centuries, was to ensure domination over much of the globe. Opportunely placed, Portugal and Spain pioneered the conquest of the East Indies and the discovery of the New World. But the large cities of Iberia, such as Lisbon, overcrowded and insanitary, proved reservoirs for nasty infections, which were transmitted wherever traders and conquerors sailed.

black slaves brought from the African coast to replace the dying Guanches. All of this constituted awful and eerie harbingers of events soon to transpire in the Americas.

It is important to note that, plague notwithstanding, the Iberians who were poised to reunite the New with the Old World were as immunologically fit as any people on earth. For aeons they had been in touch with the outside world in a way that few others had. Iberians had gone to Rome as emperors and Iberian soldiers had marched in Roman legions. From 710 onwards they were intimately involved with invading Arabs and thus with the greater Muslim empire. Indeed, Iberia became something of a melting pot of Christians, Arabs, and incoming Jews. Crusaders paused at Iberian ports on their way to and from the Holy Land (sometimes for lengthy periods as they were drawn into local political or military disputes). Iberians traded from the North Sea to the eastern Mediterranean, and their fishing fleets covered the North Atlantic. By the fourteenth century, the Catalans had built a Mediterranean empire that stretched all the way to Greece. In the fifteenth century, the Portuguese drew Africa and Africans into the Iberian sphere of pathogenic propinquity.

In short, the cities of Spain and Portugal, especially those with harbours, were clearing houses of diseases as well as bank drafts, and in them, as in other Renaissance centres, diseases flourished. Bathing was frowned upon, and clothing was coarse and changed infrequently. Hence the human body was a veritable nest of lice and fleas. Human wastes were flung into the streets to mingle with those of dogs and horses. All of this was paradise for flies that flitted from faeces to food. Water for drinking and cooking was practically a soup of microorganisms. Rats, mice, and other assorted vermin burrowed, crawled, slithered, and skulked their way through houses, shops, warehouses, churches, and taverns. The corpses of dogs, cats, and even horses were, more often than not, left to rot, adding to the stench of the streets, and providing sustenance for still more vermin.

Clearly, survivors of this milieu were equipped with very alert and agile immune systems. To reach adulthood they not only ran a gauntlet of childhood diseases, such as smallpox, measles, diphtheria and the like, but also had to weather a gamut of gastrointestinal infections along with an appalling variety of other afflictions of the skin, blood, bones, and organs seldom seen today outside of the poorest countries. The explorers and conquerors of the Americas, then, can be viewed as a sort of immunological elite, which made for a breathtaking (and deadly) contrast between them and those they conquered.

DISEASE CONQUERS THE NEW WORLD

The ancestors of those who came to be known as Amerindians were hunters and gatherers. At least 12,500 years ago, some traversed the Bering Straits from Asia to Alaska on a land bridge created by the last ice age, which had substantially lowered the levels of the world's oceans and exposed the shallow continental shelf between Asia and North America. On the basis of genetic evidence it has recently been suggested that others may have come from Polynesia. Crossing the Bering Straits was not a sunny outing. The land bridge was bleak, foggy, and cold, prompting some scholars to suspect that population pressure made such expeditions not so much a matter of human restlessness but one of human survival. In other words, the successive waves of migrants may well have been pushed into adventure.

As we have portrayed them, hunter-gatherers were relatively disease-free, and the rigours of the Bering crossing would doubtless have eliminated any that were diseased or weak. Moreover, the pioneers left the Old World before the domestication of animals, which means that (save perhaps for the dog in the later waves) they brought no other portable disease-carriers except themselves and they encountered no humans, diseased or otherwise, after their arrival.

The ice age came to a close about 10,000 years ago. Ice caps melted and seas rose to cover the land bridge and seal off the new Americans. At the same time the great glaciers covering much of North America melted, opening up an entire continent to the arrivals. If the hunter-gatherers had dreamed of paradise, this was it.

The new land, however, had a few nasty surprises. First, the Americas had a few unique illnesses to offer. Rocky Mountain spotted fever, for example, is an American ricksettial disease found today from Brazil to Canada. Although the illness, which is transmitted by ticks, was really identified only in the twentieth century, it is conceivable that it affected the continent's early pioneers as well its modern inhabitants. Those who pushed into South America may have encountered mucocutaneous leishmaniasis (uta), a protozoan disease transmitted by blood-sucking sandflies. Those reaching the Andes region risked Carrión's disease (also called Oroya fever and verruga Peruana). This illness is also spread by sandflies and its disfiguring impact is seemingly depicted on pottery thousands of years old. Another native illness of South America is Chagas' disease or American trypanosomiasis, which probably had its origin in Brazil. It is caused by a trypanosome protozoan carried by guinea-pigs and other animals and transmitted to humans by blood-sucking bugs.

In addition, there were diseases of wild animals such as trichinosis and tularaemia to contend with, and, later, some diseases of civilization made their appearance as a New World agricultural revolution got underway. The Maya, the Aztec, the Inca, and the Mississippian peoples of North America settled into sedentary agriculture and built complex civilizations complete with cities and many of the attendant problems of health that, as we have seen, accompanies such a lifestyle. Some kinds of tuberculosis developed and intestinal parasites and hepatitis passed from person to person through water and food. Pinta, one of several diseases caused by *Treponema* bacteria, seems to have been a problem wherever it was warm enough for scanty dress to permit easy skin-to-skin transmission. Other treponemal infections seem to have been present, including some sort of (apparently) non-venereal syphilis.

But the New World peoples, who were named 'Indians' by Christopher Columbus and his fellow adventurers, were 'virgin soil' for the avalanche of diseases that arrived from Europe. They had been dangerously exempted from the disease pools of the Old World, which the American scholar Alfred Crosby has listed as including smallpox, measles, diphtheria, trachoma, whooping cough, chicken-

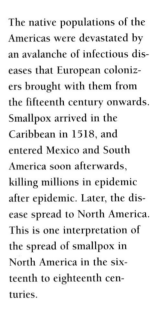

The native populations of the Americas were devastated by an avalanche of infectious diseases that European colonizers brought with them from the fifteenth century onwards. Smallpox arrived in the Caribbean in 1518, and entered Mexico and South America soon afterwards, killing millions in epidemic after epidemic. Later, the disease spread to North America. This is one interpretation of the spread of smallpox in North America in the sixteenth to eighteenth centuries.

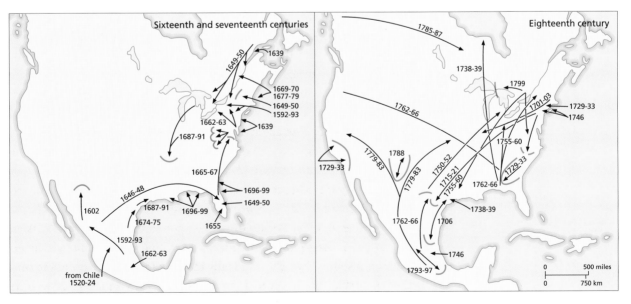

pox, bubonic plague, malaria, typhoid fever, cholera, yellow fever, dengue fever, scarlet fever, amoebic dysentery, influenza, and helminthic infestations. To this list one might add illnesses such as typhus, brucellosis, erysipelas, filariasis, mumps, onchocerciasis, relapsing fever, leprosy, and probably hookworm disease.

No one knows how many native Americans were present when Columbus and disease arrived and thus no one knows for certain the numerical magnitude of the demographic disaster they endured. Indeed, questions about the size of American populations at European contact have been among those most hotly contested by historical demographers and anthropologists throughout the twentieth century, and the subject of keen debate in the Quincentennial scholarship of 1992. But whether one is inclined to accept high estimates, of around 100 million, or a more conservative 50 million or less, there is some agreement that the hurricane of disease that swept the Americas ultimately claimed about 90 per cent of the 1492 populations.

The first American epidemic, which struck the island of Hispaniola in 1493, may well have been swine influenza. Other unnamed diseases followed so that West Indian populations were in decline even before smallpox made its official Caribbean debut in 1518. Smallpox accompanied Hernando Cortés to Mexico and raced ahead of the Pizarros into Peru, greatly expediting both conquests, while radiating outwards to kill other untold millions that the Spanish never had to conquer. Following this, epidemic after epidemic rained on the New World. One of the worst to be recorded was the typhus epidemic that reportedly killed some 2 million in the Mexican highlands towards the end of the sixteenth century.

One can only imagine the horror: young adults are frequently the chief victims of epidemics, meaning that few are left to plant, and cook, and clean, and care for children and the old. The epidemics frequently descended in pell-mell fashion, providing no time for populations to recover and immune systems to adjust. Social, political, economic, and religious life crumbled, and the wonder is that anyone managed to survive to develop immunities and pass them on. But they did, and the mainland populations of Mexico and the Andean region gradually recovered.

Population decline (and recovery) came later in North America. It took a particularly nasty downward turn in the Caribbean and in parts of Brazil where decline actually meant obliteration. The reason for these differing demographic circumstances, however, does not lie among Eurasian illnesses but rather in another group of Old World diseases whose cradle lay in sub-Saharan Africa.

AFRICAN DISEASES ENTER THE NEW WORLD

The arrival of Africans in the Americas was a tragedy begotten by another New World tragedy, the establishment of black slavery, which, in turn, was the consequence of the fall in the indigenous population. The Iberian conquerors had counted on the labour of the Amerindians to colonize the vastness of the Americas. But the rapid decline in numbers of native Americans meant that they had to look elsewhere for such assistance. By 1518 the transatlantic slave trade was well underway.

The arriving Africans bore many of the same immunities as the Europeans because, for millennia, most Eurasian illnesses had regularly found their way into sub-Saharan Africa in desert caravans and across the Indian Ocean. In addition, Africans were resistant to the resident tropical illnesses of their own part of the world, which most other peoples were not. One of these was falciparum malaria, the most dangerous of the malarial types and also a relatively new one, which, as we have seen, was spawned by the development of sedentary agriculture in Africa. It had not remained strictly an African disease and at some time in the past it had moved north to parts of the Mediterranean. Indeed, this was another lethal force that some have credited with contributing significantly to the decline of the Roman Empire. Evidence that at one time falciparum malaria was of considerable prevalence in southern Italy and Greece can be found today in the blood anomalies of many Mediterranean people that we know are genetic defences against the disease.

The incidence of such protective anomalies as the sickle-cell trait and glucose-6-dehydrogenase (G6PD) deficiency is far greater among Africans, and is testimony to their long and intimate association with falciparum malaria. Such defences also testify to an extensive and extended experience with another, more ubiquitous malarial type, vivax malaria, which has virtually disappeared from Africa. Vivax malaria is believed to be among the oldest of the malarial types. Like

From the sixteenth century, smallpox was one of the most feared diseases, partly because of it high mortality rate. Its florid spots – it was known in English as the speckled monster – deformed the sufferer while infected and often left permanent disfigurement. These pictures of infected people come from a twelve-volume compendium of Aztec history and culture compiled by a Catholic missionary scholar called Fray Bernardino de Sahagún (c. 1499–1590). His masterpiece *Historia de las Cosas de Nueva Espana* (General History of the Things of New Spain), published in 1547–69, is often called the *Florentine Codex* after the city that now houses it. The twelfth book, in which these drawings appear, describes the conquest of Mexico through Aztec eyes.

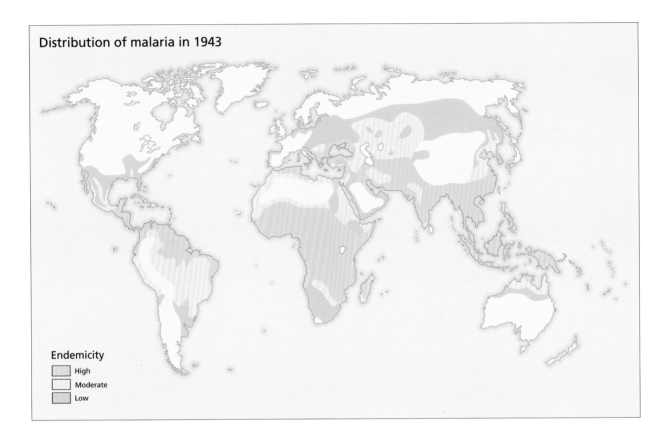

Distribution of malaria in 1943

Endemicity
High
Moderate
Low

World distribution of malaria before the era of mass travel.

the other forms it originated in Africa where the protozoan *Plasmodium*, the cause of all malarias, parasitized thousands of generations of humans. In such a process, however, close to 100 per cent of Africans acquired a genetic trait that protects them against vivax malaria and probably against falciparum malaria as well (see page 23).

With few human carriers of vivax malaria in Africa, the disease changed locales to become a scourge of much of the rest of the world, including Europe. Hence, Europeans were the carriers of vivax malaria to the New World; the more serious falciparum malaria arrived with Africans. Anopheline mosquitoes were present in the Americas to spread the protozoan infections and add them to the list of microbes slaughtering the native Americans.

Yellow fever, that other great tropical killer to emanate from Africa, was slower to make an American appearance because its principal vector, the *Aedes agypti* mosquito, was not immediately on hand. Entomological evidence suggests that slave ships brought *Aedes* from Africa, along with the yellow-fever virus. From 1647, when an epidemic in Barbados spread throughout the Caribbean, yellow fever so scourged American coastal cities that it came to be regarded as an American disease.

In discussing the fall in the Amerindian populations, it is important to note the impact of this second – African – wave of diseases. In the highland areas of the

The origin of syphilis

Columbus and his men have often been blamed for carrying syphilis from the Americas to Europe, from whence it spread around the world. The case against Columbus has seemed good, albeit circumstantial.

Syphilis broke out in 1493 or 1494 during a dispute over the Kingdom of Naples. Spain and France were the major antagonists although the French soldiers, in particular, came from all over Europe. Initially, the disease was called the 'disease of Naples', but it raged with such virulence among the French troops that France was forced to give up the campaign. When the army broke up and Polish, English, Hungarian, Swiss, and German as well as French soldiers returned to their homes, the disease quickly became known as the 'French Pox'– to everyone but the French.

The Italians seem to have been the first to note that some of the Spanish soldiers had accompanied Columbus on his second voyage, thereby giving birth to the notion of an American origin of syphilis. European physicians contradicted this idea, some claiming that the disease was a new one and others insisting that it was merely a more virulent manifestation of an older malady. It certainly acted like a new disease in Europe. It raged for a time with extraordinary virulence, became milder over time and, then, by the eighteenth century quietly assumed the form we know today. Other evidence that seemed to point towards an American cradle for the disease lay in the Spanish reports that the Amerindians experienced much milder cases of syphilis than they did.

The latter may be explained, however, by cross-immunity received from other treponemal infections that Amerindians suffered, such as pinta and non-venereal syphilis. In fact, all of the treponemal infections seem to have the same causal agent (a spirochaete bacterium); the pathogens are indistinguishable under the microscope and cannot be differentiated in the laboratory either.

This phenomenon has given rise to the theory that at least the Old World treponemal diseases – yaws, non-venereal syphilis, and syphilis – are the same disease with different symptoms and different means of transmission. For example, in tropical Africa, yaws, viewed as the oldest manifestation, is characterized by open sores on the body and is normally spread from child to child, by skin-to-skin contact. But in moving to dry North Africa, yaws gives way to non-venereal syphilis (bejel), which is also essentially a disease of children, spreading from child to child via shared drinking or eating utensils.

It was only in Europe, so the argument goes, that the pathogen was frustrated by relative cleanliness and a cooler environment, in which ample clothing prevented skin-to-skin transmission. The consequence was that the disease found another means of transmission – a venereal one, from adult to adult. According to this view, syphilis was in the process of emerging as a disease entity in European cities just as Columbus set sail.

There are other possibilities. Mutations could also account for the various treponemal illnesses. Some sort of American treponemal infection may have united with a similar one in Europe to become syphilis, with both of the earlier infections subsequently disappearing.

Syphilis, along with some other treponemal infections, leaves a signature in bone. At present, however, the findings from buried remains are inconclusive. There seems to be some evidence of venereal syphilis in the Americas before 1492. And claims have been made for the discovery of syphilis in bones of Europeans interred long before Columbus sailed. If nothing else, the story of syphilis does highlight some of the problems of historians of disease.

Alongside the horrors of smallpox, the 'great pox', or syphilis, captured the imagination in the fifteenth century. *The Syphilitic* by Albrecht Dürer, 1496.

Andes and central Mexico, the native populations staggered under the assault of Eurasian diseases, but they ultimately recovered. This was, at least in part, because they were spared the African illnesses – the mosquito vectors do not thrive at altitudes significantly above sea level. The populations of the low-lying areas of the Caribbean and the Amazon basin, however, were seriously affected by both the Eurasian and the African diseases and were almost obliterated. Other less-lethal, but nonetheless formidable, African diseases also arrived on the slave ships, among them dracunculiasis, filariasis, onchocerciasis, hookworm disease (caused by the misnamed *Necator americanus*), yaws (allied to pinta), and even leprosy, which had previously disappeared from Europe.

NEW WORLDS, NEW PATHOGENS?

The abrupt linking of the disease environments of Europe, the Americas, and Africa has come under much scrutiny by scholars. Their suspicion is that it did more than simply scatter known diseases more widely – that it, in fact, spawned some new diseases for the world. From a European viewpoint, some new diseases did seem to appear around the time of the Columbian voyages. Typhus was one of these. It appeared in Europe during the last of the wars of the reconquest, as Spain finally conquered Granada in 1492; the disease seems to have reached Spain from the Arab world. In this case, therefore, Columbus is exonerated.

Like syphilis, smallpox presents historians of medicine with a puzzle. It seems to have varied considerably in its virulence over time. There were two types of smallpox before the disease finally disappeared in the second half of the 1970s: variola major, which had mortality rates of up to 25–30 per cent, and variola minor, a much milder disease with mortality rates of 1 per cent or less. Doubtless, strains intermediate between the two also existed. Before about 1500 – in Europe at least – smallpox was not a virulent killer, but around that date it became so, causing some 10 to 15 per cent of all deaths in some countries. Investigators have occasionally voiced the suspicion that the most virulent form of smallpox originated in sub-Saharan Africa, not Asia. Recently, the argument has been advanced that it was with the Atlantic slave trade that this most deadly strain was unleashed.

These new, or newly modified, diseases served to enrich the already sizable swarm of pathogens that swept over other 'newly discovered' peoples, who, like the Amerindians, were so brutally united with the larger world. Vasco da Gama, in leading the Portuguese into the Indian Ocean (1498) and an eastern empire, also inadvertently spearheaded the spread of syphilis as far east as Japan. The voyage of Ferdinand Magellan (1519–22) finished what Columbus started by sailing west and taking the Spanish into the East. And in the wake of his ships came diseases with the crews of the Manilla galleons, as well as other explorers, missionaries, traders, and, in the eighteenth century, British and American whalers.

The inhabitants of many Pacific islands had suffered from malaria, filariasis, and tropical skin afflictions before the arrival of Europeans. But these populations

The rise and fall of tuberculosis

Tuberculosis is an ancient disease of humans, and possibly evolved with them. It flourished in the crowded and filthy cities of Europe and Asia, becoming more prevalent when plague began declining in frequency. In the nineteenth century, the disease killed millions, and in some places it affected nearly all of the population.

Medieval people seem to have suffered much from the disease but most probably had the glandular form called scrofula. In England and France, it was believed that royalty had the power to cure the affliction by touching the sufferers, and from the twelfth until the eighteenth centuries, the 'king's touch' was regularly used against the condition.

With urban and industrial development from the sixteenth century onwards, however, the virulent pulmonary form became increasingly dominant in countries as far apart as England and Japan. In many places, by the nineteenth century, 500 or more of every 100,000 people died from it each year. In the Americas, African-Americans suffered considerably more than whites, and annual death rates in some parts of the Caribbean and in Georgia, USA, approached 1,000 per 100,000 population. In part, this can be blamed on susceptibility, for the disease had not been part of the African disease environment in historical times. It was also testimony to the miserable living conditions that awaited blacks in American cities after their ordeal of slavery.

Like Europeans of the Middle Ages, slaves on the plantations suffered mostly from scrofula, as did the Amerindians of the USA and Canada during the early twentieth century. Like blacks, Amerindians revealed an extraordinary susceptibility to the disease and had little resistance once infected. For other peoples, tuberculosis began to recede in the nineteenth century and this dramatic recession continued into the twentieth century.

The retreat of the disease is mysterious because, although medicine understood the cause of the disease (a bacillus called *Mycobacterium tuberculosis*), it did not know how to treat it and had no 'magic bullet' until after the Second World War – long after the disease had faded as a problem in developed countries.

Because tuberculosis does best among the poorly nourished and makes little headway among those with sufficient high-quality protein in their diet, improving nutrition, and better hygiene and housing, has been seen by some as the most likely explanation for the widespread decline in the disease. This, however, is not a sufficient explanation, given the comeback that the disease seems to be making in depressed inner-city areas. The disease remains a major health problem throughout the developing world and is a growing problem once again in the developed world – for example, among the homeless, and those with AIDS.

Various swellings and skin conditions were well known in medieval times, notably scrofula. Scrofulous sores were treated with cleansing and ointments, as shown in these drawings from a thirteenth-century translation in Norman French of Roger of Parma's surgical treatise *Chirurgia*. In one of many epidemiological mutations, scrofula seems to have declined in the seventeenth century, being gradually replaced by the far more deadly tuberculosis.

of Asian horticulturalists, in many cases separated from the larger world for thousands of years, were 'virgin soil' for the infectious foreign diseases. However, the relative smallness of their populations, on the one hand, and isolation, on the other, would have caused most epidemics to burn out quickly.

Some idea of the thousands of small holocausts of disease that must have occurred among these populations can be gained by viewing the example of the Hawaiian Islands. First settled around AD 300, they remained 'undiscovered' until the arrival of Captain James Cook in 1778. Cook's surgeon wrote that the following year the crew deliberately introduced syphilis to the islands. Whether true or not, syphilis, along with smallpox and other illnesses, reportedly reduced the native population by 90 per cent within a century.

A similar precipitous decline of the native populations of Australia got underway after the start of English settlement in 1788. Smallpox erupted almost immediately (1789) among the Aborigines in the eastern half of the continent and, according to British estimates, destroyed half of those with any contact with Port Arthur (Sydney). After this, the disease spread into the interior with unknown consequences. A young Charles Darwin in 1836 had clearly absorbed much of this sort of mournful history when he wrote in his *Beagle* diary '[w]herever the European has trod, death seems to pursue the aboriginal'.

While Europeans were establishing their empires and carrying death to aboriginal peoples, they themselves were caught in a crossfire of disease at home. Epidemics of plague punished areas of the south and east; malaria was on the increase; in the sixteenth century, at least three severe influenza epidemics swept the continent and virulent smallpox appeared; syphilis was increasingly virulent; there were epidemics of diphtheria and scarlet fever; and typhus began to make regular appearances among armies. In fact, it was disease (in this case typhus rather than syphilis) that once more was decisive in spoiling French hopes of conquering the Kingdom of Naples. Typhus broke out among the French soldiers just as victory over Charles V seemed assured. Some 30,000 of them died before the remnants of the army were withdrawn.

On the other side of the world, new diseases such as syphilis, scarlet fever, and diphtheria entered China to join smallpox, measles, malaria, and other old ailments. Cholera was described by Westerners for the first time when the Portuguese visited sixteenth-century India, where, it seems, plague was also raging. In Japan, the first Westerners to visit in 1543 arrived during a period of great population growth, the Japanese having come to immunological terms with their most important diseases. The only new illness in their environment was syphilis, which had reached the islands from China where Europeans had introduced it somewhat earlier. The Japanese called it the 'Chinese pox'.

Europe and China were now to enjoy their own rise in population. In Europe, the winds of change stirred up by the Renaissance signalled an end to feudalism, while fostering the rise of capitalism, predatory nation states, empires, and increasingly authoritarian governments. There were strides towards industrialization and urbanization, stimulated on the one hand by growing governmental bureaucracies and on the other by the needs and fruits of empire – or by the determined quest for those fruits.

It is within this array of historical circumstances that the populations of Britain and northern Europe gradually escaped from the age-old tyranny of disease and its check on population growth. Growing cities exposed more people to disease, and increasing numbers became immunized in the process. Strong governments, by establishing quarantine measures directly, and indirectly, with the inspection of ships for tax collection, helped to keep plague and other diseases at bay (see page 79). Moreover, governments launched public-health campaigns that reduced the populations of vermin and insects, especially houseflies. Finally, attempts were made in the early eighteenth century to reduce outbreaks of smallpox by variolation, a technique that may have originated in China. Variola in pus from the pustules of infected persons was inserted into scratches on people unaffected, which gave them a mild form of the disease. The procedure sometimes proved fatal, and even resulted in epidemics, but after the 1760s safer inoculation methods were found. The strongest blow against smallpox came with the cowpox vaccination introduced in England by Edward Jenner in 1796. This was quickly adopted throughout Europe and within a few years had reached the Spanish colonies in South America and Asia.

NUTRITION AND DECLINING MORTALITY

Another important factor in this momentous demographic turnaround has to do with nutrition. If the Americas offered few pathogens to the rest of the world, they provided much in the way of foodstuffs. The increasingly widespread cultivation of the potato, which was introduced to Europe in the sixteenth century (along with squash), helped to make a better life for many, especially the poor. In addition to filling stomachs, the potato, which was easy to grow in northern climates, became an important source of vitamins (especially ascorbic acid) and minerals.

Maize from the Americas became a staple in the diet of many others, who, perhaps not enthusiastically, began substituting cornmeal cakes for the more expensive wheat bread. Maize and potatoes are staple crops that produce more calories per unit of land than any other (save cassava), and they certainly helped to sustain a growing urban proletariat. Perhaps, though, the greatest contribution to human health from maize was as animal feed. With more and more people forced from the land into cities, more space was available for domesticated animals. With hay and maize to sustain them, it became possible to carry greater numbers of animals over the winter. Thus another feature of the changing pattern of nutrition was a greater availability throughout the year of high-quality protein in the form of milk and cheese, and eggs as well as meat. Such protein would have helped people ward off many diseases more easily. A reliable supply of milk doubtless helped many more individuals to survive infancy and early childhood than had done so in the past. Improved transportation networks to deliver fresh foods more widely were also obviously vital in helping to improve nutrition.

A crossfire of debate continues over the importance of nutrition in the growth of the European population – and thus also over the importance of American crops in the European diet. It may be that answers are so entangled with and obscured by other complex forces that they cannot be teased out. Some light might be shed on the matter by examples from other parts of the world. In China, for reasons yet to be explained, there was a fall in the rate of mortality after the sixteenth-century introduction of maize and of sweet and white potatoes from the Americas. West and West Central Africa also experienced something of a population explosion after the introduction of cassava, maize, sweet potatoes, and peanuts. The irony is that the population was drained by a slave trade to the hemisphere that had provided the plants to begin with.

NEW PLAGUES – YELLOW FEVER AND CHOLERA

As we have seen, Africa also sent deadly diseases westwards. By the end of the seventeenth century, yellow fever, in addition to haunting ports in the Caribbean, Central America, and Mexico, seemed to be ubiquitous along the eastern coasts of the continent. It struck Pernambuco in Brazil in 1685, killing thousands in Recife and Olinda and spread into Ceará before it burned out some 5 years later. To the north, the disease entered New York in 1668, Philadelphia and Charleston in 1690, and Boston in 1691.

In the eighteenth century, yellow fever extended its range to become a regular visitor to the ports of Colombia, Peru, and Ecuador in the Americas; and to

Cholera – the scourge of the nineteenth century

In 1817, the first pandemic of cholera spread from the disease's endemic area in Bengal through Southeast Asia to China in the east, and from Persia to Egypt in the west. The second pandemic, which began in 1824, covered much of this same ground but also spread further by penetrating into Russia before moving west across Europe to England in 1831; it then jumped the Atlantic to engulf North America in 1832 and the Caribbean and Latin America in 1833.

The third pandemic began when cholera accompanied British troops into Afghanistan in 1839 and into China in 1840. From there it travelled to Persia and Central Asia, and then, following what were becoming well-worn pathways, it spread into Arabia and Europe before hurdling the Atlantic in 1848 to rage in North and South America.

There is some debate over whether the cholera of the 1850s represented a new pandemic or was a continuation of the third. But, whatever the case, by 1854 both the Old and New Worlds were awash in the disease. The fourth pandemic began in 1863 and burned out in 1874, visiting most of its old haunts in the interim. The fifth pandemic, which began in 1881 and endured until 1896, was widespread in China and Japan in the Far East, Egypt in the Near East, and Germany and Russia in Europe. Quick work in New York stopped the disease from spreading in North America, but South America sustained outbreaks as did East Africa.

The sixth pandemic (1899–1923) missed the Western Hemisphere and most of Europe, save for outbreaks in the Balkan Peninsula, Hungary, portions of Russia, and sporadic outbreaks in southern Europe. It did not, however, miss the Far East: China, Japan, Korea, and the Philippines all hosted the disease.

The seventh pandemic, which began in 1961, followed roughly the same pattern as the sixth. In the early 1990s, cholera returned to the Western Hemisphere, radiating outwards from Peru into neighbouring countries.

The causative agent of cholera, a bacterium called *Vibrio cholerae*, was first isolated by Robert Koch and colleagues in 1883 (see also page 184). It was one of many nineteenth- and twentieth-century discoveries that pinpointed the causative agents and the means of transmission of many of humankind's deadliest infectious diseases.

There was no known cure for cholera before the twentieth century, hence governments, doctors, and individuals had recourse to traditional modes of prevention, not least trying to keep at bay the 'miasmatics' that were supposedly responsible by purifying the air. Bonfires were believed to be disinfective, and were lit in Granada during the cholera epidemic in around 1865, as shown in this engraving (after a sketch by the British Vice-Consul, H. Stainer).

Oporto, Lisbon, Barcelona, Malaga, and Cadiz in Europe. At the same time, it attacked the now-veteran Philadelphians with six epidemics. The disease also became decisive in Caribbean military campaigns. It thwarted Admiral Edward Vernon's 1741 assault on Cartagena in Columbia – half of his original landing force of 19,000 was lost to the virus; it helped in pruning 80,000 men from the British army in the West Indies during the years 1793–6; and it accounted for a sizable portion of the 40,000 French dead in their abortive attempt to regain San Domingue on the island of Hispaniola (now Haiti).

In the nineteenth century, yellow fever was especially prevalent in the port cities of southern USA, where, before the Civil War, it hammered Savannah with fifteen epidemics, Charleston with twenty-two, and New Orleans with at least thirty-three. After the war, it resumed this assault, which culminated in the 1878 epidemic. This moved inland up the Mississippi to leave countless dead in a swathe that cut from New Orleans to Memphis and beyond. Clearly, at least as far as the USA was concerned, yellow fever evened the score for participation in the African slave trade. Its losses to the disease far exceeded the number of slaves it imported.

Yellow fever also continued to slaughter Europeans in the Caribbean, most notably Spanish troops sent to put an end to Cuba's rebellion of 1868–78 (the Ten Years' War) and Frenchmen first sent to lay a railway across Panama and then to

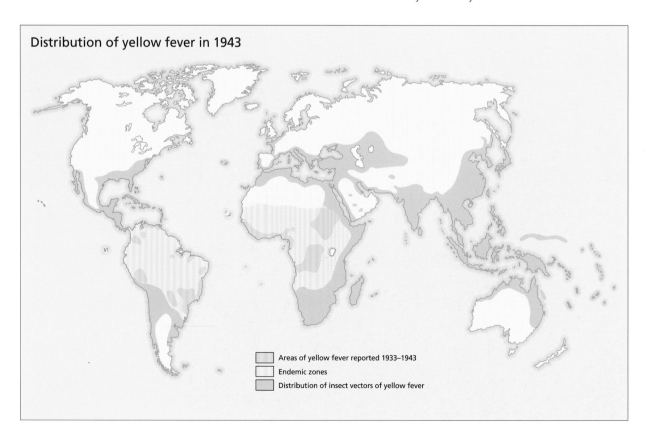

Distribution of yellow fever in 1943

Areas of yellow fever reported 1933–1943
Endemic zones
Distribution of insect vectors of yellow fever

construct a canal. It also killed Europeans at home, invading numerous cities of Spain and Portugal as well as Gibraltar, and moving north to strike at the coasts of France and England.

Save for the 1821 epidemic in Barcelona and that of 1857 in Lisbon, however, yellow fever seemed a minor disease in Europe compared to the ravages of typhus and cholera. Typhus played a substantial role in turning the 1812 expedition of Napoleon to Russia into a catastrophe, and between 1816 and 1819 the disease ravaged Ireland. The revolutions of 1848 triggered typhus epidemics in eastern Europe, which then subsided until the First World War. During that war it killed a reported 2 to 3 million soldiers and civilians. Afterwards, it continued to stalk the Russians and eastern Europeans by killing another 3 million or so.

Cholera, however, was easily the biggest epidemic news of the nineteenth century. Before that time (and thus before all the major advances in technology and transportation), the disease seems to have confined itself to India, where it had been observed and described by outsiders at least since the sixteenth century. From 1817, however, it appeared with increasing frequency outside India. By 1821, it had involved Java and China to the east and Persia to the west.

DISEASE AND IMPERIALISM

While cholera and some of the other 'old' diseases of civilization were being brought under control, civilization itself was spawning and spreading other infections. Medical advances opened Africa – previously known as the 'white man's grave' because of tropical fever – to European colonization as the nineteenth cen-

Slaves processing tobacco, an American plant that triggered perhaps the most deadly plague of all. Its toll in lives lost to cancers, heart-related diseases, and respiratory disorders continues to mount.

A child with rickets in Budapest around 1920. Rickets is a disease of children, marked by a softened condition of the bones. The result of a deficiency of vitamin D, it is chiefly found amongst the underfed children of the poor, especially in urban settings where want of sunlight contributes to the condition. It became common in the big towns of the industrialized nations in the eighteenth and nineteenth centuries. Rickets was among the earliest deficiency diseases to be described. There are, for example, Chinese accounts of the disease dating back to the tenth century and earlier. The definitive text on the subject remains that of the English physician Francis Glisson. His *De Rachitide* was published in 1650.

tury drew to a close. The discovery of the cause of malaria and the establishment of a reliable supply of quinine (derived from the bark of the cinchona tree) to protect against it simultaneously provided a green light for imperial adventure.

Once established in Africa, however, Europeans sometimes seemed intent on turning it into a black man's grave. They forced Africans into mines to extract the continent's mineral resources; they seized fertile agricultural lands formerly occupied by tribal communities; they introduced alien breeds of cattle; they transformed barter economies into monetary economies; and they built railways and roads to link them.

In this proletarianization of Africa and in rearranging ecologies, the colonists unleashed massive epidemics of sleeping sickness and did much to extend the range of other illnesses. In addition, they brought tuberculosis to Africa. Highly mobile African labourers then spread it to all corners of sub-Saharan Africa, where it smouldered in the slums of an expanding urban poor. The nutritional status of Africans also fell sharply in the face of the implementation of cash-crop economies, which were often based on monoculture (such as cocoa in Ghana).

And despite the efforts of missionaries, colonial medicine was mostly aimed at preserving the health of the oppressors, and seldom reached the oppressed.

NUTRITIONAL DISEASES

Nutritional explanations of the waxing and waning of diseases are complicated by our lack of knowledge of what constitutes good nutrition. As we have seen, our hunter-gatherer forebears consumed an amazing variety of foodstuffs, whereas we, by contrast, consume relatively few. The archaeological record leaves no doubt that humans who surrendered their hunting and gathering ways for sedentary agriculture paid a stiff price in health. They became shorter and suffered considerably from anaemias as a result of an increasingly limited diet centred around a staple crop. At the same time, their young endured what appears to have been protein energy malnutrition after weaning, which doubtless contributed to soaring rates of child mortality (see page 47).

Technological improvements in agriculture and plant breeding and the exchange of crops in the aftermath of Columbus's voyage of 1492, meant greater quantities of food to sustain more people. But for those whose survival depended on a diet centred closely on a staple crop, it meant a tremendous sacrifice in nutritional quality. Hence the appearance of the classic deficiency diseases.

The poor in the American South, Africans, southern Europeans, and peoples in India, Egypt, and the Middle East who embraced maize cultivation frequently fell victim to pellagra, a disease characterized by diarrhoea, dermatitis, dementia, and ultimately death for as many as 70 per cent of its victims. The cause of the disease is complicated, but the major factor is a deficiency of niacin. It is not that maize lacks niacin. The trouble is that it has a chemical bond that does not release the niacin to the consumer unless that bond is broken with treatment by lime – a secret that native Americans knew but it did not get passed back to the Old World.

Beriberi is another disease linked to vitamin B deficiency, in this case thiamine. The affliction is normally associated with the rice cultures of Asia. Rice husks contain plenty of thiamine, but people have, over the ages, done their best to strip away the husk to make the grain more palatable, appealing, and amenable to storage. Traditional hand-milling of rice produced the neurological and cardiovascular symptoms of 'dry' and 'wet' beriberi for many people across the world and led to infantile beriberi, which was practically always fatal for nursing babies and toddlers with thiamine-deficient mothers. The problem became especially acute after the advent of steam-driven milling, and by the late 1950s beriberi had become a leading cause of death in parts of Asia, especially for infants.

Rice, however, has not been the only culprit in the aetiology of beriberi. The disease has also been caused by diets

A diet too closely centered on maize can produce iron-deficiency anaemia. Tell-tale signs of this are perforations in the eye sockets of skulls. Early maize farmers in the Americas are among those who suffered from this nutritional disease.

St Vitus's Dance by the Flemish artist Peter Breughel the Elder. Breughel here depicts a 'fool's dance', illustrating traditional stereotypes that link folly with festive behaviour, merrymaking, and drunkenness. He may have seen 'dancing-mania', a craze affecting parts of late medieval Europe, and associated with social fears and disorder. Some historians believe that images like this represent St Vitus's dance (Sydenham's chorea, a disorder characterized by jerky involuntary movements named after Thomas Sydenham). Others have argued that ergotism (poisoning through mouldy rye bread) produced such delirious behaviour. It is more likely, however, that Breughal was simply following an artistic convention in depicting the dancers of Saint-Guy.

too closely centred on manioc meal and flour, and those confined to white bread before the adoption of enrichment procedures. Like pellagra, beriberi was particularly prevalent among institutionalized populations – for example, slaves on plantations, prisoners, children in orphanages, and inmates of ayslums – and those at sea for long periods of time.

The classic shipboard disease, however, was scurvy, triggered by a deficiency in vitamin C (ascorbic acid). Because humans do not synthesize their own vitamin C, scurvy is probably a very old disease. However, it takes some 30 weeks of vitamin-C deprivation for the classic symptoms of spongy, bleeding gums to appear, and even longer for old wounds to open and death to occur, so its appearance before the fifteenth century would have been relatively rare. But the desire for trade, exploration, and empire that accompanied the growing economic power of Europe sent ships to sea for periods long enough for the disease to develop; and it became the scourge of seamen for more than 300–400 years.

Scurvy also affected armies (especially during sieges), erupted in prisoner-of-war camps, dogged the heels of Arctic and Antarctic explorers, and tortured the Irish after the great failure of the potato crop in 1845–6, because potatoes contain vitamin C whereas the grains sent to relieve their plight did not.

In the middle of the eighteenth century it was repeatedly shown that citrus juice could prevent scurvy (see page 256). It was not until the end of that century, however, that British sailors were regularly issued lime juice to combat the disease. By the close of the nineteenth century, with medicine in the grip of the germ theory (see page 184), scurvy and the other nutritional diseases were often seen as the work of pathogens. It required the scientific knowledge generated in the twentieth century to get nutritional research back on track and to establish the concept of deficiency diseases.

All such deficiency diseases, at least when widespread, may be viewed as the consequence of nutritional problems caused by advances in civilization. The same is true for other ailments that, although not strictly deficiency diseases, are food-related. Ergotism, for example, is a disease caused by consuming cereal grains – especially rye – infected by the ergot fungus (*Claviceps purpurea*). Known since the time of Galen, it became prevalent in medieval Europe among poor people. Their bread, which constituted the bulk of the diet, was frequently made with spoiled rye, producing the 'convulsive' form when it affected the central nervous system and the 'gangrenous' form when it affected the blood supply to the extremities. The disease was often called St Anthony's fire. At least 130 epidemics occurred in Europe between 591 and 1789, and scores of thousands were killed. Outbreaks were reported from various parts of Europe as late as the 1920s.

A different kind of nutritional problem created by constricted diets is protein energy malnutrition (PEM), which, as we have seen earlier, is essentially a problem of the young and a problem that developed only as people settled into agriculture. Tell-tale evidence is seen on the teeth of early farmers, in the form of hypoplasias (growth-arrest lines) that indicate a real struggle for survival at about the time of weaning. In modern peoples, the evidence is plainly visible in the swollen bellies of kwashiorkor and the wasting away of marasmus, the two symptomatic poles of PEM.

The root cause of PEM is the weaning of a child from breast milk to a cereal pap that contains little or none of the whole protein that the child needs for its growth and development. Whereas hunter-gatherers were obliged to forage for their weaned youngsters, sedentary people concentrated on a staple cereal, which simplified the weaning process. Such simplicity, in turn, encouraged more pregnancies, so that one child was (and is) often abruptly weaned to make room for another. Thus the African word 'kwashiorkor' means the 'sickness of the deprived child'.

PEM often becomes full-blown when children acquire an infection and the latter, rather than the nutritional condition, gets the blame. Nonetheless, PEM is one of the world's great killers, especially in developing regions. It can retard the development and impair the health in later life of those that survive it as children.

The industrial revolution created the conditions for an explosion in population and for much ill health, especially in the overcrowded, insanitary slum quarters of the major cities. This engraving is from *The Builder* magazine for 14 June 1862.

DISEASE IN THE MODERN WORLD

Clearly, then, one result of the agricultural revolution – the concentration of diets on staple crops – was a mixed blessing of enabling more and more people to live but at significant costs to their health. The same might be said for the much more recent and ongoing industrial revolution, which, while creating the conditions for a further explosion in population, also produced general ill-health as well as some specific new diseases.

For example, black lung disease (coal workers' pneumoconiosis) cut life short for many coalminers; brown lung disease (byssinosis) became the curse of cotton textile workers; white lung disease (asbestosis) affected those engaged in working with asbestos; exposure to lead brought on lead poisoning; the 'phossy jaw' was an occupational risk of matchworkers who were exposed to phosphorous; and dust from stone, flint, and sand led to silicosis or 'grinders' disease'.

In 1775, London surgeon Percivall Pott pointed out that many males who had been chimney sweeps while boys later suffered from scrotal cancer. He linked this with irritation caused by soot, and thus identified the first cancer-causing occupation. Subsequently, ultraviolet light, X-rays, radioactive substances such as radium and uranium, and other irritants such as coal-tar derivatives were implicated in cancer.

Cancer, heart-related ailments, and probably Alzheimer's disease are ancient diseases of humankind. There is debate about why there seems to be a substantial increase in all three in the twentieth century, especially in the developed world. One possibility is that more people are living long enough to acquire them. Another explanation has to do with lifestyle – mass-produced and widely used tobacco products and distilled spirits, also products of the modern world, contribute considerably to at least two of these conditions.

It is probably the case, however, that a good number of other factors stemming from advances in civilization are also responsible. There may be more carbon in the atmosphere today because of forest clearance and cultivation than industrialization; but belching smokestacks and exhaust fumes from motor vehicles have put many other chemicals into the air we breathe, the foods we eat, and the water

Two views from the same spot in Widnes, Liverpool, in 1895 and 1960. Coal-smoke pollution, produced by factories and domestic heating, remained a major cause of respiratory problems in Britain till the 1960s, when smoke-abatement legislation and the introduction of smokeless fuel proved effective in producing cleaner air. Since then, however, exhaust from motor vehicles and other chemical pollutants have contributed to a rising incidence worldwide of asthma and allergies, especially among the young and elderly in congested cities.

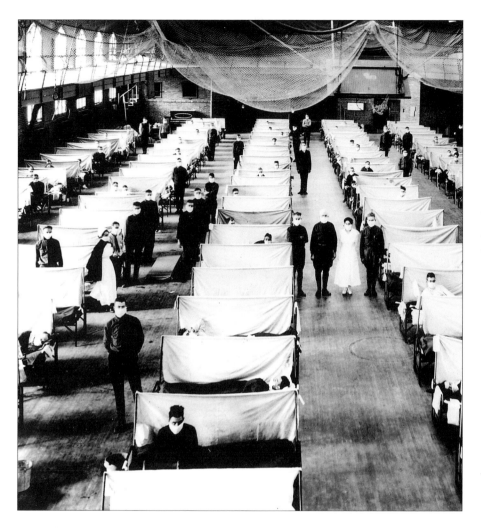

The pandemic of Spanish flu that spread around the globe in 1918 after the First World War killed more people than died in the war itself. The US Congress allocated $1 million to the Public Health Service to hire doctors and to care for the sick. Infirmaries catering for scores of people, such as this one in the gymnasium at Iowa State University, had to be set up; but there were no effective treatments for the flu sufferers.

we drink. Moreover, many suspect that the incidence of skin cancers is increasing because of atmospheric pollution, which is increasing ultraviolet intensity. Heavy use of sodium has been implicated in both stomach cancer and hypertension. And foods and water are processed with chemicals that are under increasing scrutiny by both cancer and heart-disease researchers.

Greater longevity is certainly a factor in a greater frequency of some of the genetic diseases and genetic predisposition to other illnesses. In the past, a far smaller percentage of victims of these afflictions would have survived to reproduce and pass on the traits. As some geneticists have argued, in the developed world, at any rate, the principles of rigorous natural selection no longer apply. We have entered another stage – that of 'relaxed selection', and we are having to pay for this with a greater frequency of diseases ranging from multiple sclerosis to mastoiditis.

Medicine has had the opportunity in the twentieth century to focus much of its research on genetic diseases and the chronic ailments – the new diseases of civi-

A sick child at a malnourish-
ment clinic in Sudan.
Malnutrition remains a major
source of sickness, especially
amongst the young, in the
developing world. Critics contend that international relief
agencies are able to do little
more than to palliate the
problem rather than get to
its roots.

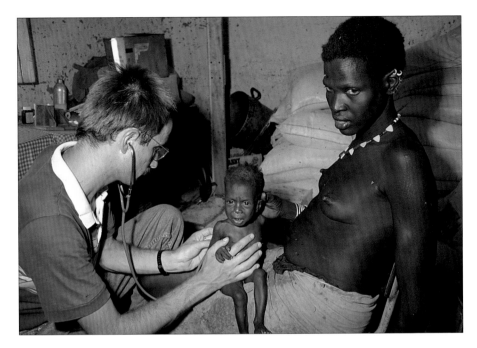

lization – because of its triumphs over the old contagious diseases, culminating with the eradication of smallpox in the 1970s. But the collective self-confidence of the medical community has been shaken on several occasions during the past 100 years. This happened, for example, in 1918–19 when an influenza pandemic of unprecedented virulence swept the world, killing between 25 and 50 million people. Hard on its heels came an epidemic of encephalitis lethargica (an inflammation of the brain and spinal cord) and another wave of killer influenza in 1920. How and why influenza suddenly became so deadly (especially to young adults) has never been satisfactorily explained – nor has its relationship with encephalitis lethargica.

The encounter of modern medicine with poliomyelitis, by contrast, has had a more satisfactory outcome. Poliomyelitis is an ancient viral disease of humankind but epidemics identified as polio became frequent only towards the end of the nineteenth century. This created the belief that it was a new disease, and the great New York epidemic of 1916 produced fears that polio was a modern-day plague – especially when what had been regarded as a children's disease began affecting adults. Such fears gradually subsided with the realization that, in the past, most children had been immunized early in life by the disease itself, which travels the oral–faecal route. Improved sanitation that in many cases had prevented this immunization was actually responsible for the upsurge of the disease. The introduction of vaccinations first by Jonas Edward Salk (1955) and then Albert Bruce Sabin (1960) has brought about a drastic decline in the disease in the developed world and much of the developing world as well. In 1994, the Americas were declared a polio-free zone after 2 years with no reported cases, and the World Health Organization hopes to elimate the disease worldwide by the year 2000.

Medicine has, however, so far proved powerless against another disease. As was the case early on with polio, acquired immune deficiency syndrome (AIDS) has seemed to be a new disease. Unfortunately, the causative agent, the human immunodeficiency virus (HIV), mutates even more rapidly than the viral agents of influenza, which has frustrated the development of both vaccines and effective antiviral drugs. Actually there seem to be two main types of the virus involved. HIV-1 was the first to be identified (1981), although in retrospect it would seem that the disease has been spreading silently for years. The principal means of transmission of most of its subtypes have been through homosexual contact and through blood and blood products. In 1985, HIV-2 was identified in West Africa; its pattern of transmission seems to be via heterosexual intercourse. HIV-1 and HIV-2 are now worldwide in their distribution, but both seem to have originated in sub-Saharan Africa where antibodies against HIV were discovered in stored blood dating from 1959, and where most of the world's cases (about two-thirds) were located as of 1995 (see page 344).

Because HIV impairs the immune system, patients often fall victim to illnesses such as pneumocystis pneumonia, tuberculosis, and other infections. Nonetheless, AIDS is a disease in itself, albeit one that can take a decade or longer after infection to manifest itself, with, what so far seems to be invariably fatal consequences. Such a hiatus, however, makes it difficult to calculate the spread of the disease, and thus projections must depend on estimates. Unhappily, even the most optimistic of these suggest that millions will die of AIDS. Some even predict that in terms of overall mortality the disease will take the lead as the biggest killer of humans in history.

Yet other deadly viral diseases have surfaced in Africa, among them Ebola, Lassa, Marburg, and Rift Valley fevers, and still others in South America such as Bolivian haemorrhagic fever and Argentine haemorrhagic fever. It is conceivable that, like AIDS, one or more of these could be unleashed on the wider world. In a sense they, too, are diseases of civilization – in this case of the developing world, where impoverished populations are swelling and chronic diseases of advancing age take second place to major infectious aliments.

Modern medicine has made it possible for increasing numbers of people to survive infancy and childhood in the developing world, but does little for them after that (except for notable campaigns such as those against smallpox or polio). However, in a world growing increasingly smaller as populations are knit ever more closely together, the question arises as to whether we can afford such neglect. Indeed, self-interest, if nothing else, may indicate the importance of cultivating health in the developing world, especially if that world continues to incubate diseases that reach out to kill in the developed countries.

The Rise of Medicine

CHAPTER 2

Vivian Nutton

Around 1570, the Basle physician and medical professor Theodor Zwinger traced the ancestry of the art of medicine back to the ancient Greeks. Even if he, a good Protestant, could not entirely believe that a pagan god like Apollo had created the healing arts to benefit humanity, he accepted the half-god Asclepius as one of founders of medicine, and the mythical centaur Chiron, half man and half horse, as the creator of pharmacology. But long before, he believed, God had placed in the world healing substances for the benefit of sick people, waiting to be discovered by subsequent generations.

One may smile at Zwinger's historical fictions, yet his recourse to legend conveys an essential truth; the evidence for healing and medicine antedates any literary text or historical event. Archaeological excavations of sites thousands of years old have revealed bodies that show signs of medical attention – broken limbs that have been set, dislocations replaced, and wounds treated successfully. Some skulls show signs of trepanation (holes drilled through the bone), a procedure that demanded technical expertise and a rationale for operating, although what that was is a matter for conjecture. We may also suppose that various plants and other substances were also used to treat those who felt ill, and that some individuals gained a reputation for manual dexterity, herbal knowledge, or ability to communicate with whatever force was causing the disease. In this sense, medicine has always been with us, and to talk of the rise of medicine is to labour the obvious.

Votive relief to the healing god Asclepius, from Thyrea, S. Greece, 350 BC. With the god, who is leaning on his staff with the entwined snake, are members of his family – his wife Epione, sons Machaon and Podaleirius, and daughters Hygieia, Aigle, and Panacea. Hygieia was the goddess of health.

The learned Zwinger was no fool, however, and his attempt to write a history of medicine was based on the secure belief that the medicine of his own day was the result of the progressive accumulation of learning over the centuries, and that those who possessed this knowledge, the doctors and surgeons, were the best (some would say the only) persons to be consulted when one fell ill. Self-medication might not be enough, while those who merely pretended to medical knowledge, frequently labelled quacks and charlatans, might kill as often as they cured. Medicine, in short, was being defined as something over and beyond mere healing, as the possession of a specific body of learning, theoretical and practical, that might be used to treat the sick. What this learning was, and how medicine came to supersede healing, are questions that this chapter will try to answer.

ANCIENT HEALERS OF BABYLONIA AND EGYPT

Although Theodor Zwinger was right to place the origins of his tradition of medicine in Ancient Greece, the Greeks were not the only peoples of the eastern Mediterranean region who could claim to have invented medicine. Ancient Mesopotamia and Egypt had medical texts and traditions that long predated those of Greece. Those of India, China, and the Far East, although impinging scarcely at all on Western medicine until more modern times, have equal claim to antiquity.

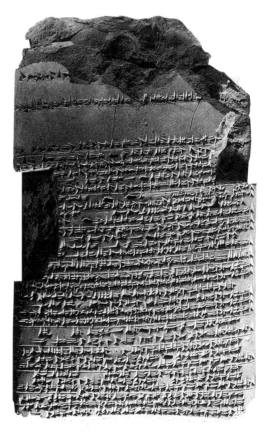

A Babylonian tablet of baked brick, around 650 BC, describes epilepsy. Each section of the text (translated on page 54) is carefully marked off from the next by a line.

The abundance of new discoveries from excavations in the Middle East, along with recent reinterpretations of fragmentary older texts, written on baked clay tablets, makes any characterization of Babylonian medicine extremely hazardous. Nonetheless, it is clear that acute observers noted down a large range of symptoms of disease, some of which can be readily identified with conditions such as epilepsy, scurvy, and bronchitis. As early as 1700 BC certain skin diseases were thought to be catching, and that direct, and even indirect, contact with a sufferer might be dangerous. But many conditions remained unknown, largely because they were associated, usually in head-to-toe order, with only one particular limb or organ.

A wide range of drugs was used, both internally and externally, and some drug lists were respected enough to be copied and commented on for hundreds of years. In several Babylonian tablets, a description of symptoms is linked to a diagnosis of the type of illness involved and, more frequently, to a statement of the likely outcome of the condition. A Babylonian medical text of about 650 BC gives a good description of some of the symptoms of epilepsy, as well as noting the more serious nature of convulsions occurring in sleep or recurring during an attack:

> If at the time of his possession, while he is sitting down, his left eye moves to the side, a lip puckers, saliva flows from his mouth, and his hand, leg and trunk on the left side jerk like a slaughtered sheep, it is *migtu*. If at the time of possession his mind is awake, the demon can be driven out; if at the time of his possession his mind is not so aware, the demon cannot be driven out.[1]

This emphasis on prediction fits in well with the Babylonians' expertise in astronomical forecasting, and in the casting of horoscopes through the examination of animal livers. Most striking of all is the frequent attribution of disease conditions to the hand of a god or a spirit, often accompanied by a prognosis of death.

It is not surprising, then, to find two types of healer mentioned in the Babylonian texts, one working largely with drugs, potions, bandages, and the like, the other akin to an exorcist in using incantations and healing rituals. Whether these groups were in conflict or complemented one another – or, indeed, whether one person could perform both types of healing – is controversial, but there is ample evidence for both being officially recognized. The law code of Hammurabi (reigned 1792 –1750/1743 BC) specifies the fees to be paid to a healer for a particular operation on a sliding scale, depending on the status of the patient (or animal), as well as draconian penalties for failure, akin to those to be imposed on incompetent architects or shipwrights.

In spite of these potential hazards of failure, it is clear that many minor surgical procedures were carried out (one text discusses a case of nosebleed incompetently treated by bandaging), and there are even records of attempted caesarian section. In short, we are far from the situation alleged for Babylonia in the fifth century BC by the contemporary Greek historian Herodotus, of a land without doctors, in which the sick were brought into the marketplace and had their cases diagnosed and treated by passers-by who had had, or who knew of others with, a similar condition.

Herodotus may simply have misunderstood the common Middle Eastern custom where the sick are placed outside the house for friends and neighbours to talk to and advise. In his comments on Egyptian medicine, however, he was better informed, and far more enthusiastic. He noted a multitude of specialists, one for each disease, and claimed that the whole country was filled with doctors, of the head, the teeth, the belly, and of more obscure diseases. He was not alone in his high regard for Egyptian healers. The king of Persia had Egyptian court doctors, and about 500 BC had sent an Egyptian physician, Udjohorresne, back to Egypt to restore the 'house of life' (a medical institution), 'because he knew the virtues of that art'.[2] Some 750 years earlier, the King of the Hittites (Central Turkey) had asked Rameses II of Egypt for a physician and an incantation-priest to attend his sister, and Egyptian physicians appear in other early diplomatic documents.

The high reputation of Egyptian doctors was owed to their skills as diagnosticians and as surgeons; in the Edwin Smith papyrus of surgery, forty-two out of fifty-eight examinations lead to recommendations for treatment. In spite of the presence of incantations, magic, and religious cures, the medical treatises are generally careful to distinguish between them and leave these to other healers. Touching, seeing, and smelling the patient (even taking the pulse) gave the physician an insight into the workings of the body, whose pathological changes were frequently ascribed to the results of putrefying residues collecting within it; heat from the anus, for example, might cause weakness of the heart. Hence the need to pay special attention to stopping the production of pus and to cleaning the body, with purges and enemas as well as washings and perfumings.

Such procedures were also followed in mummification, by which a corpse was preserved. It is open to debate whether the removal of the organs in mummification amounts to anatomy, and whether the knowledge of the mummifiers was passed on the physicians, but certainly there was not in Egypt the same taboo on handling a corpse that is found in many other societies.

Above all, the Egyptians were famous for their drugs. They ranged widely, from the humble leek, to the fat of the hippopotamus, and from pomegranate to fried mice and lapis lazuli. 'Bring me honey for my eyes and some fat … and real eye paint, as soon as possible', wrote the painter Poi to his son Pe-Rahotep around 1220 BC. 'I am weak. I want to have my eyes and they are missing.'[3] The drugs came from the Eastern Mediterranean, Africa, and Asia. To us now, the combination of identifiable ingredients and strange semi-magical substances is less important than the vast range of sources they imply.

GREEK MEDICINE

Both Egyptian and Babylonian medicine shows evidence of accurate observation, as well as hierarchies of practitioners. What their writings do not yet reveal is the questioning, argumentative, and speculative discussions that mark early Greek medicine, as found in the *Hippocratic Corpus*, the collection of some sixty tracts

A scene from an Athenian doctor's surgery of the time of Hippocrates, painted around a perfume vase. In the centre, the doctor treats a patient's arm, possibly after having let blood. Patients with injuries wait their turn.

ascribed to Hippocrates (active about 410 BC). Hence, scholars have often asserted the independence of Greek medicine from that of neighbouring civilizations, a claim more likely to be true of Greek theory than of actual therapeutic practice.

The variety of treatises in the *Hippocratic Corpus* is typical of a period when the practice of medicine was evolving in Greece from a family system, exemplified in the legends of Asclepius and his descendants, one of whom was said to be Hippocrates himself. The famous Hippocratic Oath represents a half-way stage, setting the teacher as a quasi-father figure to the student, but other evidence shows a multiplicity of competing healers – rootcutters, physicians, obstetricians, incantatory priests, exorcists, bone-setters, surgeons, to say nothing of interested laymen and laywomen, self-medication, and divine intervention. Medicine was an open art, and the speculations of philosophers such as Empedocles and Plato in the fifth and fourth centuries BC were as important in influencing and spreading medical ideas as those of more practical medical men.

In this medical marketplace, each seller could tout his or her wares, in opposition to or in cooperation with others, and the choice was left to individual patients. In such a situation, laying down rules for good practice served as both medical ethic and advertising, not only emphasizing the effective contributions of one healer but distinguishing them from the dubious or useless practices of another.

Religious healing was an ever-present alternative that was sought particularly in chronic cases. Few doctors rejected divine intervention, and most believed in a divinely ordered world, yet they were also convinced that their treatments were effective without the guidance of the gods, and could not be accused of being magical. Others might disagree. The onset of an epidemic often resulted in attempts at religious cures, by public ceremonies or by the introduction of new gods thought capable of ending the mass disease. Thus the mysterious epidemic that affected Athens and other parts of Greece in 430–427 BC helped to spread the worship of Asclepius, who superseded Apollo as the pre-eminent Greek healing god (although almost any deity could cure, and there were many local healing cults).

At shrines of Asclepius, especially at major temples in Tricca (N. Greece), Epidaurus (S. Greece), Lebena (Crete), Cos, and, later, Pergamum (now Turkey), sufferers would stay overnight (incubate) within the temple. If fortunate, they would receive healing in a dream, either directly from Asclepius or in the form of instructions interpreted by his priest and often compatible with the recipes and advice of secular physicians. Such healing was perhaps cheaper and more accessible than the services of a physician.

Numbers of healers are impossible to determine. Few towns had more than 2,000 inhabitants, and full-time healers could have existed only in Athens and other big cities or by travelling around a region. Many doctors clearly combined income from medicine with farming and other pursuits – blacksmiths with a sideline in bone-setting are not unusual even in the Middle Ages. Some went to larger towns to study as apprentices; others, especially on the island of Cos, were taught within their families; still others relied entirely on their own skills and what they could pick up by observing or listening to medical debates in the marketplace.

Some big towns, especially Athens from about 500 BC, tried to secure the services of a resident doctor by paying a retaining fee (incidentally also attesting a hoped-for competence). However, the state did not intervene in the relationship between doctor and patient, and although such civic doctors might voluntarily treat citizens for nothing, non-citizens (who were especially numerous in Athens) had to pay in full.

The medicine that these doctors practised was based primarily on dietetics – that is, regulating the whole lifestyle. Drugs were used (those from Egypt had a great reputation), but surgery was very much a treatment of last resort. Swabbing with wine reduced sepsis in hernia operations. Recommendations for the treatment of fractures, dislocations, headwounds, and uterine prolapse sound very modern, but detailed knowledge of the internal organs and arrangement of the body was lacking. Comparisons with animals or everyday objects took the place of careful observation. The internal economy of a woman, for instance, was imagined as a tube, in which the womb wandered from its normal position, to which it might be attracted back by sweet, or repelled by foul, substances introduced into the vulva or the nose.

A reconstruction of the Asclepieion of Cos. One of the main shrines of Asclepius, it was largely rebuilt around AD 60 at the expense of a doctor to the Roman Emperor Nero . Standing on a series of terraces on the hillside, the shrine would have been impressive as well as beautiful.

The *Hippocratic Corpus*

The *Hippocratic Corpus* was written by a variety of authors mostly between 420 and 370 BC. It offers advice on gynaecology, head wounds, epilepsy, and a whole range of diseases. Some of the tracts are public manifestos, others collections of case notes; some depend on close observation, others are highly speculative. A typical piece of advice in the *Epidemics* tract was

> Declare the past, diagnose the present, foretell the future: practise these things. In diseases make a habit of two things — help, or at least do no harm. The art involves three things — disease, the diseased, and the doctor. The doctor is the servant of the art. The diseases must join with the doctor in combating the disease.[4]

Although the historical Hippocrates was famous as a physician and teacher, no single tract can yet be securely identified as his, and many of the traditional details of his life are later inventions.

Hippocratic medicine, as shown in the *Corpus*, is characterized by three things: close observation of symptoms, an openness to ideas from all sides, and a willingness to explain the causes of disease. The large variety of (often conflicting) explanations offered are united mainly in considering health and disease as some form of balance or imbalance. Sometimes this is a balance of elements (the ultimate building blocks of the body and the whole universe), sometimes of fluids (or 'humours'), sometimes of 'powers' (hot and cold, sweet and sour), and sometimes of fluxes that might cause harm by settling in a wrong place. The body was viewed as inherently unstable, liable to disease, hard to diagnose, and often impossible to cure.

The four temperaments, from the *Guild Book of the Barber-Surgeons of York*, around 1500. Clockwise, from the top right, are the sanguine, the phlegmatic, the choleric, and the melancholic. The artist shows both the ages and the mental states that are dominated by the individual humours.

In many texts, the emphasis is on prognosis, which incorporates both modern diagnosis and forecasting the likely outcome of a case as seen in both Babylonian and Egyptian medicine. Hippocratic prognosis also acted as an insurance: provided the doctor distinguished between what he could and could not do, no blame was attached to subsequent failure or refusal to treat.

Two fluids above all were singled out for special concern — bile and phlegm — the ostensible cause of summer diseases such as diarrhoea and of winter colds. Many writers thought of the body as a constant battleground between the two, in which the mind was also affected — phlegm causes epilepsy, bile frenzy — and in which environment, seasonal changes, and heredity all played a part. Other authors described blood in similar terms, and the tract *On the Nature of Man* added a fourth humour, black bile or melancholy, a mysterious substance as deadly in its pure state as blood was usually beneficial.

This system of the four humours, later regarded as that of Hippocrates himself, was easily extended to cover the four elements, earth, air, fire, and water; the four seasons; the four qualities, hot, cold, wet, and dry; the four ages of man; and the four mental states (or temperaments). It offered a rationale for understanding man, in sickness and in health, against the wider cosmos, and, at the same time, for explaining the individuality of illness. The seven books of *Epidemics* bring together both individual case histories and larger surveys of disease in a community over a year; *Airs, Waters, and Places* uses environment to explain physical (and even political) differences between Greeks, North Africans, and southern Russians.

The Hippocratic Oath

I swear by Apollo the healer, by Aesculapius, by Health and all the powers of healing, and call to witness all the gods and goddesses that I may keep this Oath and Promise to the best of my ability and judgement.

I will pay the same respect to my master in the Science as to my parents and share my life with him and pay all my debts to him. I will regard his sons as my brothers and teach them the Science, if they desire to learn it, without fee or contract. I will hand on precepts, lectures and all other learning to my sons, to those of my master and to those pupils duly apprenticed and sworn, and to none other.

I will use my power to help the sick to the best of my ability and judgement; I will abstain from harming or wronging any man by it.

I will not give a fatal draught to anyone if I am asked, nor will I suggest any such thing. Neither will I give a woman means to procure an abortion.

I will be chaste and religious in my life and in my practice.

I will not cut, even for the stone, but I will leave such procedures to the practitioners of that craft.

Whenever I go into a house, I will go to help the sick and never with the intention of doing harm or injury. I will not abuse my position to indulge in sexual contacts with the bodies of women or of men, whether they be freemen or slaves.

Whatever I see or here, professionally or privately, which ought not to be divulged, I will keep secret and tell no one.

A medieval Greek manuscript of the Hippocratic Oath. In this Christian version, the first three sections have been drastically abbreviated, the names of the gods omitted, and the whole written in the form of a cross.

If, therefore, I observe this Oath and do not violate it, may I prosper both in my life and in my profession, earning good repute among all men for all time. If I transgress and forswear this Oath, may my lot be otherwise.[5]

Anatomical knowledge changed at the end of the fourth century BC. The philosopher-scientist Aristotle and his followers embarked on a massive programme of zoological and biological investigation, and his contemporary Diocles of Carystos is credited with the first book on dissection (but of animals). The breakthrough into human anatomy came outside Greece, in the newly founded city of Alexandria at the mouth of the Nile in Egypt. The conquests of Alexander the Great (reigned 336–323 BC) had brought Greek civilization out of the Aegean basin (and Sicily) to cover the whole of the Middle East, from Libya to the Punjab. Although his empire fragmented at his death, his sucessors maintained their Greek (Hellenistic) culture. Chief among them was Ptolemy, who ruled in Egypt from 323 to 282 BC and who created in Alexandria a major culture centre with a famous library and 'Hall of the Muses'.

Here, perhaps freed from some of the constraints on mutilating a corpse known in Greece, two Greek physician-scientists almost simultaneously around 280 BC began to investigate the internal body. Herophilus examined carefully the layout and organs of the body, giving names to the duodenum, and other anatomical structures. He dissected the eye, and, following his master Praxagoras of Cos, studied the pulse as a guide to illness. His contemporary, Erasistratus of Ceos, was far more radical in his claims.

Erasistratus dissected the brain, trying to establish how movement and sensation were produced, and, using analogies from Alexandrian science, described the body and its processes in mechanical terms. He challenged many of the doctrines associated with Hippocrates. He had little time for humours, and thought that the arteries contained only air, *pneuma*, a form of refined air produced in the heart. He explained the presence of blood in the arteries as resulting from seepage or from attraction following the escape of *pneuma* and the temporary creation of a vacuum. He rejected equally strongly the view of Plato and Aristotle that everything was created for a purpose (teleology), favouring a mechanical development.

Although later scholars praised Erasistratus's anatomical discoveries, especially in the brain, most doctors found them largely irrelevant. Indeed, one influential group, or sect, the Empiricists, rejected all anatomical investigation and theoretical speculation, in favour of treatments based on comparisons with what had succeeded in the past in similar cases.

The Greek world from 250 BC onwards fell more and more under the military power of Rome, which extended its control over Italy, southern France, and Spain, and, by AD 100, ruled from southern Scotland, the Rhine and Danube, to the Sahara, Israel, and the borders of modern Iraq. However much Roman chauvinist politicians might have deplored the arrival of Greek medicine and its new-fangled theories, along with luxurious furniture and silk dresses, by 80 BC Greek doctors and Greek ideas were common in Italy, especially in Rome. There even grew up a new medical sect, the Methodists, who from around AD 60 were dominant in Latin medicine. They combined a view of the body made up of atoms and pores, and of illness as an imbalance between them, with propaganda stressing the simplicity and effectiveness of their diagnoses and cures. In this they were repeating the slogans of an earlier Greek immigrant, Asclepiades, around 92 BC, who had gained a wealthy clientele by his claim to cure 'swiftly, surely, pleasantly'.

Roman practicality was shown in their public works, sewers, and aqueducts (these were also features of Greek towns by 50 BC) and in their provision of 'hospitals'. These catered for two social groups, domestic slaves (100 BC–AD 70), and soldiers in permanent forts in newly conquered territory (9 BC–AD 220). Large fortress hospitals, as at Chester (England) or Inchtuthil (Scotland), were for legionaries (not locals), and were designed on a plan of rooms opening off a square corridor. Situated usually many miles behind the frontier, they catered for the sick rather than those seriously wounded in battle. A few small forts housing non-citizen soldiers – at, for example, Fendoch in Scotland – had hospitals on a reduced scale, but a change in military strategy around 220 to reliance on a mobile fieldforce put an end to these permanent hospitals.

If in the Latin-speaking Western half of the Roman Empire, medicine was generally carried out by relatively humble immigrants, the Greek doctors who lived in the Eastern half flourished intellectually and socially. Many were among the elite of their towns, acting as magistrates or officials and serving also as civic physicians – practitioners distinguished, so lawyers declared, for 'their morals and medical experience', and also for their tax privileges. Latin medicine, even in Celsus's *On Medicine* (AD 40), an elegant handbook for laymen based on Greek sources, does not begin to compare with the Greek investigations into drugs of Dioscorides (see page 249) nor the therapeutic insights at the bedside of Rufus of Ephesus or the Methodist writer on gynaecology, Soranus of Ephesus (both around AD 110). These were in turn overshadowed by Galen of Pergamum.

Within 30 years at most, Galen's books were being studied in Egypt and somewhere near Carthage in modern Tunisia also by the Latin writer Gargilius Martialis, author of a book on garden vegetables, fruits, and herbs. Galen set a new agenda for medicine in the Greek-speaking world, from which alternative views to his were gradually extruded. As the comforting certainties of Greek city life gradually disappeared under political chaos and invasions of barbarians, Galen's apparent mastery of the medical literature of the past, as well as his achievements in anatomy and all other branches of medicine, were viewed as impossible to emulate. Medical writers continued to add their own discoveries, but more often they produced large encyclopedias of past learning or elegant restatements of

The Romans were famous for their public engineering works that helped keep towns and cities clean and healthy. A good example is the Pont du Gard aqueduct near Nimes in S. France built in the first century BC.

Galen of Pergamum

Son of a wealthy architect, Galen (AD 129–216) received an excellent education in Greek literature and philosophy before embarking in 145/6 on a medical career. He studied for 10 years (unusually long), including at least 4 years at Alexandria, where he learned more about anatomy, surgery, drugs, and Hippocratic medicine. After a spell at Pergamum as doctor to the gladiators, he moved to Rome in 162, where he quickly made a name for himself.

Galen tells how, one day out walking,

> I came upon a man surrounded by a crowd of fools. 'I have met Galen', he declared, 'who has taught me all he knows. Here is a remedy for worms in the teeth.' The quack had prepared a ball of pitch and tar, lit it, and held it smoking in the open mouth of the patient, who could not bear to keep his eyes open. As soon as they were shut, he slipped into the patient's mouth worms he had concealed in a little pot, and pretended to draw them out. The fools offered him all they had. He even went so far as to try venesection on the wrong side of the elbow. I immediately revealed myself to the crowded, saying 'I am Galen, and he is a swindler.' I then warned him, asked the authorities to summons him, and they had him flogged.[6]

In 165, he was, he claimed, driven out by his fellow competitors in medicine — others suspect cowardice in the face of the impending plague of smallpox — only to return in 169 as doctor to the emperor Marcus Aurelius. He remained in court employment for the rest of his long life.

A prolific writer and vigorous debater, Galen dominates subsequent medical history. He created a synthesis of medicine based on the *Hippocratic Corpus* (and created a picture of Hippocrates that remained almost unchallenged for 1,700 years), Plato, and Aristotle. From Plato, he took the idea of the three bodily systems — heart, liver, and brain — connected also to mental states; from Aristotle, an interest in practical investigation and in scientific logic. From all, he derived his idea of the good doctor as philosopher, and of the unity of reason and experience. These ideas he incorporated in hundreds of tracts, dictated to secretaries, and proclaimed in public debates and private conclaves.

Based on 'commonsense' notions, held together by accurate logic, and equipped with devastating critiques of alternative views, Galen's medicine was hard to contradict, and his almost miraculous forecasts (formed through shrewd observation and considerable learning) gained him patients and supporters from the highest society. His diagnostic methods included palpation, pulse-taking, and occasionally the inspection of urine, all subject to a clear-headed logic.

> I know of nothing more disgraceful than this: a man entrusted with the art of healing, who remains ignorant of alterations brought about by nature, and like those without any medical knowledge fears symptoms which laymen dread. He cannot distinguish between regular and irregular developments. This is not what Hippocrates declared.[7]

Galen's investigations into, in modern terms, stress-related illnesses are a fascinating instance of sound observation coupled with a fanciful explanation. Nonetheless, he was convinced that by using learning, logic, and experience, he could reach a sure diagnosis of any individual's complaint, and that, once made, diagnosis would easily lead to therapy or a prediction of incurability.

His other major claim was for the restoration of anatomy as the basis for the understanding of the body, a notion he traced back to Hippocrates and Plato. Trained in a revived Alexandrian tradition of dissection, he performed a series of experiments on the spinal cord, using pigs, goats, and apes, and avowedly dissected every day to gain a better feel for surgery. He attacked Erasistratus's mechanistic views mercilessly, concluding one of his anatomy treatises with a 'hymn' to the forethought and wisdom of the divine creator. Those, like Jews and Christians, who believed in miracles were worshipping a capricious deity, he said, and were to be condemned for folly, however impressive their morality.

Galen's own claims for his superiority (not entirely unfounded), his powerful rhetoric, his near impeccable logic, his abundant learning on the most unlikely of topics, and his abilities as surgeon and as bedside consultant, were recognized in his own lifetime.

Opposite: The fathers of medicine and pharmacology, from the frontispiece of a fifteenth-century manuscript by the Italian Giohanne Cademosto. Clockwise, from the top left, are Asclepius, Hippocrates, Avicenna (Ibn Sina), Rhazes (ar-Razi), Aristotle, Galen, Macer, Albertus Magnus, Dioscorides, Mésué (Yuhanna ibn Masawayh), and Serapion.

The triumph of Galen.
A fourteenth-century artist
portrays Galen surrounded by
his pupils like a medieval lord
among his retainers.

standard doctrine. Oribasius, for example, in the fourth century produced at least four separate *Synopses*.

The preservation of sound learning in an increasingly impoverished age, when medical texts had to be copied laboriously by hand and drugs and surgical instruments were hard to find, is praiseworthy. More controversial but harder to pin down are three related developments.

Between AD 200 and 600 there was formed in medicine, as in literature and philosophy, a canon of works of Galen and Hippocrates that was accorded a special place in teaching, certainly at Alexandria and perhaps elsewhere. Medicine was now becoming defined in terms of specific book-learning, and could be tested as a series of responses to questions on books. The second development was a growing split between medical theory and practice, with the former being treated with somewhat greater respect. Finally, Galen's demands for the philosopher-doctor were interpreted to mean that a doctor must first study philosophy (that is, logic and some of Plato's and Aristotle's theories of matter and the universe). This erudite paragon, found in Alexandria, Athens, or the new capital of Constantinople (now Istanbul) was far removed from, and perhaps less familiar than, the backwoods jack-of-all-trades, who offered their services to the sick – the magical healer, the peasant farmer-cum-bone-setter, the diviner, the travelling drug salesman or oculist, the amulet maker, the barmaid-cum-midwife, the teacher turned recipe writer, or the wise woman with a wonder-working hyena skin. The theoreticians became accepted as the true physicians, even though their opponents might allege, sometimes with justice, that their intellectual expertise was confined to words and not to therapy.

THE CHRISTIAN VIEW OF THE SICK

More significant than any of these internal changes within medicine was the recognition, from 313 onwards, of Christianity as an (later the) official religion of the Roman Empire. Like Judaism, from which it took much, Christianity had an ambiguous attitude towards medicine. Some preachers, expounding the healing miracles in the Gospels, emphasized the power of faith to cure disease (although few went so far as to claim that that was sufficient), and, especially from 370 onwards, the shrines of saints and martyrs became places of pilgrimage for the sick, vying with, and ultimately replacing, the pagan temples of Asclepius.

Both Christianity and Judaism also believed in the notion of a whole community bound together by religion, in which everything, including medicine, had its

place, and where religious doctrines and religious authority might rightly intervene in what had earlier been purely secular affairs. It was, for example, important
to prepare the patient for a good death, leading to an eternal life in heaven, and
hence to involve a priest at the bedside as well as a doctor.

Irksome though this intervention might occasionally appear, the church
viewed medicine positively on the whole. True, some of its most eminent practitioners in the fifth and sixth centuries were unrepentant pagans, but Galenic medicine, with its appeal to a monotheist creator, could easily be assimilated, and
the workings of drugs and the skills of the surgeon held up as prime examples
of the bounty of God towards humanity. Although church institutions offered
a potential source of conflict with medicine, this was outweighed by the ways
in which, increasingly, the church acted as the preserver of learning, including
medicine.

Nowhere was this more evident than in a new institution, the hospital, the
product of Jewish and Christian ideas on charity. Ancient charity had been narrowly defined, limited to particular groups, usually of male citizens. The Jews and
Christians broadened this to include their fellow-believers and, in the case of
Christians, all who might be in need, for all were potential Christians. By AD 60
the Jews had built hostels for those on pilgrimage to the Temple at Jerusalem, in
at least one of which medical assistance was available. Christianity extended these
hostels geographically. By 400 they were common in Asia Minor (modern Turkey)
and the Holy Land, and by 450 had spread to Italy, North Africa, and southern
France. At the same time, church laws throughout the Middle East specified that
each community should set aside a room for looking after those in need.

Most 'hospitals' were small, but in Constantinople or Jerusalem they had 200
or more beds. As the variety of names used for them shows, they catered for many
different groups – the sick, the old, the poor, and the stranger; sometimes
together, sometimes not. Some institutions specifically excluded the maimed and
sick, others treated them in separate wards. Increasing size brought administrative
specialization, into wards, by sex, and, by 600 in one hospital at Constantinople,
by illness. Medical assistance was available in the biggest hospitals, but most provided only care (food, warmth, and shelter), although this should not be despised
as an important component of the process of cure. Some hospitals were run
almost as family businesses, others as extensions of a bishop's role as father of his
flock. They were all examples of Christian charity in action.

From the fourth century onwards, doctrinal splits within the Christian church
contributed towards the very gradual political and military disintegration of the
Roman Empire. The Western half, Latin-speaking and centred on Rome, had by
570 become an amalgam of barbarian states. In the East, the central government
of Constantinople continued to exercise control over the eastern Mediterranean
until the Arab conquests of the seventh century restricted it largely to the Aegean
basin and Asia Minor.

A fourth-century Christian painting from a Roman catacomb, showing a lesson in philosophy, an essential part of medical training.

In a region stretching from Egypt through Syria to Persia, a local language, Syriac (akin to Hebrew), competed with Greek, as the language first of the church and then of advanced culture. By 531 the texts of Galen that formed the basis for the Alexandrian medical curriculum had been translated into Syriac, and medical compendia were being written in Syriac of a standard comparable with those in Greek. The ready availability of Syriac translations of Aristotle helped to confirm the authority of Galen, so often an Aristotelian in his ideas and prejudices. Once again Greek medicine was transplanted into another linguistic society.

THE ARAB INFLUENCE

The Arab conquests of the seventh century grafted a new political order onto a basically Christian, Syriac-speaking society. Although the Arabs had their own medicine, based on herbs and chants, they were not numerous enough to impose it on their new subjects. Besides, the Koran and the traditions that soon grew up around the figure of the prophet Mohammed said very little about medicine; and the little there was could easily be reconciled with Galen's teleological monotheism and, at least at first, impinged little on a conquered Christian population.

Here, the practice of medicine long continued as a non-Muslim speciality, families of Christian or Jewish physicians attending the ruling families for centuries. A specifically Islamic medicine, the so-called 'Medicine of the Prophet', does not appear important until the tenth century.

Of medicine under the early Caliphate, we know little. Only with the transfer of power from Damascus to Baghdad in 762, and under such rulers as the Caliph Harun ar-Rashid (reigned 786–809), does light return again. This period saw in the Middle East a conflict between Islam and those who believed in Manichaeanism, a religion with many adherents in Iraq and Iran. Manichaeanism had long been attacked by Christianity as a dangerous heresy, and Islamic authorities turned to their Christian subjects for assistance against a common enemy. This is the background to a massive takeover of Greek philosophy and science, whose Aristotelian insistence on the purposefulness of the divine creator struck at the Manichaean notion of a world divided between good and evil. Texts on logic and philosophy were translated into Arabic, and were followed by medicine, often at the behest of government officials and with government support.

The major ninth-century medical figure in Baghdad was a Christian Arab, Hunain ibn Ishaq, an amazingly accurate and productive scholar, who travelled to the Greek Byzantine empire in search of rare Galenic treatises. In all, he, his pupils, and a few contemporaries translated 129 works of Galen into Arabic, often making a translation first into Syriac. His labours provided the Arabic world with more Galenic texts than survive today in their original Greek, and with versions that are both technically accurate and stylistically elegant.

In an eventful life (he was once imprisoned by his royal master), Ibn Ishaq also wrote a major tract on eye diseases and a summary of Galenic medicine in the form of *Questions and Answers* (c. 850). The group of Christian doctors to the Caliph (including for four centuries members of the Bakhtishu'a family) all engaged in similar tasks of translation or reinterpretating their Galenic heritage for Arab patients and patrons.

This successful transfer of classical knowledge into yet another language (there are contemporary translations also into Armenian and Hebrew) led in the tenth to thirteenth centuries to a massive expansion of medical writing in Arabic. Ar-Razi, or in Latin Rhazes, described smallpox and measles accurately, as well as his chemical experiments; al-Biruni wrote at length on the plants and herbs he had seen in his travels in Afghanistan and India; and the Syrian physician Ibn an-Nafis argued strongly against Galen for some form of circulation of the blood (Galen had argued that blood produced in the liver was all used up as nutriment and its residues excreted). But these new discoveries, however impressive they might now seem, were unusual (and Ibn an-Nafis reached his conclusion by logic, not experimentation).

More typical were attempts to develop and systematize Galenic ideas. Galen had once suggested ranking drugs according to their degrees (or grades) of action,

GENTILIS·FVIGINAS·SPECVLATOR

PRINCEPS

ABINSCENI

The *Canon of Medicine* of Ibn Sina (Avicenna), 'prince of physicians', was widely read, and, in Latin translation, formed the foundation of university medical courses in Europe from 1250 to 1600. In this edition (Venice, 1522), Avicenna is pictured as a medieval professor dictating to a student – the later commentator, Gentile da Foligno (d. 1348).

but he himself had suggested grades for only a third of the medicinal substances he discussed. Arabic pharmacologists extended his system to a wider range of substances, which they then combined in complex mixtures designed for the individual patient. Elsewhere, as with Galen's ideas of the eye or on urines, his opinions were scattered throughout his enormous works, and it was Arabic authors who brought them easily together. Finally, there were compendia, of all sizes, expanding what Galen had hinted at and amalgamating a variety of diffuse observations into a coherent whole. Thus it was Arabic authors who first wrote about the three spirits ruling the body (Galen had accepted the psychic spirit in the brain and nerves, and possibly the vital spirit in the heart and arteries, but his reference to a natural spirit in the liver and veins was at best muted), and who developed his ideas of a physicalist psychology.

The most important of such compendia were those by ar-Razi, al-Majusi (Haly Abbas), and Ibn Sina (Avicenna). Ibn Sina's *Canon of Medicine,* which still retains its primacy within this tradition as it is taught today in the Muslim world, displays a wondrous appreciation of all Galen's medical writing, and is tightly structured by Aristotelian logic. It is no coincidence that Ibn Sina, like Ibn Rushd (Averroës) and the Jewish physician Moses ben Maimon (Maimonides), active in twelfth-century Muslim Spain, North Africa, and Cairo, was famous as a philosopher as well as a physician, for Galen had encouraged the study of philosophy and logic, and his method of argumentation invited philosophical enquiry just as it did experimentation. Others took Galen's insistence on book-learning almost to excess: the wife of Ali ibn Ridwan at his death in 1068 is said to have dumped all his huge Galenic library into the fishpond, as she did not wish any longer to share the house with her late husband's great love.

This bookishness, possible only in a wealthy and learned society like that of medieval Islam, may have helped to downgrade manual skills such as surgery; the best doctor was the one who could diagnose correctly without even seeing the patient. But that did not prevent some writers – for example, al-Zahrawi (Albucasis) – from producing excellent surgical textbooks, in which they reported details of complicated abdominal operations. New techniques were invented for the treatment of cataract and other eye complaints, just as other scholars promoted new theories about the mechanics of vision. But the sheer danger of surgery may have been the greatest handicap to its further development.

How far the Islamic world took over the medical institutions of the Greek world is an open question. Certainly, by the eleventh century, there were large hospitals in every major Muslim town (and with a Muslim religious bias to match that of a Christian hospital). Medicine was also being formally taught within the hospital setting, with certificates granted for attendance. Theoretical treatises on the duties of the 'Market-superintendent' imply that this official had to examine candidates in medicine and surgery before they could practise, but evidence for theory translated into action is hard to find.

More plausible is a picture of a variety of overlapping types of healing, in which the learned Galenic tradition was but one part, alongside the medicine of the prophet, astrological and magical healing, and, by the eleventh century, healing at the shrine of famous Muslim 'saints'. In spite of the traditional picture of a unified Islam, Jews, Christians, and other groups still continued to offer their own forms of healing, within and without their own communities.

The Mongol invasions of the early thirteenth century devastated the eastern half of the Islamic world, and civil war, and the increasing success of the Christians, pressed hard on the Islamic communities of Spain and North Africa. The openness to Hellenism of ninth-century Baghdad was replaced by a more fundamentalist Islam, in which adherence to tradition, both religious and medical, was enjoined on the community of the faithful. Even so, medicine in thirteenth-century Cordoba or Cairo had arguably reached a higher level of sophistication and effectiveness than anywhere in the Western world, with the possible exception of Constantinople.

MEDICINE IN THE BYZANTINE WORLD

In Constantinople, as the Byzantium Empire shrank to become little more than the area around the capital, professors argued, taught, and perhaps even demonstrated in the Galenic tradition of learned medicine. There were hospitals, like the Pantokrator, a royal foundation in 1136, whose fifty or so patients (and outpa-

Inventory of the Pantokrator Hospital, Constantinople

The hospital (*xenon*) of the Pantokrator was founded in 1136 by the Byzantine Emperor, John II, as part of a religious complex, which included a monastery, an old folks home (*gerokomeion*), and, 4 miles away, a leper house.

It was said to cater for fifty inmates and had an outpatients dispensary as well. Its foundation charter lists in detail its ward furnishings, its staff, and the food to be provided:

● **Leper house** has provision for food, but no medical assistance

● **Old folks home**
Twenty-four residents; one master (monk); six servants. Should one of the old men fall ill, the *nosokomos* of the hospital to be notified; patient treated in home or, if necessary, in hospital, to return once recovered

● **Hospital**
Fifty beds in five sections, with five extra beds:
Section 1: ten beds, wounds or fractures
Section 2: eight beds, diseases of eyes or stomach
Section 3: twelve beds, women only
Sections 4 and 5: ten beds each, for men
Each bed has one mattress, one pillow, sheets, cover; two winter blankets
Also six special 'commode' beds
Bedding replaced annually, and stuffing in mattresses and pillows carded annually
Three fires; two latrines (1 male, 1 female)
Baths available in monastery for a twice-weekly wash

● **Meals**
Daily, 850 grams of bread, two vegetable dishes with oil, two onion heads (3,300 calories daily); money to buy extra food and wine

● **Staff**
Abbot superior
Four monks with abbot to form board of management, responsible for finance and administration
Nosokomos: hospital administrator and medical superintendent
Meizoteros: deputy; in charge of food supplies and drugs
Primikerioi (2): chief physicians
Protomenitai (2); in charge of section 2
Doctors (2) in charge of section 1
Doctors (4) in charge of sections 4 and 5

Doctors (2) in charge of section 3
Doctors (2) attached to monastic infirmary for monks
Surgeons (2) and doctors (2) in dispensary
Possibly other doctors could be brought in for consultation; all work alternate monthly shifts
Each male ward has three medical assistants, two supernumeraries, and two servants
The female ward has one female doctor, four female medical assistants, two female supernumeraries, and two female servants
The dispensary has four medical assistants, and four supernumeraries

● **Other staff**
Five pharmacists; one teacher of the children; one usher; five laundresses; one kettle-keeper; two cooks; one groom; one porter; one purser; two priests; two lectors; two bakers; four pallbearers; one funeral priest; one latrine cleaner; one miller; also money for craftsmen to keep surgical instruments in repair, and a specialist in hernia surgery.

The entrance to the church and hospital of the Pantokrator in Constantinople (now Istanbul), and the groundplan.

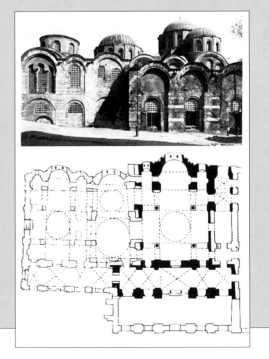

tients) were, according to the charter, to be provided with a more than adequate diet and treated by a trained medical staff with a wide range of drugs and therapies. But, even if the demands of the charter were fulfilled, the hospital itself could have made only a tiny contribution to the health of the city, its population then numbering some 300,000. Outside Constantinople, there was much less provision for the sick. In 1185, Thessalonica, the second city of the Empire, had only one hospital.

For all its failings, however, the medical services of the Byzantine Empire were far superior to those of the contemporary West, and the capture of Constantinople by the Crusaders in 1204 may have led to the copying in Western Europe of some Byzantine medical institutions. For example, from 1250 in some towns in France and northern Italy hospitals had up to 200 beds and a large medical staff, and became the focus of community care for the sick.

MEDICINE IN THE DARK AGES

The situation in Western Europe in the preceeding centuries – during the so-called Dark Ages (roughly 500–1050) – was very different. Here the crumbling of Roman imperial power brought about a catastrophic downturn in economic prosperity, most noticeably as expressed in the life of towns. Although doctors continued to practise medicine in some of the more important towns, there is evidence for a massive decline in the number, and quality, of medical writings available. Short handbooks replaced learned disquisitions, digests their original tracts, drug lists academic pharmacopeias. Although law texts continued to repeat rules for civic physicians and the costs of slave physicians, they were legislating for the past, not present reality.

Two features stand out in this decline. The first is the preminence of 'do-it-yourself' handbooks, primarily of dietetic medicine, which presented a small amount of basic theory with a concise exposition of a few diagnoses and treatments. By contrast, only a handful of Hippocratic and Galenic texts were available in translations made in northern Italy around 550, and even Latin Methodist medicine was poorly represented. The second feature is the ecclesiastical takeover of medical learning – and learning in general, for few could read outside the ecclesiastical community.

Probably only within monasteries or, from the ninth century, the schools that grew up around certain major cathedrals, such as Laon and Chartres in France, were medical texts in Latin being copied and studied. Only about 150 manuscripts of medicine survive today from the period 800–1000, and in the latter year there may have been no more than 1,000 in all Europe, and these were confined to a small number of centres. Yet there was some preservation of classical learning. Medicine in Anglo-Saxon England, almost unique in being written in a vernacular language, shows traces of Greek learning, and uses some drugs and drug recipes from the eastern Mediterranean.

Six miracles of Christ on an ivory diptych of about AD 475 from Rome. The miracles of healing reported in the Gospels served as a model for the Christian physician and encouraged those whom human aid had failed to place their faith in Christ and his saints.

This relatively learned medicine was supplemented by the healing offered at shrines and by holy men. Tales abound of so-called miraculous cures, and, by 1000, shrines were competing among themselves in the number of their cures. Some saints were almost specialists – St Dymphna was favoured for mental diseases (page 289), St Roch for plague, St Hubert for rabies sufferers, and St Blaise for throat complaints. Others serviced a locality – for example, the shrine of St Godric at Finchale (County Durham) was mainly visited by sufferers from northeastern England. Only a few shrines, like that of Roquemadour (southern France), drew pilgrims from all over Europe. Nor were the cults necessarily directed against secular healers. They might advise patients to rely on God and the saints, and, in turn, St John of Beverley or some other saint knew which diseases could be treated by secular means and by secular healers. Besides, in an age when secular healers were few, the sick needed to rely on a variety of resources.

The change from Dark Age medicine is generally located around 1050 in the region of Salerno, southern Italy. Here was a thriving medical community in touch with the Greek and Arab worlds, as well as the wealthiest and intellectually most advanced abbey of Europe, Monte Cassino. From 1080 or so, the Salernitan masters reintroduced theoretical speculation into medical teaching. Aided by contacts with Constantinople, and, from 1200 onwards, by Latin translations of some Arabic texts by Constantine the African, they re-established Galenic academic learning, combining commentary on a few set texts with philosophical discussion of wider issues and, by 1250, with practical demonstrations of animal anatomy. Galenism was reintroduced in Arabic form, in particular via the medical compendia of al-Majusi and the so-called *Introduction of Johannitius* (an abbreviated version of Hunain ibn Ishaq's *Questions and Answers*). The *Rule of Salerno* (*c*. 1300), a Latin poem, translated later into many languages, helped to spread a knowledge of classical dietetics throughout Europe.

The Arabic basis of Latin medicine was further strengthened by a series of translations made in Spain by Gerard of Cremona and others of such texts as Ibn Sina's *Canon*, and *On the Grades of Drug Action* by al-Kindi. By 1190 many texts of Galen had been translated, largely from the Arabic, along with most of the major Arabic works of medicine: by 1350, thanks to the South Italian Greek Niccolò da Reggio, many minor Galenic works became available in Latin, although few bothered to read them. There were three consequences of this translation movement. First, the amount of learned medical material suddenly burgeoned beyond all recognition. Second, the language of medicine was heavily arabized (for example, *siphac* for peritoneum), and its therapeutics depended heavily on Arabic sources, especially in pharmacology and surgery. Third, there was now a heavy philosophical component, based on Aristotle, whose Latin revival, also from Spain, helped and in part determined the character of medieval learned medicine. Nobody could properly understand the new medicine without some knowledge of the technicalities of Aristotelian science (or natural philosophy).

DEVELOPMENT OF UNIVERSITY MEDICINE

Translation accompanied the development of university medicine, first in northern Italy, in the wealthy towns of Bologna and Padua, and then in France (Paris and Montpellier), and in England (Oxford). Germany lagged behind, but by 1400 many areas of Western Europe had their own institutions of higher learning. Medicine came late into the universities. Professional associations of medical teachers, as at Salerno, joined universities only when they saw the advantages of the new institutions' ability to secure their own rights and privileges in law and theology, and many universities, especially in France, never had a medical faculty.

Once in the universities, the doctors readily adopted university procedures – lectures on set texts, such as *The Introduction of Johannitius*, Ibn Sina's *Canon*, and some Galen, debates on medical questions, and a theoretical (heavily Aristotelian) bias – and university prejudices. Because their medicine was based on texts, they increasingly argued that proper medicine depended on such knowledge, and that they, as university graduates, alone had the right to decide who should or should not practise medicine – a textual examination supplemented, and at times replaced, practical instruction by apprenticeship.

The ceremony of dissection

The teachers in late twelfth-century Salerno were the first to introduce animal dissections into their courses. The first teaching involving a human corpse is credited to Mondino dei Liuzzi in Bologna around 1315, but it spread only slowly outside Italy, and even there was carried out irregularly, save at Padua and Bologna. At Pavia, although in theory there was an annual dissection, none was held between 1457 and 1465. When one took place, it was as much spectacle as instruction; the university teacher endeavoured to set the anatomy of man (rarely of woman) in the whole context of creation, while a dissector, usually a surgeon, cut up the body in an order designed to reduce putrefaction.

The supplementation of animal by human anatomy was the result of several developments. The newly translated Galenic texts emphasized the importance of anatomy; the taboo on mutilating corpses was reduced by the custom, frowned on by the Church, of cutting up and boiling the bodies of pilgrims and crusaders for their bones or heart to be transported back home. From 1250 onwards, there are increasing records in Italy of autopsies, performed by surgeons to establish causes of death. The corpses chosen for university dissections were also those of criminals (or witches) and, especially, non-locals — in other words, of those on the margin of society.

Although some believed that such dissections were opposed by the Church, there is little evidence for this. Provided that the corpse was given a reverent burial, ecclesiastical proprieties were satisfied. Besides, the whole pomp and ceremony of the dissection, occasionally held indoors to keep the 'vulgar multitude' away, marked it out as something more than voyeurism.

The numbers of medical students were tiny (not surprisingly, since a medical degree took at least 7 years of study, including a full course in the arts): most universities, except for Bologna and Padua, saw only one or two medical graduates a decade. But by appealing to an increasingly university-educated elite of administrators, they often succeeded in imposing themselves and their own qualifications on the medical community. A popular saying on the prospects of university doctors and lawyers in about 1250 was 'Galen gives riches, Justinian offices'. The view was held that if only graduates could practise, there was legally no place for Jews

Roger of Parma, around 1160, examines a patient with a headwound, while assistants prepare an ointment in his dispensary. From a thirteenth-century translation in Norman French of Roger's surgical treatise *Chirurgia*.

Tombstone of the Pistoris family, 1527, in St Thomas's Church, Leipzig, Germany. The family served as doctors and university professors of medicine in Leipzig for at least three generations. Their memorial shows their symbols of office and their coats of arms.

and women (who might even perform surgery and often attended male patients), and a potential source of conflict with other organizations, especially medical guilds or colleges, who took a more realistic view of medical competence.

Medieval university medicine is indeed often speculative and highly theoretical. Yet its claim that a proper understanding of health and disease required an understanding of the fundamental structures of the body is not foolish, neither is its attempt to relate questions of medicine to wider 'scientific' ones. In the thirteenth century, teachers such as Taddeo Alderotti at Bologna and Arnald of Villanova at Montpellier were expert physicians as well as expositors, and could call on a formidable range of learning. Their fifteenth-century successors went further in emphasizing the practical basis of therapeutics, and in linking the medicine of the classroom to that of the bedside. Many university statutes, especially in Germany, demanded a period of supervised practice before granting a degree; whether they were enforced is another matter.

Below the university doctor in the medieval medical hierarchy stood the surgeon. In Italy and Germany, he might have been trained in part at a university, although a guild-apprenticeship was more common, and, even in London, the surgical elite had more in common with physicians than with their lower competitors, especially barber-surgeons. They had their own books, and some of their successful treatments – of abdominal injuries, anal fistulae, bladder stones, and cataracts – are impressive, and are far more than mere burning and bleeding. There were innovations, such as in the treatment of inguinal hernia, and in some artificial limbs, and even university men might have been forced to acknowledge the expertise of itinerant bonesetters or tooth-extractors. Bleeding, a favoured remedy and prophylactic (see page 122), was often carried out, especially in spring, by a local barber, who might also attend to cuts, bruises, and the ubiquitous ulcerations.

Others also offered their services. Although excluded as non-Christians from universities, Jews were often favoured as practitioners, especially among the aristocracy. The drug trade was in the hands of apothecaries and spicers, importers of drugs from far afield, who might also offer medical advice to their clients. Women were often attended by female healers or midwives, but it would be wrong to imagine that womens' diseases were left entirely to women, or that women with healing skills confined themselves only to women and children. Although regulations might endeavour to restrict them in this way, they were never universally enforced.

This situation reflects the multiplicity of institutions and organizations with pretensions to authority over medicine – the church, guilds, medical colleges (usually, but not always, of medical graduates), town councils (increasingly involved from 1200 or so in selecting a public doctor), and magnates of all descriptions. Sometimes authority was mediated through an individual (for example, a royal physician), sometimes through a committee. In fifteenth-century Brussels, midwives were licensed by a board of ecclesiastics, doctors, and midwives themselves; in Bruges in 1486, the town council had authority over them. 'On 24 March, paid by order of the council to Mary, widow of Henry Craps,and two other midwives, for having at the council's request questioned and examined a woman seeking to show knowledge in that field…twelve gros and three solidi each.' The conflicts, common in the sources, between doctors and surgeons, or medical men and lay administrators, are typical of this fragmentation of authority in Europe. Effective resolution of these conflicts reflects far more the growing effectiveness of the state than any public consensus about the suitability of types of healing.

An English artist around 1200 shows a surgeon cutting out a nasal polyp while the patient holds a bowl to catch the blood.

Explanations of the Black Death

The Black Death evoked a variety of overlapping (or competing) responses, from religious penitential processions and mass panics, to isolation, and the preparation by university physicians of a great caudron of theriac (a famous antidote with over a hundred ingredients, including snake venom) for distribution to the population of Florence. Explanations of the epidemic, like all other diseases, involved a hierarchy of causes, each with an appropriate response.

At the top was God, whose anger might be assuaged by prayer and contrition. Beneath Him were the heavens, configurations of stars and planets that affected the weather and the individual. Shrewd doctors (or astrologer-astronomers) could predict potential changes, and take appropriate preservative action.

The surrounding air could be altered by the heavens or by the noxious vapours (miasmas) given off by the sick or unhealthy swamps and cesspits. These could be improved by cleaning, avoiding forms of contact, or reducing one's intake of bad air.

Finally, all disease was an individual phenomenon. Even if one came into contact with a leper or walked in the hot sun, one fell ill only if one's natural constitution could not resist the changes imposed on one's humours from these external phenomena. Besides, one could fall ill in the same way just by eating the wrong food or failing to take appropriate exercise, for the natural humoral balance between illness and health was precarious. Writing in 1401, Lapo Mazzei, a Florentine doctor, gave this advice for avoiding plague:

> Let not the sun go down behind the hill without your having gone out, or if you cannot, take before meals a little exercise, without, however, causing you to sweat … and it would help you to drink, a quarter of an hour before your repast, a full half-glass of good red wine, neither too dry nor too sweet.[8]

Hence the need above all for prophylaxis, ways of strengthening resistance to harmful change, and, if all else failed, for restorative medicines and diet. But this last, strictly medical, intervention was only one (and the final) way of coping with disease.

The Black Death and subsequent recurring epidemics of plague ravaged Western Europe until the eighteenth century. How terrible the initial onslaught was can be seen in this miniature from a contemporary chronicle by Giovanni Sercambi in Lucca, Italy. A variety of remedies was proposed, as in this *Directory for the Poor Against Infectious Disease*, published in the great Plague of London, 1665.

The growing state involvement is shown by the Health Boards, which were first developed when the Black Death arrived in Europe in 1348. Originally temporary creations, even in small communities, to face the plague, they had become permanent in most major towns of Italy by 1500. Composed of laymen, with medical advisers and often large staffs, they could impose quarantine (first at Dubrovnik in 1377), remove the sick to isolation hospitals, ban goods from entering or leaving, clean the streets, unblock waterways, and compile lists of the dead. Their information networks sometimes stretched far, and their powers of punishment were draconian. In effect, the sophisticated northern Italian towns faced the great challenge to their lives by effective administrative measures, in which a directly medical response formed only one part.

The Black Death – bubonic plague with complications – first noted in Asia in 1346, was the greatest medical disaster of the Middle Ages, killing in its first wave, from 1347 to 1350, perhaps 25 per cent of Europe's population (see also page 28). It also became endemic, with possibly even graver consequences. Between 1350 and 1400 the average European lifespan may have shrunk from 30 to a mere 20 years, and Florence lost almost three-quarters of its population between 1338 and 1447. (Reasonably accurate figures for population and mortality begin in Italy around 1350, but are absent from much of northern Europe for two centuries more.)

The Black Death differed from earlier epidemics in its extent and in its ubiquity. Leprosy, which was widely feared in the twelfth and thirteenth centuries and which was explained in the same way as plague, affected fewer individuals, who could be easily segregated from the community in a leper house in a form of living death. But plague struck both more extensively and with harsher results. Death might be swift, and the imposition of rule by a Health Board might bring financial ruin.

How healthy was medieval society? In a crowded Italian city in 1480, the poor rarely lived beyond thirty, and even in the countryside few attained the age of forty. Diarrhoeas, smallpox, tuberculosis, typhus, measles, and meningitis were common, colics and the ubiquitous 'fever' frequent, and winter chills carried off many of the old and malnourished. Accidents, drownings, and burnings were often recorded, as were malarial fevers, kidney and bladder stones, and intestinal disorders. Degenerative diseases, such as cancer, were less common, because the population died at a relatively young age. The evidence of skeletons shows that few, even among the young, escaped without some debilitating disease.

The process of childbirth was particularly hazardous. Medical texts, largely based on Greek ideas, emphasized that woman was a weaker (and wetter) version of man, and hence more prone to disease, never more so than in pregnancy. The delivery itself was made without forceps or effective anaesthetics (although some opium-based drinks might have reduced pain a little). Although caesarian section is mentioned, evidence for its use is disputed. All that could be done was to

A medico-astrological chart from Germany, about AD 1450. Each part of the body is linked with a sign of the zodiac, which would help to decide on good or bad times for treatment. Such medical astrology goes back to the Roman period, and often demanded a good grasp of mathematics as well as of medicine.

A midwife attends a woman in labour, from an English manuscript of around 1400. The pictures of the possible positions of the child at birth go back to late antiquity and were well known throughout medieval Europe. The birth process was usually left to the supervision of a midwife, assisted by the woman's female friends and relatives, and took place at home. However, many books on obstetrics, like this one, seem to have been owned by male surgeons, who may well have been called in to attend extremely difficult cases of labour.

ensure, as far as possible, that the child in the womb lay in the best position for an easy birth – a recommendation far from simple to achieve. There are agonizing stories of women dying in labour, or from later complications, and although many of the recommendations for the care of the newborn are eminently sensible, the *Books of the Dead* reveal a veritable massacre of the innocents.

Mental diseases were treated in a variety of ways. Doctors generally believed in a strong link between physical and mental well-being, and paid attention, even in fevers, to the general psychological state of the patient. For some sufferers from mental diseases, physical remedies might be suggested – good food, healthy walks, and very occasionally drugs to change the overall humoral balance. Others sought a cure from God or the saints, by pilgrimage to a shrine or a holy dance, or indeed saw some conditions as 'holy folly', a special mark of grace, far beyond the love-madness sung by the medieval troubadour. Although we hear of the mad locked up in chains – in fifteenth-century Nuremberg (Germany) one could hire a cell in the town gaol – they were mainly looked after at home, within their own community and frequently given tasks that would integrate them with society and reduce the frightening aspect of their disorder.

The borderline between madness and divine inspiration is narrow and it is hard for modern scholars to interpret the narrative of a mystic or madwoman like Margery Kempe without using anachronistic categories. Yet it is fair to note that she lived in the world, bore fourteen children, travelled to the Holy Land and Germany, and was certainly aware of the different types of psychological experiences that she felt over many decades.

Margery Kempe, who was born in England in 1393, was a wealthy woman, familiar with practical medicine. After a period of insanity, she made pilgimages to Jerusalem, Rome, Germany, and Spain and described them and her spiritual experiences in *The Book of Margery Kempe* (c. 1423). This narrative, which is one of the earliest autobiographies in English literature, reveals the interaction between medicine and late-medieval society. It describes a learned medicine with roots in the Greek past but not unintelligible to the lay person: the good housewife might be more effective in providing healthy remedies than many an expensive physician or surgeon.

To some of her companions she was a sick woman, a nuisance with her interminable wailings; to others, she had been chosen as a mouthpiece of God. Her account describes her relationship with others in society, and gives an insight into how her condition was viewed by others at the time.

> Many said there was never saint in heaven that cried as she did, and from that they concluded she had a devil within her which caused that crying. And this they said openly, and much more evil talk. She took everything patiently for our Lord's love, for she knew very well that the Jews said much worse of his own person than people did of her, and therefore she took it the more meekly.[9]

Margery lived to a ripe old age, and cared for her husband when he, too, was senile.

The picture that Margery Kempe portrays is very different from that of modern medicine. It is not that many diseases were hard, if not impossible to cure – although medieval drugs may have worked more often than we think, and they certainly would have wrought little harm

Leprosy, which would have have included other serious skin conditions, was common in the Middle Ages. Lepers would have returned to their towns from isolated leper hospitals to beg for alms, or importuned passing travellers.

– but the whole context of medicine has changed. The Galenic – Arabic tradition stressed a holistic form of medicine, and, whether we are dealing with Islam, Christianity, or the scattered Jewish communities of medieval Europe, there was a social involvement that is often lacking today. Birth was a process attended by the women of the village; cleaning the streets might be a task imposed on all citizens; and death was an occasion for an assertion of communal values as well as private grief.

Yet medicine, and medical institutions, were also challenging some of the older ways. A new vocabulary of medicine, the growth of medical inquests and autopsies, Health Boards, Death Books, public physicians (and official pharmacopeias), and the isolation of lepers and plague victims, all gradually contributed to a move away from a communal consensus within medicine. Some might argue that this was a move towards a more effective system of health care; others that in 1500 this was centuries in the future; and others that an important part of the healing process, the interaction of patient and therapist, was being subverted to a medical monopoly.

Whichever point of view is adopted, medieval medicine was far from being static, unchanging, or entirely given over to the contemplation of past authorities. It was, in fact, capable of responding effectively to the challenge of disease within its own terms, and by invoking communal and religious responses, by involving caring and curing, it may have done as much as was possible until the therapeutic revolution of the late nineteenth and twentieth centuries to maintain health.

CHAPTER 3   *What is Disease?*

Roy Porter

Perceptions of sickness have varied greatly over time and place. According to the tradition of Greek medicine, which continued to have currency into the Renaissance, melancholy was the sickness that resulted from an excess of the bodily fluid known as black bile. This is depicted not merely in the depressed, lethargic sufferer but in the wider symbols of finitude and disintegration, including the setting sun and the hour-glass – symptoms of the decaying world. Albrecht Dürer's *Melencolia I*, 1514.

Understanding the history of medicine presents many challenges. Not only has medicine itself undergone profound change in its encounters with disease and death, but the very conception of illness – its nature, causes, and meaning – is complex and enigmatic. Perceptions of sickness have varied greatly over time and place, shaped by diverse circumstances. Different social groups conceptualize illnesses disparately. In Shakespeare's time, melancholy was called the 'courtier's coat of arms' and regarded as an eligible, fashionable disorder of the elite; but a poor person suffering similar symptoms – what we might call depression – was considered 'mopish' and rebuked for being sullen. Gender has counted too: the condition that in 1800 would have been called 'hysteria' in a woman might have been diagnosed as 'hypochondria' in a man. Not least, illness may be regarded differently by patients and practitioners. Sufferers experience the personal side of being sick; doctors, especially those with scientific pretensions, are more likely to emphasize its objective aspects, the facts underpinning diagnoses and prognoses.

DISEASE AND ILLNESS

Chapter 1 dealt with 'disease' as a biological force in the economy of Nature, showing humans and microbes locked in a Darwinian struggle for survival; this chapter looks at 'illness'. The terms are often used interchangeably: 'he's got a disease', we say, or 'he's suffering from an illness'. Yet they may also be differentiated.

After all, it makes perfect sense to say of somebody with a tumour: 'he's got cancer, but he's not feeling ill'. 'He's sick' is said of someone with a hangover, without generally implying that any 'disease' is involved – although we might think he was also suffering from alcoholism, a rather particular species of disease.

In modern English parlance, disease is normally an objective thing, often triggered by a pathogen, such as a bacillus or a virus, and marked by telltale symptoms – a rash or a raised temperature. Illness, on the other hand, denotes something subjective, feelings of malaise or pain. They may be two sides of the same coin, but not always. This may seem semantic quibbling, but words are often revealing symptoms of underlying realities. And our habit of distinguishing between disease and illness itself betrays historical transformations. For the term 'disease' has developed from 'dis-ease'; similarly, malaise from 'mal-aise' (ill at ease, a state of discomfort). Thus, within the modern, scientific concept of disease lurk softer, more subjective, and historically antecedent connotations. The emergence of the neutral, scientific concept of 'disease' from earlier ideas of 'dis-ease' (akin to our 'illness') offers a insight into different cultural perceptions and changes over time.

HEALING AND HOLINESS

First, it is worth glancing, for contrast and comparison, at conceptions of sickness in what might be called traditional societies; groups without an indigenous written culture, ones in which medical skills are orally transmitted. It would be entirely wrong nowadays to accept the derogatory Victorian verdict on the medical beliefs of such societies, condemning them as primitive, superstitious, and irrational. We feel confident that we have 'progressed', and science certainly furnishes Western healing with powers that the medicine-man or witchdoctor lacks. But tribal medicine 'makes sense' no less – and, in some ways, far more – than Western medicine.

It is easy to spot similarities between the traditional medicine of Africans or Australian Aborigines today and the religious framework that cradled illness and

Traditional concepts of sickness

There are glaring hazards in venturing generalizations about the beliefs of myriad such societies from the Nuer to the Navajo. However, it can broadly be said that, unlike modern Western medicine, traditional healing is disposed to see much sickness (especially that of a spectacular, unusual, or fatal nature) as essentially personal, in two senses.

First, sickness is typically regarded as an affliction deliberately visited upon a victim by some individual force — perhaps a witch or sorcerer, or maybe a ghost, ancestor, or demon. Falling sick is thus a curse or possession, malevolently inflicted through magic or spells. It involves an act of will, often an act of war. Second, such sickness does not strike randomly. It is targeted against a specific individual, family, or tribe, in retribution for some act of commission or omission: forefathers have been slighted, taboos breached, ceremonies neglected, the gods not propitiated, and so on. Illness is thus a reprisal or a punishment. Because illness is thus regarded as

the outcome of personal, social, and religious beliefs and behaviour, healing is no mere technical, clinical procedure. It involves kin and community, and requires rituals that ceremonially cleanse the polluted, offer reparations, and lay ghosts. Rituals, incantations, and sacrifices are thus indispensable to healing. Wrongs inflicted by sorcery may be exorcised by rite.

What could be further from our official medicine? Indeed, Western doctors have routinely condemned folk and tribal medicine as mumbo jumbo — not medicine but its pretence. The contrast may be less real than we care to think; reversing the binoculars, medical anthropologists have pointed to parallel rituals nearer home, including the stethoscope 'necklace', the symbolic white coat, and the magic of the placebo pill through which Western doctors reassure and even fob off patients for whom they may be able to do remarkably little.

Detail of an effigy jar showing a shaman healing a woman, from the Mochica period (AD 1–600), coast of N. Peru. Among native Americans, priests, shamans, medicine men, or sorcerers were entrusted with the rituals of diagnosis and cure. Supernatural agencies were believed to cause illness, often as a punishment for evil, and Amerindian cultures in Mexico, the Yucatán, and Peru identified specific diseases with particular deities.

Throughout the Middle Ages and beyond, Christianity offered a range of explanations of suffering and death. Disease could be regarded as God's punishment for the wicked. But the Old Testament figure of Job struck down with pestilence, as depicted here in a sixteenth- or seventeenth-century woodcut, served as an illustration of how the Lord might visit the righteous with afflictions by way of a special test of their faith. Pain was broadly viewed as the inevitable state of fallen man, whose body had been corrupted by Original Sin.

healing in medieval Europe. Medical magic was then explicit within folklore, the Church, and learned medicine alike. Religion and medicine shared a common orientation in the Middle Ages – that of making whole. Etymologically, 'holiness' and 'healing' stem from a common root (the idea of wholeness), as do salvation and salubrity, and also cure, care, and charity (from the Latin, *caritas*). But our culture (being literate and analytical) has also developed demarcations between the body on the one hand and, on the other, the soul, mind, or spirit. Such dualisms have fostered a differentiation of medicine from faith, and of doctor from priest, the one attending the cure of bodies, the other the 'cure of souls'. Such distinctions have been contested, and physic and faith have continually crisscrossed or collided, engaging in border disputes. Although often complementary, there remains potential for conflict; while separate, there remains scope for unification.

Not least, Western medicine developed within dominant value-systems established by the Church (until quite recently, medicine remained a junior, subaltern profession, less prestigious than the cloth). Like other great faiths, Judaeo-Christianity proclaims a dualistic cosmology that ennobles the soul or mind while disparaging the body, which is often viewed as the soul's prison house. Spirit is immortal; the flesh, by contrast, is weak and corruptible, and, thanks to Original Sin, theologically depraved. It was Adam and Eve's disobedience in the Garden of

Eden at the Fall that created vile bodies and brought sin, suffering, and death into the world.

Anxieties about the corruptions of the flesh are registered in the strict body regulation demanded of the Chosen People in the Pentateuch and upheld ever since within Judaism's elaborate rituals concerning hygiene, diet, and sex. Cleanliness had to be defended against such defiling pollutions as the blood of a menstruating woman. It was a Talmudic requirement that Jews should not live in a city without a physician. Mistrusting the fallen body, early Christians responded with defences of their own. Drawing on traditions of Eastern asceticism, the Desert Fathers mortified the flesh and exalted continence. The lusts of the flesh had to be tamed to free the spirit. In the Middle Ages, chastity, fasting, and self-flagellation became hallmarks of holiness.

The disciplining of the flesh has been a key element in many faiths. Christianity, however, encodes especially complex attitudes towards the body. It personalizes the Deity (God the Father), and weaves Him into the plot of the terrestrial world. God has an only son, who is born in the flesh, before being crucified in bodily agony. Incarnation and sacrifice are in turn commemorated in the Eucharist, whereby, for Roman Catholics, sacramental bread and wine are literally transubstantiated into the Saviour's body and blood. Through divine propitiation, believers are promised bodily resurrection at the Last Judgment. While abhorring the flesh because tainted by sin, Christianity, in short, also emphasized a certain sanctity immanent within it. While asceticism was prized, mortification was never to be pursued to the point of self-destruction. Suicide was a mortal sin: being God's creature, how could man be free to dispose of his own body?

CHRISTIANITY, PAIN, AND SUFFERING

To modern medicine, pain is an alarm bell, part of a system that warns of trouble within; it is thus a necessary evil. To some churchmen, it has been a positive sanctification: it was not unusual for evangelists to follow St Paul and commend the 'thorn in the flesh'. The great Victorian Baptist preacher, Charles Haddon Spurgeon, was convinced that 'the greatest earthly blessing that God can give to any of us is health, with the exception of sickness … A sick wife, a newly made grave, poverty, slander, sinking of spirit, might teach us lessons nowhere else to be learned so well'.[1]

The man in the street has been less enthusiastic about pain – Christian zealotry may seem to verge on masochism – and philosophers have felt obliged to confront the problem of pain. What is it for? Should it be enjoyed or endured? If shunned, how? A prime aim, for example, of the Epicureans (followers of the Greek philosopher, Epicurus) lay in devising damage limitation, designed to curb self-inflicted exposure to agonies: the simple life would avoid giving hostages to fortune. Stoicism similarly recommended soaring above worldly passions, for they brought disappointment not pleasure.

Detail from *The Procession of Flagellants* by Goya, 1816. The figure of the flagellant was common in the Middle Ages. Since the time of the Desert Fathers in early Christianity, holy individuals had been encouraged to mortify the flesh. Especially at times of civil crisis, plague, and pestilence, groups might gather for collective mortification, flagellating themselves and others, by way of expiation and propitiation of sins. By Goya's time, Enlightenment intellectuals were regarding pious mortification as a symptom of collective religious mania or derangement.

Christianity taught that pain and sickness were not original to God's design. Agony had entered the world through Original Sin, through which man was condemned to labour by the sweat of his brow and woman to bring forth in pain; after the Fall mankind would thereafter suffer disease and death. Thus the Bible construed pain as the penalty for disobedience – a notion reinforced by etymology, the word pain being derived from *poena* (the Latin for punishment).

Scripture further showed God visiting woe upon the wicked through pestilence, while chosen individuals were devoutly to rejoice in the Cross of illness. As Job's trials showed, the pious response to divine affliction was to be long-suffering. Martyrdom to disease in this vale of tears might be as glorious as martyrdom to the infidel. Especially within Catholicism, expiatory mortification of the flesh, with goads, hair-shirts, and fasting, struck a blow for holiness.

Yet caution was always urged upon Christians, lest they fetishized pain, glamourizing the man of sorrows. And charity also required succour for the sick and relief of distress. Thus Christian doctrine regarding welfare, philanthropy, and medicine grew extremely complex. Suffering was a blessing, yet it was also to be alleviated by medicine and charity. Ambiguities similar to these are also mirrored in the casuistry of the Churches' teachings towards war: Christians should turn the other cheek, but just wars may be holy.

MEDICINE WITHIN CHRISTENDOM

Over the centuries, certain fundamentalist Christian sects have condemned medicine as more or less impious. Some Calvinists in Britain and North America rejected smallpox inoculation and vaccination on the grounds that implantation of diseased material into a healthy person risked breaking the Sixth Commandment. Jehovah's Witnesses originally denied the germ theory, and still refuse blood transfusions, convinced that they contravene Scripture (Genesis 9:4) – although, somewhat eccentrically, they today accept organ transplants. Nevertheless, the main Christian churches have routinely accepted that medicine has a valid role. Was not the Evangelist Luke 'the beloved physician'? And did not Christ himself, while instructing physicians to heal themselves, give proofs of his divine powers by some thirty-five such curative miracles? The apostles exercised healing as 'a gift of the spirit' (1 Cor. 12:9). From the start, Christianity was a healing faith.

Christianity has always been a healing religion. According to St John's Gospel, at the Pool of Bethesda just north of the Temple in Jerusalem, Jesus said 'Rise, take up thy bed and walk', and thereby immediately cured a hopeless cripple. This depiction of the healing miracle was painted by William Hogarth (1735–6) for the main staircase up to the Great Hall of St Bartholomew's Hospital in London. Only the central part of this large painting is shown here.

Christianity's vision of the body – fallen, yet God's instrument – suggested a division of labour between the churches and the medical profession. Priests were to tend the salvation of the soul, while the ailments of the body became the physicians' prerogative. The Fourth Lateran Council (1215) in Rome forebade clerics to shed blood through the practice of surgery, and warned against immoderate involvement of clerics in treating physical complaints. Doctors and priests thus mapped out 'separate spheres' – in principle, a mutually acceptable *modus vivendi*. Matters pertaining to the soul were rendered unto the Church; and the body was rendered unto the 'Caesar' of the doctors. Peaceful coexistence was the norm but border flare-ups were inevitable.

For one thing, Catholicism energetically involved itself in healing rituals, championing recourse to relics, offerings made in fulfilment of vows, pilgrimages, holy waters, and, above all, shrines and cults. Saints won reputations for special healing powers: for example, to cure toothache, you prayed to St Apollonia (d. 249), who had been martyred by having her teeth yanked out. Some other examples are noted in Chapters 2 and 8 (see pages 73 and 289).

Down the centuries, holy people have claimed healing gifts. In Restoration England, the Irish gentleman Valentine Greatrakes healed by prayer and laying on of hands; a century later, Bridget Bostock from Cheshire cured with holy spittle; in mid-nineteenth-century France, the visions of Bernadette Soubirous, the miller's daughter, led to Lourdes becoming a leading healing shrine, today visited by around 3 million pilgrims a year. 'Miracle' healing has commanded a mass appeal, and the less the medical profession and even churches countenance marvellous cures, the more faith-healing falls into the hands of hucksters.

Epidemics often excited confrontations between the Church and the medical profession, public authorities and the people, as to the meaning of diseases and the measures required. Plague above all provoked such problems, for bubonic plague was lethal, rapidly fatal, and spread like wildfire, imperilling whole communities. Laden like leprosy with Scriptural associations and moral metaphors, plague was typically interpreted as a visitation, requiring public atonement. In the fourteenth century, the Black Death (see pages 28 and 78) led to expiatory flagellant movements and anti-Semitic pogroms. Faced with plague, Church authorities in Renaissance Italy proclaimed mass intercessions and propitiatory prayers. The municipalities, for their part, counterordered quarantine and isolation, sometimes banning religious processions. This prompted tests of strength, the populace typically siding with the priests (for public-health decrees like quarantine were commercially ruinous). On one occasion the entire Florentine Health Board was excommunicated.

In Tudor and Stuart times, plague led to tussles in England between royal health policy and protesting Puritans. The Crown and city corporations responded to epidemics by containment, bolting city gates, banning markets, and quarantining sufferers and suspects. Preachers condemned such measures as misguided, medically worthless, and (because they seemed to fly in the face of Providence) impious. 'It is not the clean keeping and sweeping of our houses and streets that can drive away this fearful messenger of God's wrath', wailed the Puritan pastor, Laurence Chaderton, 'but the purging and sweeping of our consciences from … sin.'[2] True Christian fellowship demanded not hygiene but holiness, not sequestration but trust in God.

Witchcraft became a prime bone of contention between the medical and religious outlooks. The baselines were well established. Almost all agreed (here pre-industrial Europe mirrors modern tribal societies) that the Devil and his minions could wreak bodily evil: sickness and death were indices of such diabolical power. When someone fell ill without obvious cause, accusations of *maleficium* (malice) might follow. But could one be sure that the victim was bewitched? Faced with such symptoms as fits, vomiting, confused speech, or delirium, there seemed three possible explanations: disease, fraud, or demonic possession. Doctors developed examination procedures to decide the matter. Were there unambiguous wounds or ulcers? Could the Devil's stigma (*stigmata diaboli*) be discerned? Priests had trials of their own: how did the victim respond to prayer, to display of the Cross?

In most instances, religious and medical experts concurred. But not always. In 1602, Mary Glover fell sick with fits and Elizabeth Jackson, a London char-

Bubonic plague was a medical catastrophe of almost unimaginable proportions; some 80,000 people died, for example, during the Plague of London in 1665. Such outbreaks were widely interpreted as divine punishment for sins or ungodliness, leading to calls to penitance and religious reform. Solomon Eccles (or Eagles) was a Quaker fanatic who ran naked through the streets of London during the Great Plague with a dish of burning sulphur on his head, preaching repentance and prophesying catastrophes. This engraving is from a painting by Paul F. Poole (1807–79).

woman, was accused of bewitching her. Testifying in court, the physician, Edward Jorden, contended that her disorder was organic. Puritan counterwitnesses protested that this was a case of demonism, a view upheld by the judge, Sir Edmund Anderson, a noted hammer of witches. Overruled, the angry Jorden published a book called *The Suffocation of the Mother* (1603), arguing that the accepted signs of witchcraft were generally produced by a somatic disease that he called 'the Mother', an old term for hysteria.

Jorden did not deny the reality of diabolism in general, he merely claimed that it did not apply to Glover. Nor did the case produce a clear line-up of physicians versus priests. Leading Anglican ecclesiastics supported Jorden, for the bishops wanted to put a damper on witchcraft accusations, which they saw as being exploited by Roman Catholics and Puritans alike in their battles against the Church of England. Although to us it might seem paradoxical, Anglican bishops were eager to wash their hands of devil-dabbling, and were happy to consign cases of 'possession' to the doctors.

In the long run, governments, church establishments, and ruling elites throughout Europe, terrified by the anarchy of the witchcraze, 'medicalized' demonism. Indeed, in the eighteenth century, in the rationalist atmosphere of the Enlightenment, belief in diabolism, once so orthodox, became condemned as bigoted or even psychopathological, a mark of the lunatic fringe. This in turn spotlighted a new malady, religious insanity (see Chapter 8).

THE MEDICAL VIEW OF ILLNESS

Alongside Christian beliefs about sickness, suffering, and healing – with their transcendental visions of providence and punishment, trial, and tribulation – medicine was all the time offering its own theories of the nature and meaning of sickness. The medicine of the Greeks and Romans bequeathed a complex message. On the one hand, the Hippocratic tradition, laid down in writings thought to be by Hippocrates of Cos (see page 58), insisted that sickness was of the body, and that the body formed part of the comprehensive economy of Nature (*physis*): hence, physicians should study physis. Hippocrates – or, more accurately, one of the anonymous authors of the *Hippocratic Corpus* – poured scorn on the superstitious view that sickness was a supernatural visitation.

Behind this Hippocratic onslaught was a push towards the creation of a more coherent professional identity. In early Greece, there were no state privileges or legal safeguards for the medical art, and anybody was free to jockey for trade in the medical marketplace. In such circumstances, the Hippocratic doctors strove in various ways – witness the celebrated Hippocratic Oath (see page 59) – to elevate themselves above other healers. Imposters and disreputable healers 'who first attributed a sacred character to this malady', a Hippocratic author complained, 'were like the magicians, purifiers, charlatans and quacks of our own day, men who claim great piety and superior knowledge. Being at a loss, and having no treatment

Opposite: *The Transfiguration* by Raphael (1517) illustrates a scene recorded in the Gospel according to St Matthew (17:15) in which a sick boy's father cries (as translated in the Authorized Version) 'Lord, have mercy on my son: for he is lunatick, and sore vexed: for ofttimes he falleth into the fire, and oft into the water'. The boy is undergoing an epileptic seizure; Jesus as the source of healing floats in a sea of light. From early times epilepsy, on account of its extraordinary manifestations, was known as the 'sacred disease'. Within Christendom many religious cures were attempted. It was widely believed that St Valentine, St Sebastian, and St Vitus assisted epileptics. In Greece, however, Hippocratic physicians judged that epilepsy had natural origins, like all other diseases.

The healing god Asclepius (or in Latin Aesculapius), seated on the throne in this bas-relief, was in Greek mythology the son of a god, Apollo, by a mortal mother, variously Arsinoe or Coronis. He was taught herbal remedies by Chiron the centaur and healed mortals with them. In anger at his rescue of men from death, Zeus killed him with a thunderbolt, but he was later enrolled among the gods. Many temples and shrines were dedicated to Asclepius (see page 57): this fragment from the fourth century BC (a cast of the original) was found in Athens. The Ancient Greeks believed that from Asclepius's family, the Asclepiads, descended all doctors, and the family of Hippocrates traced their origin back to him.

which would help, they concealed and sheltered themselves behind superstition, and called this illness sacred, in order that their utter ignorance might not be manifest'.[3]

Naturally, the Hippocratics also thought they knew more than other people; but their claim to unique expertise lay in appropriating the organic. As pioneered by the Hippocratics and passed down through the great Galen (see page 62), medicine was expertise in the body. Greek medical theory thus plucked sickness from the heavens and brought it down to earth. Historians have regarded the Hippocratic programme as, symbolically at least, constituting the foundation of scientific medicine, through denial of a supernatural causation of disease and concentration on the body.

Yet, as emphasized in Chapter 2, if Graeco-Roman medicine was secular and naturalistic, it was also holistic. It focused upon what it called the humours, those fluids whose equilibrium was vital for life: the body must not become too hot or too cold, too wet or too dry. It emphasized 'animal spirits', superfine fluids mediating between the body and the mind. And it postulated various 'souls' that governed bodily functions – a 'vegetable soul', directing nourishment and growth (that is, autonomic processes and metabolic regulation); an 'animal soul', governing sense, feeling, and motion (similar, in our terms, to the sensory/motor system); and an 'intellectual soul', regulating the mental powers (that is, what Renaissance theorists of human nature later designated as reason, will, memory, imagination, and judgement). In short, the human animal was presented as a complex, differentiated integrated whole. The humours formed one facet, and their balance was reflected in the 'complexion' (or outward appearance) and the 'temperament' – or, as we might say, personality type. Humours, complexion, and temperament constituted an interactive system.

Greek medicine was thus 'holistic' or 'whole person' in two crucial ways. First, it assumed that health and illness were 'organic' or 'constitutional' in the sense of deriving from inner processes. It did not see illness as typically caused by invasive pathogens: the cause of sickness was largely internal. Second, all aspects of the person were interlinked. The body affected the mind, as with fever causing delirium. Equally, however, passions and emotions influenced the body, producing what we would call psychosomatic complaints.

Thus Greek medicine – and by extension the learned medicine espoused by bookish physicians through the Middle Ages and the Renaissance – adopted a constitutional or 'physiological' doctrine of sickness. It was the product of physical processes, not of spirit possession or sorcery. It was an expression of changes, abnormalities, or weaknesses in the whole person; peculiar to the individual, it was 'dis-ease' rather than disease. Such a person-centred view could underwrite a certain therapeutic optimism: relief was in the hands of the 'whole person'. Classical medicine taught that the right frame of mind, composure, control of the passions, and suitable lifestyle, could surmount sickness – indeed, prevent it in the first place: healthy minds would promote healthy bodies.

MECHANICAL SCIENCE

Medical thinking took its cue from the Ancients for a long time: Galen of Pergamum, in particular, was deified throughout the Middle Ages. But the tradition was to be challenged by the Scientific Revolution, especially its onslaught on the person-centred and vitalistic views ingrained in Greek, and especially Aristotelian, science. Champions of the 'new science', such as the seventeenth-century philosophers René Descartes and Thomas Hobbes, denounced Aristotle for falsely endowing Nature with vitality, proclivities, appetites, will, consciousness, and purposes ('final causes'). In reality, they argued, Nature was made up of particles or corpuscles of inert matter. The motions of planets, or of balls falling from the Tower of Pisa, were not to be explained in terms of any 'desires' but through the laws of mechanics, of matter in motion, which found ideal expression in the language of geometry and number. Nature was in truth a machine.

This view of Nature – seen as particulate matter uniformly moved by immutable, universal laws (Hooke's Law, Boyle's Law, and such like) – had momentous implications not just for understanding the Solar System or the trajectories of cannon but also for the conceptualization of living beings. Were animals machines? Were humans machines? These were tempting if perilous possibilities pondered on by the fashionable members of London's Royal Society and its equivalents in Paris and Florence. During the seventeenth century, scorn was poured on the 'humours' – they were dismissed as empty verbiage. Thanks to dissection techniques rendered prestigious by the Flemish anatomist Andreas Vesalius, attention was refocused on the solid body parts. Arguing for the circulation of the blood, the London physician William Harvey depicted the heart as a pump. Dissection and experimentation spurred inspection of muscles, cartilage, fibres, vessels, and interpretation of their operation by analogy with levers and springs, pulleys and pipes in man-made mechanisms like mills and clocks.

Analysis of the transformations in anatomy and physiology arising from the Scientific Revolution is provided in Chapter 5. They had the profoundest implications for conceptions of health and disease: wellbeing became compared to the running of a well-tuned, well-oiled machine, and sickness was depicted as a mechanical breakdown, due perhaps to a blockage, fuel shortage, or excessive friction.

The mechanical outlook's appeal was enhanced by the new dualistic philosophies associated above all with Descartes. He postulated two radically different

In the seventeenth century the body became widely viewed as a machine and sickness as a form of mechanical breakdown. The pioneer of this way of thinking was the philosopher and natural scientist René Descartes (1596–1650). French-born, Descartes spent his creative years in the Dutch Republic, developing a dualistic philosophy that postulated the essential distinction between mind and matter. His naturalistic approach demystified the human body and laid it completely open to scientific analysis.

After the publication of Andreas Vesalius's massive *De Humani Corporis Fabrica* (On the Fabric of the Human Body) in 1543, anatomists developed an ever more sophisticated grasp of the basic bodily systems. This new understanding was broadcast by means of sumptuous anatomical atlases on which medical men and distinguished artists collaborated. Knowledge of anatomy (structure) paved the way for a better grasp of physiology (function). This illustration of the structure of the armpit, or axilla, is taken from the *Traité Complet de l'Anatomie de l'Homme* by J.-B. M. Bougéry and N. H. Jacob, 1831–54.

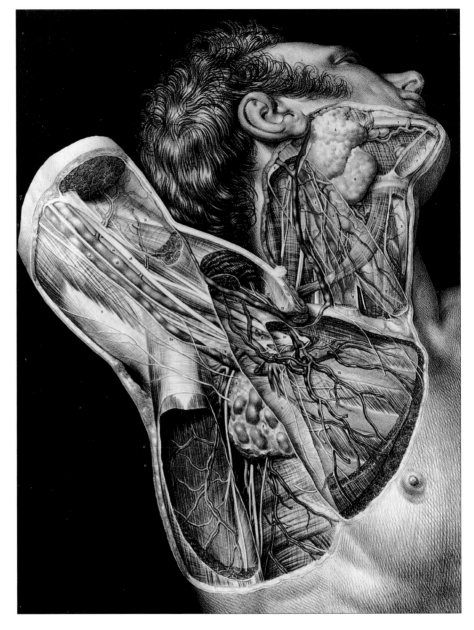

entities, extension (material) and mind (immaterial). Only the human soul or mind possessed consciousness. Literally everything else in Nature, including the human body and all aspects whatsoever of all other living beings, formed part of the realm of what Descartes called 'extension' (obeying the laws of mechanics). 'Extension', which included all other living creatures, was a legitimate terrain for scientific investigation. By Descartes' deft manoeuvre, mind had, so to speak, been mystified, while the body was laid bare.

Such a demarcation clearly had attractions for medicine. If the body's workings were purely 'mechanical', its territory must be the exclusive property of medical science. A huge KEEP OUT notice had, as it were, been pinned to the body, excluding theologians, moralists, and any one else considering fishing in medicine's pond. Moreover, if the flesh truly were a machine – no more, no less – it should prove as comprehensible as the workings of a clock. Reductionism now, for the first time, loomed large in medicine's agenda: explaining the whole in terms of its parts, the complex in terms of the simple, the biological in terms of the physical or chemical.

The mechanical world-view with its attendant mind–body dualism unleashed an extraordinarily productive programme of anatomical and physiological research that bore exceptional fruit, in the nineteenth century, with experimental physiology and cell biology and, in the twentieth, with molecular biology. Nineteenth-century medical scientists felt increasingly certain that for each sickness they would find, under the skin, tangible localized lesions: an inflamed organ, an obstruction, a tumour, or pathogens and parasites. Material interventions – drugs and surgery – would relieve or cure. Confident professional articles of faith proclaimed the autonomy and authority of biomedical science. Such developments imparted a new scientific aura to nineteenth-century professional medicine. Biomedicine claimed an explanatory monopoly over the body, its exploration, and its treatment. Proponents of scientific medicine, such as the German bacteriologist Robert Koch, discoverer of the cholera bacillus, believed they had cracked the secret of disease.

So the core medical project over the past two centuries has lain in exploring the workings and the malfunctions of bodily tissues and cells. Chapter 5 examines the role in this of the laboratory and the medical specialisms it has sustained. For example, thanks to the microscope and the rise of cytology, cancer and other cellular diseases could be investigated for the first time. On the microscope slide were exhibited the bacteria and viruses responsible for infections: disease organisms became visible. Furthermore, biochemistry has examined deficiency and digestive diseases, endocrinology has explained hormonal imbalances, neurology has revealed the basis of behavioural disturbances in the central nervous system, and modern genetics is cracking inherited conditions such as Huntington's chorea.

Alongside the laboratory, the hospital played a major part in establishing disease as objective ('ontological'). As the French thinker Michel Foucault emphasized in his study *The Birth of the Clinic* (1963), the vast nineteenth-century expansion of hospitals created disease showcases. The presence under a single roof of scores of cases of tuberculosis or typhus switched attention from the individual to the type. What seemed significant in the hospital was not the slightly diverse symptoms of this or that patient but the fact that diseases routinely followed essentially the same course in case after case, and that clinical regularities could then be confirmed in the morgue through postmortem pathological examination. Nicholas Jewson, a British medical sociologist, has spoken perceptively of the 'disappearance of the sick man' in the nineteenth century: doctors directed their gaze not on the individual sick person but on the disease of which his or her body was the bearer.[4]

Hospitals also became sites for surgery; and the progress of surgery – especially after anaesthetics and antiseptics made abdominal surgery feasible and safe (see Chapter 6) – proved the capstone and ultimate vindication of the programme of medical research and thinking espoused from the seventeenth century. For surgery was human engineering; as with car maintenance, one peered under the bonnet and repaired faulty parts. Nowadays, transplant surgery permits, for the first time, replacement of parts that are beyond repair. Mechanical and reductionist approaches found their culmination in spare-part surgery.

BODY AND GUT

The laboratory and the hospital created and confirmed a viewpoint disposed to think of disease as an objective, physical entity, and so contributed to a shift from 'dis-ease' to diseases, or from 'physiological' to 'ontological' conceptions of disease. So, too, the emphasis changed in general practice and bedside medicine. In premodern medical consultations, the doctor's job was mainly to manage the patient's condition – generally with some pretty ineffectual drugs washed down with a hefty gulp of the placebo effect. With the advent of scientific medicine, it was transformed to attacking the disease. The mark of this shift was the emergence of physical examination and its accompanying diagnostic technology – a topic fully examined in Chapter 4.

Before the turn of the nineteenth century, when a patient saw a doctor, the physician first had to be put in the picture. This was achieved through the sick person relating his 'history': when and how the complaint had started, what might have precipitated it, the characteristic pains and symptoms, and whether it was new or recurrent. The patient would also recite the main features of his lifestyle – eating and sleeping habits, bowel motions, details of emotional upsets, and so forth.

The practitioner would appraise this history in the light of prior experience. He would also conduct some kind of physical scrutiny of the body, but, by today's standards, this was cursory. It would be conducted by the eye, not by touch, paying attention to such features as skin colour and lesions (rashes or spots), swelling, and inflammation. Doctors would commonly feel the pulse with the finger, making a qualitative assessment (was it languid or racing, regular or erratic?), look at the tongue, listen to coughs, and sniff bad odours.

Physical examination was perfunctory. For one thing, too much touching or exposure of the patient's body was liable to be thought indelicate. Groping beneath the clothes was undignified to a genteel physician. For another, traditional medicine had no diagnostic instruments to augment the senses. Stethoscopes, ophthalmoscopes, and other gadgetry were not introduced till after 1800, and even then they met resistance from patients and practitioners alike. To the end of her days, Queen Victoria was noted for her 'great aversion' to the stethoscope. In all the 20 years he attended her, remembered the Queen's last physician, Sir James Reid, 'the first time I had ever seen the Queen … in bed' was when she was actually dying, and it was only after her death that he discovered that she had a 'ventral hernia, and a prolapse of the uterus' – proof that he had never given her a full physical examination.[5]

In traditional medical consultations, the physician was reliant on what the sick person said and his skill in interpreting the patients' words. This did not leave him in too parlous a state, because lay people, both educated and illiterate, had entrenched notions of their own about their systems and what made them ill. Letters and autobiographies from earlier centuries reveal deep preoccupation with matters of health and with attempts to plumb the sources of sickness.

Samuel Pepys, for example, still subscribed to a humoral theory of illness, stressing 'cold' and therefore the role of phlegm. Cold was dangerous because it 'clogged the pores' and thus impeded healthy expulsion of 'peccant humours'. For

The preoccupations of Pepys

In the diaries that he kept for 10 years from 1660, Samuel Pepys referred to his health well over a thousand times; and often his point in noting his condition was to record sickness episodes for future prophylactic purposes.

One of his great bugbears was cold. On no fewer than 102 occasions he recorded taking cold. He generally blamed it on the weather (which also bred such other complaints as itching, pimples, tickling, and pissing pains). But his own carelessness was often at fault: leaving off his wig, having a bare head, bare legs, standing in draughts, being underdressed, wearing unaired clothes. Every move might be full of peril:

> [2 November 1662] Then up into my new rooms, which are almost finished, and there walked with great content and so home and to bed, with some pain in making water, having taken cold this morning in staying too long bare-legged to pare my cornes.[6]

Pepys mainly treated himself but it is clear that, when he did consult a physician, he would not

have lacked details of his complaints to tell the doctor. On 31 December 1664, Pepys balanced his books:

> So ends the old year, I bless God with great joy to me; not only from my having made so good a year of profit, as having spent 420*l.* and laid up 540*l.* and upward.
>
> But I bless God, I never have been in so good plight as to my health in so very cold weather as this is, nor indeed in any hot weather these ten years, as I am at this day and have been these four or five months. But am at a great loss to know whether it be my Hare's foote, or taking every morning of a pill of Turpentine, or my having left off the wearing of a gowne.[7]

In the final scene of Colley Cibber's play *The Careless Husband* (1704), the good wife, worried about his catching cold, covers her faithless husband's shaven head. His wig has fallen off, doubtless during his dalliance with the maid – a Pepysian scenario! The painting is by Philip Mercier.

Cupid's arrows had struck from antiquity and lovesickness was recognized as a disease from medieval times. But it was only later that the figure of the physician became erotically charged, associated with physical examinations and especially the rise of the ambiguous figure of the man-midwife. The doctor was sometimes seen as a secret seducer – or, more grossly, he was a figure of fun, being cuckolded by his young assistant. Whether there was any medicine for love was much debated. Coloured mezzotint by W. Ward, 1802, after J. Opie.

commonsense humoral thinking, the key to health lay in the body functioning as an efficient throughput system. Abundant food and drink were necessary to stoke the vital fires (the 'flame of life' was a popular metaphor). But regular evacuation was equally needed to prevent blockages. Hence people set great store by taking vomits, letting blood (venesection or phlebotomy), undergoing 'sweats', and, above all, in purging themselves (see Chapter 4). Regular and energetic evacuations helped maintain good 'flow'.

Dis-ease in eighteenth-century Saxony — the fluid body

In line with humoral assumptions, the medical common-sense of earlier centuries regarded the innards — a sort of 'black hole', out of sight and known only indirectly — as extraordinarily fluid. This can be seen from a remarkable study by the German medical historian Barbara Duden of nearly 2,000 women from the town of Eisenbach in early eighteenth-century Saxony. The illness experiences of the women were logged in the casebooks of their physician, Johann Storch.

Dr Storch's patients regarded their insides as a sites of astonishing changeability. They might claim, for example, that the disappearance of freckles caused their breath to smell; their sweat sometimes smelled of urine; if they failed to menstruate, they said, they developed diarrhoea or the delayed discharge came out as bloody sputum. Almost any bodily process could thus turn into any other — the interior was a kaleidoscope. Bodies had to flow to be healthy.

In an agrarian society preoccupied with changes in the weather, soil and seasons, the system beneath the skin was equally viewed as fluid, a succession of transactions: digestion, fertilization, evacuation, parturition. What counted was not structures but processes. (A parallel might be seen in traditional Chinese medicine, which has often seemed, to Western doctors, puzzlingly indifferent to the fixed anatomical parts basic to modern science.)

Aware of the processes going on out of sight in their insides, the Saxon women gave Dr Storch very 'subjective' accounts of their illnesses. They complained, Barbara Duden notes, of the following ailments:

> Slight headache, darkness of the eyes, a feeling that their hair was falling out or sight was fading or hearing was disappearing, a tearing in the jaw, a dizzy and dull headache, heavy tongue and speech, toothache, nosebleed, a flux in the ear, hiccups, a sore throat, a rising in the throat and constriction of the same, contraction of the throat, withdrawing of the gum, bilious vomiting, choking, hoarseness and coughing, phlegm dripping from the head onto the throat, neck pains, tightness of throat, sweating of the head, gloominess of thoughts, sadness. Searing pain in the limbs, numbness in the arm, trembling, tingling in the limbs, numb hands, cramped hands, crushed limbs, heaviness in the arm, stirring in the arm, apoplexy in the right arm, tearing fluxes in the limbs, fright in the limbs, painful gout. A rising of the blood toward the breast, shortness of breath, a tight shortness of breath, choking in the breast, stinging pains around the breast, anxiety, fearfulness, a wooden stake in the heart, squeezing in the pit of the heart, heart anxiety, a pain in the breast that felt as though something was eating inside, anxiousness, throbbing of the heart, burning under the breastbone. Painful womb colic, womb fear, womb anxiety, womb trouble, cramps, a cold womb that was open too wide, a knot in the womb, a closed-in wind turning toward the womb, a womb cramp manifesting itself mostly in the mouth and in the tongue and rendering the latter useless for speaking. A swollen body, thick belly and rumbling, upward rising wind, downward moving wind, stagnating wind, stomach cramps, a rising from the stomach, rattling in the body, griping in the body, a feeling as if everything was turning about in the body, a fluttering sensation in the lower body, a body full of wind and water, burning the stomach, constipation, burning pain in the side, pain around the area of the liver, pleurisy, spleen fear, pain in the soft part of the belly like a cold stone, fits of the evil thing, stone colic, raging pain in the hip, urge to urinate, knots on the buttocks, lameness in the back, sensitive pains in the back, loins, and hips, stoppage of urine, pressing of feces. Feet and knees that are stiff and lame, sensitive pain in the shin, heat in the feet, swollen legs, swollen varicose veins, pains in the foot as though the blood itself was trying to force its way out, cold feet, a bad foot.[8]

It is an exhausting list, and that is the point. These women experienced practically no discrete 'diseases' of the kind identifiable by the diagnostic tests that modern medicine runs. Rather they noted highly personal changes they could feel and which, being strange and painful, incommoded and frightened them. They suffered 'dis-ease' but not 'diseases'.

In time, such a labile view of the body came to be regarded by the medical profession as suspect, partly because better scientific knowledge of anatomical structure and specialized physiological function tended to localize pain and disease. In due course, pains that flitted randomly around the body were described as 'hysterical'.

During the nineteenth century the 'hands-on' approach became the model for the caring physician, and the 'physical examination' was the centrepiece of his art. His close attention to children – at a time when the young were especially vulnerable to infectious diseases – marked him out as a trusted family friend, not just a skilful professional. Those were the days when extensive house visits were still *de rigueur* for the general practitioner, as depicted in this painting by Norman Rockwell, early 1900s.

The situation was to change, and the development of physical examination was an important factor and marker. Emerging during the nineteenth century, it revolved round a sequence of highly stylized acts performed by the doctor – feeling the pulse, sounding the chest, taking blood pressure, inspecting the throat, taking the temperature, and so forth. The patient would commonly be made to lie on a couch and loosen or remove clothing. Many procedures involved touching body zones not normally exposed or handled. From the stethoscope through the X-ray to the biopsy and the CAT- or PET-scanner, mechanical means have successively permitted scientific medicine to peer right through the body, and see disease independently of the individual who happens to be its carrier.

Through such means, physical and symbolic, the medical profession has radically transformed its viewpoint. With its costly technology, its research and laboratory programmes, modern medicine promotes its claim to be scientific, and hence to be as attentive to the objective laws of disease as, say, physics is to particles. This minute concern with cells and pathogens, has, of course, risked the wrath of uncomprehending critics, asking: *cui bono*? Two centuries ago, Samuel Coleridge damned doctors for such debasing and blinkered somatism: 'They are *shallow* animals', judged the poet, 'having always employed their minds about Body and Gut, they imagine that in the whole system of things there is nothing but Gut and Body.'[9] Yet clutching the coat-tails of science has also lent medicine immense authority and prestige – as well as greatly advancing medical knowledge and its capacity to vanquish disease. Many now have cause to be grateful that medicine knows so much about the gut.

SCIENCE AND STIGMA

This tale of the rise of medical science is, however, only one side of the story. For one thing, the science of disease long remained and still remains in key respects less an accomplished reality than a programme. There has always been rivalry over concepts of scientificity and contention concerning models of causation. As is explored in Chapter 5, experimentalists, epidemiologists, public-health experts, and clinicians have been at loggerheads regarding the classification and causation of individual diseases and of whole divisions of disorders.

In the eighteenth century, controversy raged over the value of disease classification, or nosology: were there truly different species and varieties of disease that could be classified taxonomically? Or, as the radical Scottish doctor, John Brown and his followers (called Brunonians) claimed, was there but one disease that struck at different levels of intensity in different ways? Disputes about the part played by 'nature' and 'nurture' and 'seed' and 'seed-bed' were to the fore in the late nineteenth and early twentieth centuries – controversies given greater edge by the founding of movements aiming to curtail the fertility of alleged hereditary 'degenerates'.

Tuberculosis was the scourge of early industrial society. Was it a hereditary malady? Was it a self-inflicted condition that the indigent brought on themselves by their squalid habits? Or was it the consequence of the wretched urban environment in which the labouring poor were forced to live? Competing theories were fiercely debated through the Victorian era in Europe and North America. All were wrong: tuberculosis proved to be caused by a bacillus, discovered in 1882 by Robert Koch.

Thus the pretensions of medical science to penetrate the causes of disease – and hence to direct preventive and remedial action – have often run ahead of copper-bottomed knowledge. And it would be simple-minded to believe that discovery of the presence of harmful bacteria finally settled all issues. For tricky questions remained as to why the tubercle bacillus precipitated the disease in some people, yet not in others. Medicine still seemed different from physics, for evidently bacteria did not cause disease in precisely the way that lightning caused thunder. The same debate now rages about the human immunodeficiency virus, HIV. From 1984, the official line has been that HIV was the 'cause' of AIDS, but some medical researchers now believe that this is far too simple a model for understanding AIDS, and think that 'co-factors' are equally important. Some – a minority – even claim that the presence of HIV is no certain indication that a person will develop AIDS.

The cause of epidemics led to the keenest debate from the Renaissance into the bacteriological era. Why did certain fevers ravage communities? And why did some individuals succumb to infections while others escaped? Stressing internal balance, Greek humoralism was effective at explaining why an individual fell sick, but theories seeing sickness as principally constitutional only went so far. They hardly explained Black Death or smallpox – or the seemingly 'new' diseases on the march, such as syphilis which appeared at the close of the fifteenth century (see page 35). Some said it was brought back from the New World; others that it spread from Italy or from France (the 'French disease'). Whichever, rotting genitals bore tell-tale marks of a disease communicated by direct and intimate contact, and speculations abounded. In the sixteenth century, an Italian physician, Girolamo Fracastoro, advanced the first influential 'contagionist' theory of disease: syphilis, he contended in *Syphilis, Sive Morbus Gallicus* (1530), was spread by 'seeds' sown by human contact.

Thus sexually transmitted diseases and 'contagionism' arose at the same time and became melded in the mind. Certain consequences followed. If disease was contagious, could not its spread could be halted by taking sufferers and suspects out of circulation? Renaissance Italy accordingly developed quarantine systems; not least, the hospitalization of those new moral lepers, syphilitic prostitutes.

The notion of contagion became familiar, fearsome, but contentious in the early modern world, because of its weighty moral as well as medical overtones. For it was already powerfully associated with infection by the Devil and with magic's invisible arrows. Everyone knew that diabolical *maleficium* was transferred from person to person: what else was 'possession'? Witchcraft could similarly involve the power of charms or the evil eye. In other words, the notion of a

Venereal disease was widely viewed as just deserts for sexual transgression. From the beginning of the sixteenth century, the syphilis epidemic, probably brought back by Christopher Columbus from the Americas, rendered venereal infections far more severe and even fatal. The most powerful method of countering syphilis was mercury, taken both externally and internally, often in conjunction with exposure to extreme heat in steam baths or dry furnaces. It was jested that an hour with Venus might require a lifetime of mercury. The dramatic scene here was drawn by John Sintelaer for a treatise on venereal disease published in 1709.

'contagious disease' was, from the start, connected in the popular mind with magic and diabolism.

Residual associations between contagion, astrology, magic, and the occult explain the appeal of a counter-theory of epidemics that rose to prominence in the eighteenth century – the notion of 'miasma'. 'Miasmata' were atmospheric exhalations given off by stagnant ponds, rotting vegetable and animal matter, human waste, and all that was filthy and putrescent. Miasmatism seemed to explain why it was slum districts and the poor who were most severely stricken in times of epidemic. Moreover, with its palpable linking of soil, environment, atmosphere, and sickness, 'miasmatism' seemed scientific, open to empirical investigation.

Faced with the raging epidemics of early industrial cities, vehement struggles ensued between contagionists, miasmatists, and many other '-ists'. Arguments were medical; but they were also implicitly or explicitly political, economic, and moral. Insofar as the contagionist position was linked with calls for quarantine, for example, it roused the wrath of commercial interests fearful of the interruption of trade. Alternatively, insofar as the wretched habitations of the poor were thought to breed disease-bearing miasmata, miasmatism could become a fatalistic doctrine (the destitute created unhealthy environments) or a call for change (slum clearance and public-health measures would reduce sickness).

If bacteriology finally settled those debates, questions of the origin and nature of disease still arise. Even today, major, widespread, and often lethal diseases still elude full scientific elucidation. Most cancers fall within this category. The involvement of hereditary factors, environmental elements, and viruses in carcinoma remains deeply contested amongst cancer specialists. We await full elucidation of many degenerative diseases, from arthritis to senile dementia, and, as Chapter 8 explores, mental disorder continues to divide professional doctors, neurologists, psychiatrists, and psychoanalysts. Medicine may express confidence about the 'medical model'; within that model, however, enormous scope remains for disagreement and controversy. This is nowhere better seen in our own time than with the question of AIDS.

Some religious fundamentalists have contended that AIDS is a divine punishment for sin. Early in the epidemic speculation was rife that it might be the consequence of disastrously injurious lifestyles: drug abuse and rampant sexual promiscuity, notably amongst the male homosexual community ('the gay plague'). Once again, medical hypotheses and moral judgements had seemingly become confused. There was therefore great relief when a viral source (HIV) was identified in 1984. Not God, not lifestyles, but a neutral, scientific microorganism was responsible – one that could fell the supposedly

This AIDS poster, produced by Charles Michael Helmken in 1989, refers back to a Renaissance painting of the martyrdom of St Sebastian by Tanzio da Varallo. The beauty of art helps counter the view of AIDS as a dirty and disgusting disease and holds out sympathy for the sufferer as a 'victim'.

'innocent' (such as recipients of blood transfusions) no less than the 'guilty' (promiscuous gays).

Once AIDS was recast as a communicable disease, however, a Pandora's Box was opened, loosing all those destructive fears that fester when diseases are regarded as being caused by unseen agents spread by 'other people'. In particular, punitive, guilt-ridden fantasies have been rampant, associating AIDS with a sexual malaise in our midst (a 'social cancer') that needs to be controlled, policed, segregated, and eradicated.

Notions of contagion evoke spectres of pollution and defilement. In a study of the representation of disease, the American historian Sander Gilman has drawn attention to pervasive tendencies to construct schemes of Self and Other, Us and Them, in which self-definition is strengthened through stereotyping and scapegoating of those who are 'different' and (therefore) dangerous. It is easy to cast the sick as Other and label the Other as sick. This has happened throughout history, especially with disease conditions involving peculiar appearances, for visible abnormalities are held to bespeak moral defects – the marks of Cain, Ham, or the Devil. Regarded as singled out by God, lepers, for example, were forced to the fringes of medieval society, beyond contaminating contact, made to wander, ringing bells: they were 'unclean' or even socially 'dead'.

On leprosy's decline, the stigmata of uncleanness became transferred to syphilitics – moral lepers who wore their pocky skin like a convict's uniform, advertising their carnal sins. Lunatics, too, were similarly stigmatized. In art, medical texts and the popular imagination, maniacs were standardly shown as savage, bemired, unkempt, locks dishevelled and straw-matted, near naked or raggledy-taggledy: William Blake depicted King Nebuchadnezzar, demented by God, reduced to shaggy brutishness, lower than the animals. By setting the sick apart – in our mental pictures, but also behind institutional walls – we uphold the fantasy that we are whole. Purity is maintained by driving away pollution. In other words, 'scientific' disease theories can frequently reinforce, yet hide, collective moral prejudice and personal stigma.

When cholera swept Europe and the Americas from the 1830s, physicians blamed the outbreaks on the low morals and drunkenness of the poor. Writing in the late eighteenth century, a leading American physician, Benjamin Rush, suggested that blackness (negritude) was a disease, akin to leprosy. Victorian doctors proposed that women with robust sexual appetites were suffering from 'nymphomania' and sometimes recommended surgical cures – removal of the ovaries, womb, very occasionally, the clitoris. Published case histories reveal all too clearly the sexual atrocities committed on female patients in the name of medicine. For a nineteenth-century German physician, Gustav Broun, physical 'anomalies' in the female genitalia were caused by an overactive sexual sensibility: 'Under the influence of a salacious imagination, which is stimulated by obscene conversations or by reading poorly selected novels, the uterus develops a hyperexitability which leads to masturbation and its dire consequences', he wrote. With one 25-year-old patient, Broun's concern was to prevent her from touching her outer genitalia, as had been her custom:

> on November 11, 1864, a good part of the labia minora and the foreskin of the clitoris were cauterized with a cauterizing instrument. To limit the copious discharge from the uterus, the uterine cavity was cauterized with Chiari's caustic solution. At the same time, the patient was given Lupulin, in dosages of three grains to combat her sexual excitement, and lactic iron.

When that and other treatments brought no benefit, 'the amputation of the clitoris and the major portions of the labia minora was proposed to the patient as the only possible cure'.[10]

Ever since the Greeks, medical writers have implied that the female gender is, in itself, an abnormality (Aristotle called women 'monsters'), and that, on account of their gynaecological disorders, women were inherently pathological. In short, physicians' accounts of the causes of diseases have, in reality, doubled as sagas of condemnation.

The aim here is not to ridicule or castigate doctors: blaming doctors for victim-blaming would be singularly futile. Rather, two points deserve consideration. First, we must remain sceptical about claims that medicine has ever been, or has finally become, 'value-free' in its accounts of diseases and their causation. For one thing, medicine has largely embraced the model of the physical sciences, a materialist reductionism – which is by no means self-evidently right for comprehending the true character of all kinds of human sickness. For another, as the graveyard of discarded 'diseases' shows, medicine has often stuffed into disease envelopes strange collections of clinical symptoms, social phenomena, and prejudices. Second, we must see that this apparent 'frailty' of medicine arises from the fact that sickness is not simply the work of pathogens; it is a function of social relations. For this reason, physic necessarily goes beyond the bounds of the paradigms of physics.

STORIES OF DISEASE

It is easy to come across evidence of the medical profession weaving moral fantasies around the sick and around diseases: if you masturbate you will go blind or mad (medicine has often been guilty of creating this kind of pseudoscientific folklore). It has enabled doctors to sound off their prejudices, and also to camouflage their ignorance behind plausible fabrications and just-so stories.

The need to cope with ignorance is all the greater with the sick themselves, especially those suffering from mysterious, incurable, and fatal conditions. It may appear doubly dreadful (reflected the American writer Susan Sontag in her book *Illness as Metaphor*) to succumb to a virus if it seems a bolt from the blue, without rhyme or reason, for life is thus reduced to an irrational chapter of accidents. And so the dire explanatory void ('Why me? What have I done to deserve it?') is filled by fabricating stories of the meanings of disease. The diseased organ may be deemed 'bad', or one's personality may be accused of precipitating the malady. Thus, Susan Sontag argued, it has commonly been said that such-and-such person got cancer due to a 'cancer personality', a supposed proclivity to bottle-up feelings and drive anger inside, the thwarted passions finally taking self-destructive vengeance on the flesh. It is no accident that the most feared disease of our century, the 'Big C' (significantly, the disease cannot speak its name) has been associated with 'dirty' parts – the colon, rectum, womb, scrotum, and breast – or that, in the popular imagination, AIDS has acquired an identity as a disease associated with anal intercourse. Another instance is offered by tuberculosis.

Nineteenth-century physicians regarded tuberculosis primarily as a female disease. Simply being a woman was itself 'a condition favourable to the development of tuberculization', said one doctor. The tubercular state was the female ideal taken to the limit. Romantic fashions expected ladies to be slim – their delicacy expressed a child-like air. Satirists insinuated that young belles or their mothers even courted tuberculosis by swanning around in flimsy attire or deliberately undereating, so as to grow slender enough to snare a husband. Around 1800, the English physician Thomas Beddoes bantered that tuberculosis had become *à la mode* amongst the fair sex. 'Writers of romance', he grumbled, 'exhibit the slow decline of the consumptive, as a state … in which not much more misery is felt, than is expressed by a blossom, nipped by untimely frosts.' The preposterous idea had thus got about, he protested, that 'consumption must be a flattering complaint', radiating mystery and allure.[11]

Yet chic tubercular cadaverousness was not wholly confined to women of a Pre-Raphaelite look. Because leanness betokened high-minded refinement, the triumph of mind over matter, male poets and poseurs equally liked to display an aetherial presence. 'When I was young', recalled the French writer Théophile Gautier in the mid-nineteenth century, 'I could not have accepted as a lyrical poet anyone weighing more than ninety-nine pounds.'[12] Ideally, flesh simply melted into the imagination.

The consumptive look signalled the becoming petiteness of the feminine, but, paradoxically, it also conveyed a thrilling eroticism. Consumptive beauties like Mimi in Puccini's *La Bohème* and Marguerite Gauthier in Verdi's *La Traviata* were fragile, yet they were also feverish with passion. It was part of the mythology, confirmed by doctors, that tuberculosis was an aphrodisiac. The tubercular woman was bewitching in appearance, with her prominent eyes, pallid skin, and the hectic flush of the hollow cheeks. And the disease supposedly triggered inner erotic cravings too. For public-health experts, tuberculosis was, alongside syphilis, the principal disease of the prostitutes thronging Paris – the result of 'venereal excesses', according to René Laënnec, the leading hospital physician in Paris in the early nineteenth century.

The transience of consumptive beauty

Tuberculosis was the staple fare of Romantic tragedy: consumptive heroes and heroines spat blood and wasted away in scores of melodramas and sentimental novels — for instance, Henri Murger's *Scènes de la Vie de Bohème* (1851), which provided the inspiration for Puccini's *La Bohème*. Murger's heroine Francine (Puccini's Mimi) is a typecast fictional consumptive; young, full of beauty and *joie de vivre*, yet touched with melancholy passion. Slight and delicate, she is 'as pale as the angel of consumption'; yet, wrote Murger, 'the blood of youth runs hot and fast in her veins', and she had a 'rosy tint to her skin, transparent with the whiteness of a camelia'.

The transience of consumptive beauty was brought out even more in Murger's heroine. Francine almost became her illness: sickness served as a metaphor for the 'sad passions' of the waif, poor in everything but the grace of youth. On her deathbed, knowing she will soon pass away 'because God does not want me to live any longer', Francine asks Jacques to buy her a fur muff to keep her hands warm for the better times ahead. The last remaining leaf from the tree outside is blown through her window and onto her bed; the two sweethearts spend their last night together, and at dawn she breathes her last, clutching her muff for warmth. The radiance on the consumptive's face gave her 'a saintly glow, as if she had died of beauty'.

In Mimi, Puccini reproduced Francine's divinely beautiful death. Puccini's Mimi also suggests Marguerite Gauthier, the heroine of *La Traviata*, adapted by Verdi from Alexandre Dumas' *La Dame aux Camélias* (1848). Dumas *fils* perfectly captured the Romantic associations of consumption with femininity. The disease's wasting effect was portrayed as enhancing female beauty; in sickness, Marguerite, the fallen woman, paradoxically became purer than her prim and proper judges. Disease represented the impossibility of innocent love in a wretched world. Dumas' consumptive courtesan thus became a motif for Woman herself — seductively simple, desirable yet doomed.

These associations of tuberculosis were not purely the figments of Murger and Dumas, Puccini and Verdi. They reflected the convictions of the age, as expressed by physicians no less than poets and artists.

The disease that dominated the nineteenth-century artistic, literary, and moral imagination was tuberculosis, the 'white plague' that was for long the greatest killer of young adults. In this painting, *Too Late*, by William Lindsay Windus (1858), a lover returns, only to find the woman of his dreams dying of consumption (as the disease was then called), pale and white, supporting herself with a stick. The battle between love and consumption also formed the theme of Puccini's *La Bohème* and Verdi's *La Traviata*.

A victim of gout caricatured by George Cruickshank (1818). Gout was a disease that carried a complex set of moral messages. It was regarded as the reward of overindulgence. Yet it was also a disease that struck High Society – or ran in their blood as a hereditary disorder. Hence it was, in some ways, a highly eligible disease, being a mark of good breeding and superiority. Unlike certain maladies, such as tuberculosis, the gouty sufferer was always depicted as being male.

It was thus poetic justice that tuberculosis was lethal, yet it was an affliction that destroyed in a distinctive way. There was something serenely rapturous about the consumptive's deathbed. The body, it was said, almost vanished away, the flesh dissolved, leaving just the parting smile, freeing the spirit. The sufferer died, but his or her agony was the relinquishing of mortal flesh that permitted the soul to breathe. So death was not just an end, it was atonement; suffering was morally redeeming.

Such moralizing with sickness (what I have said applies equally to many diseases, not just tuberculosis) has a *prima facie* appeal: it rationalizes menacing maladies and render adversity less mysterious. Compensatory comfort was thus offered by the Romantic myth that bodies wasting away with tuberculosis were actually being refined into pure, angelic 'spirituality'. Better a tale with a barbed moral and a tragic ending than no story at all. Yet such labels may mainly serve to 'blame the victim': disease fantasies are usually punitive.

It is worth glancing at a different condition and a separate set of metaphors: gout, a condition chronic and painful, though rarely fatal. Gout was widely esteemed as a disease, because of the myth that the gout-ridden were thereby protected from worse disorders. Gout was thus a kind of immunization. A gouty foot might even be a sign of health, since the big toe typically affected was far distant from the vital organs. Secure in his 'gouty bootikins' (slippers), the mid-eighteenth century English man of letters Horace Walpole thus recommended sitting it out stoically. 'It prevents other illnesses and prolongs life', he maintained: 'Could I cure the gout, should not I have a fever, a palsy, or an apoplexy?'[13]

Influential here was the old saw that diseases were jealous of each other and mutually exclusive. So long as gout was in possession, no deadlier enemy could gain invade. 'To the Gout my mind is reconciled', Samuel Johnson informed his friend, Mrs Thrale, for he had been assured by his physician 'that the gout will secure me from every thing paralytick.'[14]

Paradoxical as it may seem, gout was thus regarded as a disease that protected – a prophylactic. Charles II's Archbishop of Canterbury, Gilbert Sheldon, reportedly offered '£1,000 to any person who would "help him to the gout", looking upon it as the only remedy for the distemper in his head, which he feared might in time prove an apoplexy; as in time it did and killed him'.[15] In short, being gout-ridden was preferable to being rid of gout. All that needed to be ensured, according to Jonathan Swift, was that it never got deep into the innards:

> As if the gout should seize the head,
> Doctors pronounce the patient dead,
> But if they can, by all their arts;
> Eject it to the extreamest parts,
> They give the sick man joy, and praise
> The gout that will prolong his days.[16]

Gout is thus an exemplary case of how disease is rationalized. In these sufferers' accounts, gout is neither the focus of a Romantic, punitive, or sadomasochistic fiction, in the manner of the 'cancer personality'; nor is it reduced to a laboratory specimen, alien and meaningless. Rather, gout is a malady that is humanized, accepted as the other face of life, and integral to the human condition.

A radical critic of modern medicine, Ivan Illich, argued in *Limits to Medicine* (1977) that the progress of scientific medicine, or at least the success of its propaganda, has been creating Promethean expectations of an almost infinite prolongation of healthy, fit, and fully functioning existence. Cosmetic and spare-part surgery feed these fantasies. Such dreams, Illich argued, are, finally, unrealistic: all must age and die, and longer life may mean greater pains. Hence these utopian myths of perfect, endless health are disabling, because they impair our ability to come to terms with fates that are inevitable. Moreover, they prove heartless, because they provoke the young, healthy, fit, sexy, and beautiful to distance themselves from the aged, decrepit, and dying.

Illich's analysis may suggest, in short, that we have moved – partly thanks to the philosophy of scientific medicine and partly because of genuine health improvements – from the morbid sickness culture of medieval Christianity to one in which disease is denied, becoming either meaningless or featuring only in punitive moral tales. By contrast to the traditional myths of gout, the triumph of scientific medicine, reinforced by the inflation of unrealistic health expectations (above all in the USA), has challenged the legitimacy of traditional stories of sickness and discounted our capacity to cope.

THE SICK ROLE

Modern life thus creates various binds. It produces claims, or illusions, of freedom from sickness and positive health, thanks to the benign intervention of the medical profession. Yet that also fosters preoccupations with sickness. Indeed, the growth of medicine has encouraged what has been called 'medicine-mongering'.

Medicine enjoyed a golden century from around 1850. Before the Victorian era, medicine had but paltry power to cure disease and save the sick, and few entertained great expectations of it. Thereafter, surgery leapt ahead, thanks to anaesthetics and antiseptics; public health improved hygiene; bacteriology explicated aetiology; laboratory medicine flowered; and, at long last, sulphonamides and antibiotics wrought a pharmaceutical revolution. Lethal diseases were overcome, life expectations soared. Medicine and society enjoyed a honeymoon era.

Since around the 1960s, however, the marriage has soured. Cancer and many other major diseases remain embarrassments, even scandals; medicine itself is increasingly held responsible for pain and sickness, through 'iatrogenic' (doctor-created) complaints. Above all, modern critics accuse medicine of embarking upon what Ivan Illich has called the 'medicalization of life'. For various reasons – some would say genuine compassion, others would blame professional 'imperialism' – medicine is allegedly set on course to put all aspects of living into the hands of the doctors. Pregnancy and childbirth are nowadays seen, if not precisely as diseases, at least as conditions requiring professional medical attendance, by law in advanced Western societies. Many geriatricians argue that ageing is a pathological process; and, like birth, dying is becoming routinely hospitalized. During the past couple of centuries, all manner of personal habits, vices, and idiosyncrasies have been redefined by the medical profession as ailments or medicopsychiatric disorders; for instance, heavy drinking has been medicalized as alcoholism.

Such medicalization requires subtle interpretation. In some ways, it might be viewed as emancipatory, as it has been for suicide. Traditionally, the Church regarded self-murder (*felo de se*) as a mortal sin. From the late seventeenth century, doctors, with public approval, began to contend that suicide was typically, almost by definition, committed in an unbalanced state of mind. Thereby the censure of sin and crime was avoided, as also was forfeiture to the state of the suicide's property.

Often, however, medicalization has involved stigmatization, as feminists have noted, protesting against medical accounts of menstruation, menopause, and anorexia nervosa. And it may be particularly perilous as medicine increasingly serves as an arm of the state, through com-

The hypochrondriac became a figure of fun from the seventeenth century when Molière, the French playwright, satirized the complaint in *Le Malade Imaginaire*, a title also given to this nineteenth-century lithograph by Gabriel Aubert. Hypochrondria was originally understood as a physical infirmity of the lower abdomen. But with the new psychologival theories of the eighteenth century, increasingly its characteristic pains were attributed to an overstimulated imagination. Hypochondria was commonly judged a male equivalent of hysteria.

pulsory health insurance, the National Health Service, and the use of medical records to monitor employment, criminality, delinquency, and so forth. Political dissidence has been called 'sick' and subjected to medical and psychiatric correction as a matter of policy in the former Soviet Union and Communist China. In subtler ways, similar pressures exist elsewhere.

In part, medicalization spreads because the public colludes in it: medicine promises benefits. Moreover, in a secular society where the Church no longer explains fate and directs behaviour, the culture of sickness offers a surrogate. Being ill becomes a way of life accorded social sanction and medical encouragement. Two facets are worth examining: the sick role and the psychosomatic complaint – frequently, it is obvious, two sides of the same coin.

The idea of the sick role was formulated in the 1950s by the American sociologist Talcott Parsons, who regarded it as a tacit deal between sufferer and society by which John or Joan Citizen would be allowed occasionally to retire from social demands under the cover of being ill. Temporarily relieved of social responsibilities, he (or she) could stay off work, take to his bed, and luxuriate in tea and sympathy. In return, he must abstain from drink, sex, sport, and other pleasures, and would be honour-bound to recover as quickly as possible, so his 'well role' could be resumed. A legitimate 'time out' was thus offered, a sort of joyless extra holiday or Scottish Sunday, begirt by conventions of reciprocity.

Parsons's account of 'legitimate deviance' affords insight into society's perennially ambiguous attitudes towards the sick. It also expresses a 'victim-blaming' of its own, reducing the social actor who avails himself of the role to a sort of *malade imaginaire* or at least a manipulative game-player.

The existential side of playing sick is psychosomatic illness, whose intriguing history has been traced by Edward Shorter.[17] He focused on what he calls 'somatizers' – that is, people suffering from 'pain and fatigue that have no physical cause'. These are patients frustrating to no-nonsense physicians such as the early-twentieth century Kentucky doctor who thought a 'good spanking, sometimes even a good "cussing"', was the surest way with such evident hypochondriacs'. Most of those suffering in the past two centuries from conditions variously called 'nervous spine', 'neurasthenia', 'fits', and nowadays myalgic encephalomyelitis or ME (also called 'yuppie flu' or chronic fatigue syndrome) and perhaps repetitive strain injury (RSI) have had nothing intrinsically organically wrong with them, argued Shorter, but have been consciously or unconsciously seeking solace, attention, or social excuses. Such somatizers have produced a fascinating succession of phantom diseases, Shorter suggested, the

LE MÉDECIN DE DAMES.

Neurotic and depressive disorders became highly conspicuous amongst the genteel and the affluent in the nineteenth century, especially young ladies with little to occupy them, whose need for attention might be gratified by being sick. From the 1860s nervous complaints were widely termed 'neurasthenia', a condition of collapse marked by symptoms of fatigue, weakness, lowness of spirits, and even paralysis. Widely recommended was the health-farm rest cure in which the patient would be well fed, would receive massage, and other physical stimulus, and would be removed from everyday cares. Other physicians recommended the pursuit of amusements as a way of reviving melancholy spirits. Lithograph by Ch.-E. Jacque.

The Baths of Caldas da Rainha in central Portugal, famous for their warm sulphur springs. Spa resorts became favourite places for invalids and valetudinarians in the eighteenth and nineteenth centuries, combining taking the waters with amusements and a stimulating social round. The most commercialized and fashionable of the early spa resorts was Bath in the west of England; its social life was depicted by novelists from Tobias Smollett to Jane Austen. In the nineteenth century, continental resorts grew in sophistication, notably Carlsbad and Baden Baden, famous not least for their gambling casinos. The waters were touted as curing all known diseases, but probably were genuinely useful for arthritis and other joint complaints.

'unconscious', selecting convenient suits of somatoform manifestations from a wider 'symptom pool'.

Early in the nineteenth century, motor disorders were prominent. Archetypal Victorian ladies collapsed on their beds, literally incapable of standing on their own two feet, from fits, convulsions, spasms, or paralysis. By 1900, such operatic displays softened into a symptomatological chamber music, and motor defects were superseded by more discreet sensory complaints: neuralgia, headache, and fatigue. Each made sense in context. In the claustrophobic milieu of the Victorian family, only a melodramatic acting out of abnormalities could command attention. Amidst the twentieth-century 'lonely crowd', by contrast, the introspective ego finds expression in private pain.

Somatizers act ill, and a melancholy collusion has entangled 'somatizers' and doctors – above all, those physicians grasping or cynical enough to spy rich pickings in pandering to insatiable, well-heeled valetudinarians. And in the succession of medical alibis tacitly negotiated between profession and patient in the Victorian era and subsequently, the constant was a gentleman's agreement that the complaint was truly physical. Sufferers were relieved to hear that their ailments were organic, requiring medical or surgical treatment. For the entrenched 'medical model' presupposed that a somatic malady was real; all others might be fictional and fraudulent. With an organic complaint, patients lost no face: there was no hint that they were shamming, and no risk that they be thought crackers. Medical men maintained the charade by cooking up innovations in minor surgery, spa regimes, coloured waters, and health-retreat regimes, relying on the desperate gullibility of patients prepared to believe that each and every organ could spawn dozens of defects.

The presence – indeed, growing incidence – of psychosomatic disorders, and hence of people enacting the sick role and reaping its secondary gains, speaks volumes about the profound ambiguities of disease concepts and sickness strategies. In our secular, atomized environment, illness is one of the relatively few ways of expressing social complaints and the ambiguities of self. Yet it is riven with ambiguity: publicly distrusted, freighted with stigma, and often mocked by the very professionals who massage it.

ALTERNATIVE MEDICINE

One apparent escape from such impasses lies in positing radically different ideas of disease, sickness, and healing. Over the centuries, alternative medicine and holistic theories have tended to reject materialist, ordinary (allopathic), or mechanical theories of disease, and to espouse the belief that health and sickness involve the whole person – often the whole cosmos. Sickness is a malady not of the body but of the complete self; within that self the cure lies, through acts of will or lifestyle changes. Such ideas were extensively developed in nineteenth-century North America, through such movements as Christian Science. Health reform was championed not by regular physicians but by lay people, disaffected equally with official churches and with regular medicine, and seeking to replace both with a unified, holistic philosophy of spiritual and bodily health, carved out of personal experience.

Among the medical botanists (called Thomsonians after Samuel Thomson, an early Victorian health reformer in New Hampshire) and similar sects, certain convictions were widely shared. They promoted a medical version of original sin, arguing that civilized man had 'fallen', bringing disease on himself by greed, speed, excessive meat-eating, and alcohol abuse. By way of remedy, they advocated a return to 'natural' living – vegetarianism, sexual restraint, temperance, abandonment of such stimulants as tea and tobacco, and an end to artificial drugs,

The founding of homeopathy

The founder of homeopathy, Christian Friedrich Samuel Hahnemann, was born in Meissen, Germany, in 1755. He studied medicine at Leipzig and then practised for 10 years in Leipzig and Vienna. After experimenting on the curative power of cinchona bark (the source of quinine) for 6 years, he concluded that drugs produce a very similar condition in healthy persons to that which they relieve in the sick. This was the origin of his famous principle, *similia similibus curantur* ('like cures like'), which he contrasted with the belief of ordinary, or allopathic, medical practitioners.

Hahnemann's own infinitesimal doses of medicine pro-voked the apothecaries, who refused to dispense them; accordingly, he illegally gave his medicines to his patients, free of charge, and was prosecuted in every town in which he tried to settle from 1798 until 1810. He spent much time undertaking the 'proving' of drugs that then entered the homeopathic pharmacopoeia. Many of these were herbal in origin, and subsequent homeopaths have continued to emphasize natural remedies. By the time of his death, his system had been taken up by practitioners throughout Europe and North America, although their relations with ordinary doctors were often bitter.

This homeopathic pharmacy in Philadelphia around 1890 illustrates the great range of herbal cures widely in use before the antibiotic revolution of the 1940s. If they possessed relatively little power to cure, they certainly made an impressive show. Along with many other fringe and unorthodox medical movements, homeopathy took a particular hold in the USA, because there was little medical regulation and the democratic ethos favoured patient choice. The pharmacist in the photograph is C. A. Otto Vischer.

trusting to herbal remedies. Homeopaths for their part insisted on ultra-pure medicaments, taken in minute quantities.

Influenced by the teachings of the mystic Emmanuel Swedenborg, some groups went further, discarding medicines altogether, and trusting to the healing powers of Nature, aided by water, prayer, self-control, and spiritual illumination. With its 'a plague on both your houses' attitude, the Christian Science movement exemplifies all these features. Its founder, Mary Baker Eddy, spent much of her New Hampshire youth in the 1830s sick with obscure nervous disorders. She rejected her parents' strict Congregationalism. Regular physicians did her no good. Relieved by homeopathy and mesmerism, she then undertook self-healing, and her success led her to adumbrate her own system, in which 'there is but one creation, and it is wholly spiritual'. Matter therefore was an illusion; hence, there could be no such thing as somatic disease, the marrow of medical science. As explained in her best-selling *Science and Health* (1875), sickness and pain were illusions that true 'mind healing' would dispel.

In England, the Moses of alternative medicine at the dawn of the Victorian era was James Morison. A businessman first in Aberdeen and later in London, who had suffered gastric disorders and consulted numerous ordinary doctors, he despised regulars with evangelical fervour. Doctors, he contended, were not merely ignorant and mercenary, but also dangerous. Their polypharmacy and heavy dosing habits were little less than criminal. Morison proposed new institutes for medicine, encapsulated in Ten Commandments:

- The vital principle is contained in the blood.
- Blood makes blood.
- Everything in the body is derived from the blood.
- All constitutions are radically the same.
- All diseases arise from the impurity of the blood or, in other words, from acrimonious humours lodged in the body.
- This humour, which degenerates the blood, has three sources – the maternine, the contagious and the personal.
- Pain and disease have the same origin; and may therefore be considered synonymous terms.
- Purgation by vegetables is the only effectual mode of eradicating disease.
- The stomach and bowels cannot be purged too much.
- From the intimate connexion subsisting between the mind and the body, the health of the one must conduce to the serenity of the other.[18]

There was a single cause for all disease – bad blood – and a single therapeutics: heavy and frequent purgation, using vegetable laxatives. In 1825, Morison marketed the perfect purge, his 'Vegetable Universal Pills', that would cure all diseases.

The early Victorian age saw myriad medical movements, such as homeopathy, naturopathy, medical botany, and spiritualism. Phrenology – the belief that char-

The American Mary Baker Eddy (1821–1910), founder of the Christian Science movement. She suffered a multitude of ailments as a child and young woman before, at the age of forty, being cured of hysterical paralysis through faith healing.

WONDERFUL EFFECT OF MORRISONS VEGETABLE PILLS
*They told me if I took 1000 pills at night I should be quite
another thing in the morning*

Many nineteenth-century alternative medicines combined a popular, anti-orthodox message with the colourful appeal of the skilful advertiser. In Britain, the early master of this was James Morison; he was later outstripped by Thomas Holloway. 'Vegetable' cures had a great appeal to the highly earnest, anxious, and desperately busy Victorian middle classes (as with today's 'herbal' remedies). They seemed gentler and more natural than the 'artificial and 'chemical' remedies often prescribed by regular physicians – above all, their fiercely purgative antimonial and arsenical pills. Alternative medicine could thereby claim for itself that exaltation of the natural made popular by the Romantic poets.

acter is determined by the relative size of the different parts of the brain and hence can be known by feeling the bumps of the head – and mesmerism (and their hybrid form, phreno-mesmerism) were others. All made a break with regular medicine. Each argued in its own language that the whole system of allopathic medicine was radically wrong. Characteristically, they accused the orthodox of striving to blitz disease with poisonous drugs. Each offered a new plan of life based on Nature's way, and claimed to use more natural modes of healing – using herbs alone or pure water. Each professed to invest the individual with new control over his health as part of a culture of self-improvement and realization. Medical heretics typically doubled as heretics in politics and faith as well, while cultivating unorthodox lifestyles.

Holism is back in fashion. Promising not the 'pill for every ill' approach but rather positive health, alternative healing holds out glowing prospects: life-enhancing organic gentle remedies fresh from Mother Nature's bosom – therapies free of hi-tech impersonality. But, as is evident, in attacking the scientific simplicities of regular medicine, alternative medicine creates a simplistic, black-and-white philosophy of its own. *They* are threatening your well-being with chemicals and pesticides, processed food, and pollution. *You* can safeguard it by following Nature – eating natural fare and, in so doing, discovering your natural energies and vital forces.

What is this but junk rhetoric? Moreover, alternative cults often carry unsavoury, victim-blaming hidden agendas. Sickness proves you are not in touch with yourself. So the fault lies within. Luckily, you can put youself right by working on yourself. But this turns out to be another variant on sturdy Protestant self-help, masquerading as a radical alternative: working-out is the old Protestant work ethic in a new guise.

WHAT IS DISEASE?

It might be thought that we live in an age in which the questions of illness and disease should be sewn up as never before. Medicine has enjoyed exceptional success: of special symbolic significance was the final global eradication of smallpox in 1979. Life expectations continue to rise. The realities are, however, more murky. Many diseases continue to thwart scientific medicine. Public dissatisfaction grows; dreams fade, promises are broken, people vote with their feet and try alternative medicines and psychotherapies. New conditions appear, such as ME, which do not merely resist ready cure but which challenge the categories of established medicine. Faced with 'yuppie flu', chronic fatigue, strange allergies, and today's sickness salad-bar, the medical profession has made hostile and dismissive noises: all was psychosomatic, whingeing. Then the doctors jumped on the band-waggon, medicalized ME as a real condition, and railroaded it. Yet they proved no nearer to resolving its nature or satisfying its sufferers.

Such developments offer windows onto history. The past presents a changing disease panorama, in several senses. For one thing, diseases, like empires, rise and fall: plague has declined – although occasional localized outbursts remain severe – but cancer has worsened. For another, there have been shifts in perceptions of diseases. One does not need to embrace a modish sociological scepticism to recognize that diseases, like beauty, are somewhat in the eye of the beholder: people see what they want or are programmed to see. Particular anxieties, academic training, new technologies, and so forth cause conditions to come into focus and create pressures to create labels. People doubtless died of heart complaints in earlier centuries, but it took the outlooks and diagnostic apparatus of modern medicine to create the modern categories of the heart attack and coronary thrombosis, or to perceive how the condition long seen as 'dropsy' (oedema) was actually due to heart disease; weaknesses depicted in earlier medicine became crystallized into diabetes. Diseases become 'framed' at particular times and for particular reasons.[19]

'Disease', and its complex interplay with sickness, has its history, too. Different circumstances lead to different facets of life – pains, fevers, bad habits, impairments – being called disease. The fit between what someone experiences as sickness and what doctors deem disease may be close or it may be loose. Wider issues are often at stake: quests for research funds, insurance company regulations, medical exoneration before the law or at the workplace, social excuses. This volume examines the rise of medicine. But it must be remembered that medicine has always been embedded both in human cultural milieux and in the diverse needs of intelligent warm-blooded bodies.

CHAPTER 4

Edward Shorter

Primary Care

The first doctor that one sees when one is ill offers 'primary care'. The doctor might be in a hospital emergency room or in a local clinic, but, historically, general practitioners have been the first point of call. This is a story of how patients and general practitioners have collided and colluded over the past two centuries. The story could, of course, be extended much further back in time than the late eighteenth century. Yet that is when the practice of medicine, which had been fairly constant in its humoral theories and drastic treatments over the centuries, began to change. Although medical theories had been in flux over the seventeen centuries from Galen of Pergamon to Herman Boerhaave of Leiden, the actual practice of medicine, or primary care, had changed little. With the infusion of science into medicine late in the eighteenth century, however, the story begins to change. Many of the subsequent travails of primary care may be understood as the confused efforts of doctors and patients to come to grips with the ever-changing realities of medicine imposed on them by science, on the one hand, and by subjective views of 'medical correctness' on the other.

WHAT THE TRADITIONAL PATIENT WANTED

In the past (and even today in countries lacking a National Health Service), doctors competed against one another for the custom of patients, for they practised

In the nineteenth century, the general practitioner emerged as a family friend no less than a medical professional. The sick set great store by familiarity and trust. By modern standards the family doctor still had little science at his disposal. Most of his diagnostic methods were old tried and tested ones, such as taking the pulse. Modesty inhibited extensive physical examination, especially with female patients. *The Doctor*, by Arthur Miles, *c.* 1860.

medicine to make a profit. To attract patients, they often felt obliged to offer whatever it was the patients wanted. As George Bernard Shaw wrote in his preface to *The Doctor's Dilemma* (1911),

> The doctor who has to live by pleasing his patients in competition with everybody who has walked the hospitals, scraped through the examinations, and bought a brass plate, soon finds himself prescribing water to teetotallers and brandy or champagne jelly to drunkards; beefsteaks and stout in one house, and 'uric acid free' vegetarian diet over the way; shut windows, big fires, and heavy overcoats to old Colonels, and open air and as much nakedness as is compatible with decency to young faddists, never once daring to say either 'I don't know', or 'I don't agree'.[1]

This desire to placate patients' ideas of what constitutes good medicine is one of the basic motors of change in primary care.

'Traditional' means the prescientific phase of medical practice, before doctors became 'men of science' and before patients acquired respect for that science. Traditional patients often had (to us) bizarre notions of what was wrong with them and how it might be fixed. One popular idea in the eighteenth century stressed ridding the body of the poisons that cause disease by drawing them out through the skin. This entailed sweating cures, and patients cherished the idea – as did physicians to a lesser extent – of sweating a patient with a fever. Edinburgh physician William Buchan wrote in his best-selling medical guide *Domestic Medicine* in 1769, 'It is a common notion that sweating is always necessary in the beginning of a fever … The common practice is to heap clothes upon the patient, and to give him things of a hot nature, as spirits, spiceries, &c. which fire his blood, increase the spasms, and render the disease more dangerous.'[2]

How else might one get those poisons, or bad humours, out of there? Bleeding was much beloved by the common people, extending past the time when it lost popularity with physicians. There were many other popular strategies for eliminating toxins. One was vomiting, relinquished relatively early by academic medicine but cherished until the twentieth century by patients.

Taking emetics was intended to produce therapeutic puking, ridding the stomach of toxicity that was supposedly making the whole body sick. The German physician Adolf Kussmaul himself took emetics therapeutically until around the age of forty in 1864. He recalled many patients whose faith in their efficacy was deeply held. One day a peasant in the practice of Kussmaul's father sent word that he was ailing, weak, losing weight, and unable to arise from bed. The father, busy

Debate ranged in pre-modern medicine as to the curative properties of sweating as a cure. Free perspiration was claimed by some to be necessary for removing poisons from the body (especially syphilitic contagions). Homeopathic principles in any case regarded fever sweats as therapeutic rather than harmful. Followers of Thomas Sydenham, by contrast, were advocates of 'cool' methods with fevers – plenty of ventilation and cold drinks. By 1800, the sweating cure was becoming an object of satire. Caricature by Johann Wenzel Zinke after J. Cajetan, 1848.

at that moment, sent on by messenger some remedy containing a sweet syrup that could at least do no harm.

Arriving at the peasant's cottage, the doctor found the man restored, at that very moment delecting a roasted dove and drinking a glass of wine. 'Herr Doktor, you prescribed that very well. It was really tough medicine but it cleaned me out and drove out the illness. But I don't think I could get the ants down a second time.' The ants? Apparently, the messenger had fallen asleep *en route*, and as he snoozed under a tree the cork had popped out of the bottle, giving a local ant colony a chance to check out the syrupy prescription by climbing into the bottle. The peasant, so implicitly convinced of the restorative powers of emetic therapy, had vomited heartily after downing the ants – and was well again.[3]

The point is that sweating, bleeding, and vomiting, in addition to salivating, urinating, purging, and many other ways of getting the bad humours out, had a hold on the popular mind that reached back for centuries, existing alongside medical doctrines of belief in such procedures. Thus the patients arrived in primary care with their own definite views of what was needed.

WHAT TRADITIONAL PHYSICIANS OFFERED

Before the threshold of the twentieth century, physicians in primary care were surrounded by fever. Fever, a symptom of the body's response to invasion by bacteria and viruses, occupies a minor role in Western medicine today, mainly in the form of initial childhood encounters with common microorganisms and of colds and coughs (upper respiratory infections). Being a doctor before 1900 meant spending the bulk of one's time on fever. Fever was the axis about which the traditional consultation turned – the hot bedridden patient, his pulse quickened and respiring rapidly, the doctor making a house call.

The diary of Richard Kay, a doctor who lived near Bury in Lancashire in the mid-eighteenth century, shows how immersed in fever was the typical practitioner.

> *July 10.* Kay visited Mrs. Chippingdale at Ewood, 'she being very bad', ill apparently with typhus, a tick-born bacterial infection characterized by malaise, severe headache, and sustained high fever.
>
> *July 11.* 'In the evening as I returned home I visited Miss Betty Rothwell at Ramsbottom who is dangerously bad of a miliary fever [one causing skin eruptions, again, probably typhus].'
>
> *July 13.* Mrs. Chippingdale was now dying.
>
> *July 14.* Miss Rothwell was now dead. 'I visited a young man in Rossendale who is dangerously bad of a fever.' Another patient, John Mills, was also ill with fever.
>
> *July 15.* He visited John Mills again.
>
> *July 16.* 'This last night about midnight a messenger came with a letter ... I was

to come to Manchester to visit Mr William Blythe.' 'I found Mr Blythe very dangerously bad of a miliary fever.' Dr Kay also received word that Mrs. Chippingdale and John Mills were dead.

July 17. William Blythe had now died of the fever.[4]

By the time another year would pass, the author's father, his sister Rachel, and his sister Elizabeth were also dead of fever. Dr Kay himself died of fever in October 1751.

Infection means pus. Late in the nineteenth century Arthur Hertzler, a small-town doctor on the Kansas frontier, was called to a case of empyema, or pus in the lungs. 'To answer the call eight miles from town I battled mud for three hours. As I entered the sickroom I saw a boy fourteen years of age half sitting up in bed in deep cyanosis [caused by lack of oxygen], with grayish-blue skin and heaving chest, his mouth open and his eyes bulging. It seemed that each gasp would be his last.'

Dr Hertzler threw down his medical bag and sat flat on the floor with his legs under the bed.

> Grabbing a scalpel I made an incision in his chest wall with one stab – he was too near death to require an anesthetic. As the knife penetrated his chest, a stream of pus the size of a finger spurted out, striking me under the chin and drenching me. After placing a drain in the opening, I wrapped a blanket about my pus-soaked body and spent another three hours reaching home.[5]

The nineteenth-century physician was regarded and often idealized as a wise, grave man who was a friend, even to the poor. He was a man to whom his patients would be duly deferential. Lithograph by F. van Loo after Édouard de Jans.

Bloodletting – getting rid of poisons

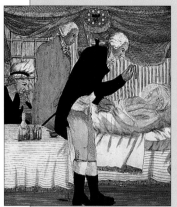

Bloodletting took the form of using a knife to open a vein, when it was called venesection or phlebotomy, or applying leeches to the skin above a supposed lesion, and letting the leech engorge itself with the bad blood thought to dwell below. Isabella Beeton in her *Book of Household Management* (1861) gave instructions for doing one's own bleeding 'in cases of great emergency'. 'Place a handkerchief or piece of tape rather but not too tightly round the arm, about three or four inches above the elbow'. Once the veins had swollen, one should 'take the lancet in his right hand, between the thumb and first finger ... then gently thrust the tip of the lancet into the vein'. Further directions followed on bandaging the wound and also on what to do if the patient fainted, for often the patient was supposed to be bled 'until syncope', or fainting.[6]

Towards the mid-nineteenth century, Philadelphia surgeon Samuel Gross remembered individuals, ill or not, who so trusted bleeding that they would request it as an annual spring tonic: 'I recollect it was the custom thirty-five years ago, in the spring, for scores upon scores of people, especially in the rural districts, to go to the doctors to be bled', he wrote in *Then and Now* (1867). 'Sometimes non-professional men performed the operation on a large scale.'

> One day a stout, hale-looking Irishman came up to [Mr Hazard, a lay bloodletter] to be bled.
> The Irishman said, 'Mr Hazard, and how much do you charge for takin' a pint o' blood?' Drawing a pint was customary.
> 'Nothing', was the reply.
> 'Then, by St Peter', said the Irishman, 'you may take a whole quart from me.'[7]

Top: Bloodletting was especially popular in North America around 1800, where the leading physician Benjamin Rush advocated heroic levels of venesection. Some critics of the technique believed that George Washington was bled to death in his last illness on Friday 13 December 1799. Right: Eighteenth-century equipment for bloodletting and cupping.

Venesection required for its performance a nearby superficial vein. A gentler and more desirable form of bleeding was to put a leech on the affected part. Leeches secrete a protein (hirudin) in their saliva that blocks the body's natural clotting mechanism and keeps blood flowing from the capillaries. They may be placed anywhere on the body to extract supposed excess blood.

Europeans and Americans imported leeches in bulk from Russia where they were commercially raised. Consequently, leeches were a rich man's remedy. As Richard Arnold, a doctor in Savannah, wrote in 1838 to a friend in Philadelphia,

> I will in return beg a favor of you. Leeches sell here at the very high price of 50 cents each and there is not a regular leecher here to apply them. The Medical Society made a contract with a druggist to supply the public at not exceeding 25 cents each. Before he complied with his contract, he sold out ... If leeches were not so dear many more would be used. At present they are only in the reach of the rich.[8]

In medical practice well into the twentieth century, fever was omnipresent. Pneumonia, for example, counted as 'the old person's friend', because it was so common in the elderly and often fatal after a short illness. And few physicians would not face the sadness of death in the young from the epidemic diseases of childhood. James Herrick, a doctor in Chicago, recalled what it was like to treat diphtheria before the introduction of the antitoxin to the USA in the early 1890s. In diphtheria, the growth of bacteria in the throat interferes with breathing.

> In the case of an attractive seven-year-old child in whom the disease had invaded the larynx, I had inserted an O'Dwyer intubation tube [Herrick had practised the technique in the morgue of the Cook County Hospital]. This gave relief for several hours; then it was evident that the tube was becoming clogged. The parents begged me not to let the child strangle. I explained the desperate nature of the trouble, the extreme weakness of the circulation due to the toxaemia, and the danger of even mild manipulative treatment. They understood. The mother left the room, the father took the child in his arms, and with little difficulty the tube was removed. As the father uttered a 'Thank God', the child gave a feeble gasp and was gone. In memory I can still see the room, the exact location of the bed, the chair, the limp child in the father's lap, the adjustment of the light.[9]

Herrick himself was so upset at the loss that he nearly broke into tears.

Before the twentieth century, therefore, infectious diseases dominated over all others. Tuberculosis, syphilis, diphtheria, plague, meningitis, malaria, and postpartum sepsis were the diseases against which medical graduates and physicians everywhere had to struggle. That is what primary care was all about.

For this task, the doctrines of traditional physicians had singularly ill-equipped them. In the middle of the nineteenth century, medical theories about the causes of disease would be turned inside out. But before that time notions of disease causation were constructed along 'humoral' lines, attributing illness to imbalances of the fluids, or humours, which the Ancients believed to be the constituents of the body: black bile, yellow bile, phlegm, and blood (see page 58). By the eighteenth century, these Galenic humoral doctrines had undergone considerable modification.

The Dutch physician Herman Boerhaave, for example, added to the ancient theories baroque elaborations that distinguished between disorders of 'the solids' and those of 'the blood and humours'. Tuberculosis was an example of weakness of the solid parts, thrombosis and blood clots examples of overly rigid fibres. Give milk and iron for weak fibres; do bloodletting for rigid ones, Boerhaave counselled in the early eighteenth century. Yet virtually all theorizing about the mechanisms of disease before 1800 was like a castle built in the air: it had little empirical foundation and was completely false in modern scientific terms.

Therapies derived from these humoral theories were almost without exception injurious to the patient. Little was cured and much damage caused by depleting

This title-page of one of Herman Boerhaave's works shows him addressing a large audience at the University of Leiden. He was appointed to lecture on the institutes (i.e. theory) of medicine at Leiden in 1702, became professor of medicine and botany in 1709, and he also assumed the chair of clinical medicine in 1714. In 1718, he was further appointed to the chair of chemistry. Boerhaave was the quintessential scientific physician and medical teacher of the early Enlightenment. His introduction of the study of the natural sciences into the medical curriculum was especially innovative.

the body of its natural physiological constitutents and dosing it with toxic metals. Bloodletting was a mainstay of medical therapy in treating fever. A variety of mechanical contrivances, from the little folding knife called the 'lancet' to the elaborate 'scarificators' of the early nineteenth century – fiendish devices whose multiple blades would cut simultaneously into the skin – testify to its commonness. To be a surgeon or 'medical man' before the 1870s meant bloodletting.

A proper physician (as opposed to a surgeon or an apothecary) might disdain such procedures as bloodletting and setons in favour of giving 'physic', or medicine. The aim of traditional therapeutics was getting the bowels open. To the extent that the traditional pharmacopoeia used drugs that were active in the body at all, the medicines were mainly laxatives, or purgatives – a more powerful laxative. One treated fever with laxatives, getting those bad humours out of the bowels by procuring an 'opening'.

Towards 1800, Edward Sutleffe, a medical man of long experience in London's Queen Street, called on Mrs. W. of Finsbury. Her fingers were painful and swollen, 'thickly studded with eruptions, from which issued a semi-transparent excoriating ichor. I suspected the latent cause, and told her she had neglected her bowels in particular'. She confessed to having done so. Sutleffe prescribed for her 'a tepid bath and mild aperients [laxatives]'.[10] Quite dramatic substances were used to get those bowels open, those bladders peeing. Philadelphia's Benjamin Rush popularized the use of mercury, calling it in 1791 'a safe and nearly a universal medicine'.[11] Calomel, or mercurous chloride, appeared in every physician's bag throughout the nineteenth century, and was an active ingredient in the 'blue pills' that distinguished nineteenth-century English therapeutics.

Traditional medical therapeutics therefore amounted to making patients anaemic through bloodletting, depleting them of fluids and valuable electrolytes via the stool, and poisoning them with compounds of such heavy metals as mercury and lead. Even some contemporary physicians had the wit to notice what damage traditional therapeutics inflicted. Boston's William Douglass observed in 1755: 'In general, the physical practice [giving medications] in our colonies is so perniciously bad, that excepting in surgery and some very acute cases, it is better to let nature under a proper regimen take her course (*naturae morborum curatrices*) than to trust the honesty and sagacity of the practitioner ... Frequently there is more danger from the physician than from the distemper.' When Douglass had first arrived in New England he had asked a colleague, 'what was their general method of practice; he told me their practice was very uniform, bleeding, vomit-

The battle against 'inflammation'

Related to the humoral theories was the technique of irritating the skin, or counter-irritation. Further elaborations before it died at the end of the nineteenth century included the use of 'moxas', or cotton wool soaked in a flammable substance and permitted to burn down to the skin causing a scar. There were also 'setons', threads inserted under the skin with a surgical knife to excite a continual discharge of pus. Getting deep-seated poisons out of the body could be done by irritating the skin. Here is Glasgow surgeon John Burns in 1800 on counter-irritation in the battle against 'inflammation': 'If the internal parts be inflamed, the action of the surface is diminished; and, by increasing this action, we can lessen or remove the disease below.' How was this done?

- With blisters, for 'deep-seated inflammations of the breasts, bowels, or joints'. Physicians used blistering agents such as cantharides (spanish fly) or acetic acid to raise a serum blister on the skin.
- With 'rubefacients' – reddening the skin without blistering it. 'When the stomach, intestines or kidney have been very irritable', said Burns, 'I have known a sinapism [mustard plaster] to act like a charm.'
- With 'issues' – placing some caustic substance such as potassium hydroxide ('caustic potash') in a hole in the middle of a bandage to form an open sore. Burns said, 'The utility of issues, in diseases of the lungs, the liver, and the joints, is to be explained on the same principle [as that of blisters]. In these cases, we find that issues do little good unless they be somewhat painful, or be in the state of healthy ulcers.'[13]

This composite illustration from the seventeenth century depicts surgical practice. On the left, a barber-surgeon is cauterizing, to cleanse and seal a wound; on the right, another is applying a seton. Bloodletting bowls hang from the ceiling.

ing, blistering, purging, anodyne [relieving pain], etc. If the illness continued, there was repetendi, and finally murderandi'.[12] These murderous methods were characterized in general as 'heroic medicine'.

Patients, generally speaking, adored some bloodletting and some purging. But heroic medicine went beyond the bounds of what patients found acceptable. It was the excesses of traditional therapeutics, not its basic principles, that caused unease among sufferers, making primary care seem more a last resort than a route to wellbeing. 'If we look into the profession of physic', said Joseph Addison in *The Spectator* in 1711, 'we shall find a most formidable body of men. The sight of them is enough to make a man serious, for we may lay it down as a maxim, that when a nation abounds in physicians it grows thin of people.'[14]

The brusque physician on the right is a caricature by Charles de Villiers of the distinguished early nineteenth-century French doctor, François Broussais. Broussais' instructions for the patient are 'Another ninety leeches ... and continue the diet'. It was his belief that almost all disease was caused by inflammation, especially in the digestive tract. The application of leeches was thought to reduce such inflammation. Broussais' zealous faith in his theories and remedies became objects of fun.

Two centuries later Baltimore physician Daniel Cathell, in an 1882 work aimed at fellow physicians called *The Physician Himself and What He Should Add to the Strictly Scientific*, captured less laconically this loathing of the excesses of traditional medicine: 'So great, indeed, is the popular dread of what doctors *might do*, that in choosing an attendant from among regular physicians, the nervous and the timid, who constitute nine-tenths of all the sick, are greatly inclined to shun all who treat heroically, and seek those who use moderate, even though less efficient, means.' Hence the popular fondness for 'irregulars', such as homeopaths, who, Cathell mocked, 'cure by Mild Powers or Harmless Methods'.[15]

At the outset of the story of primary care, therefore, we find the doctors in the grips of (to us) ludicrous and dangerous theories, the patients terrified, and in search of alternatives. Science, however, brought the two opposing parties together.

THE MAKING OF THE MODERN DOCTOR

The modern general practitioner, the guarantor of primary care in the USA until the 1920s and in the UK until the present day, evolved more from surgery and pharmacy than from academic medicine, and was called into being as much for social as scientific reasons. Before the Napoleonic years most medical care in Britain was furnished by men who were not qualified physicians but had trained as apprentices and passed the examinations of the Society of Apothecaries or the Company of Surgeons. With an act in 1815 these surgeon-apothecaries began to be recognized as general practitioners, a term legitimized in 1826 when the Association of Apothecaries and Surgeon-Apothecaries renamed itself 'The Associated General Medical and Surgical Practitioners'.

Among middle-class families, the demand was rising for a single practitioner who would be able to fulfil all of the family's medical and surgical needs, from bleeding and lancing boils to dispensing physic. These families, according to one observer in 1815, 'had long wished for a class of the faculty to whom they could apply with confidence in any description of case in which medical or surgical aid was necessary'.[16] Thus, 'medical man' came to mean apothecary-surgeon or general practitioner, and 'doctor' meant a qualified member of the Royal College of Physicians in London, a tiny elite of physicians who supplied health care to the rich and consulted in difficult cases.

A Medical Reform Act of 1858 created a single overseeing council for the entire UK, and stipulated that only the universities and the established corporations (Surgeons, Apothecaries, Physicians) of England and Wales, Scotland, and Ireland could grant medical licenses (and no longer the Archbishop of Canterbury, for example). Henceforth only those registered by a General Medical Council, which the Act set up, would be considered 'qualified medical practitioners'. This Act

Traditional quack medicine, involving spectacular theatrical performance, remained common till the close of the nineteenth century. As this illustration suggests, the similarities between the charlatan and the itinerant preacher were close. Quackery throve on the exotic. Many itinerants pretended to come from Eastern parts, with its implications of mystique and magic. Others, like 'Sequah', who was active in late nineteenth-century England, masqueraded as an American Indian, to evoke the folk wisdom of the New World. He sold 'Prairie Flower' oils, curing rheumatism and removing teeth. In reality, he was a certain William Hartley, born in Yorkshire in 1857, who picked up the tricks of the medicine shows in America and Australia and made a fortune touring England in the 1880s. Here he is on Clapham Common, London.

gave general practitioners the same legal though not social status as the elite consultant physicians of London, and established the framework within which primary care would grow for the next century.

In the USA, the regulation of physicians remained chaotic until far later in time. Until the beginning of state licensing in the 1880s anybody could call him- or herself a 'doctor' (for there were numerous women doctors as well). Typically, these doctors would apprentice for 3 years to a 'preceptor', who would supply books, equipment, and a certificate at the end. In the first half of the apprenticeship the aspirant would read basic medical textbooks and help compound drugs; in the second, he would go riding with the doctor on house calls. Medical schools had existed in the USA since the middle of the eighteenth century, but they tended to be 2-year affairs, the students repeating in the second year the lectures they had heard in the first. There was little opportunity to do dissections or to see patients. Once medical licensing systems were established, many of these earlier medical men, who had qualified without undergoing examinations, came to be known under the embarrassing title of 'Y-of-P' men, standing for years of practice – their sole qualification for the practice of medicine.

There were scientific reasons, too, for the emergence of the modern family doctor. Awareness was dawning that medicine was something more than an art, that it possessed a scientific basis with a corpus of knowledge from such disciplines as physiology that must be mastered before one could diagnose or treat patients effectively. And this *prise de conscience*, in addition to the social needs of the middle classes, also drove forward medical reform on both sides of the Atlantic. Once medicine had something to teach other than anatomy and get-those-poisons-out-of-there-style therapeutics, medical competence would be acquired in a stepped programme of study and verified with qualifying examinations. The point about the onrush of science is important, because the physician's new scientific attainments transformed the nature of the relationship between doctor and patient and thus the nature of primary care.

Consider how the style of practice changed under science. The traditional physician was casual about history-taking; he limited himself in the physical examination to looking at the tongue, feeling the pulse, and inspecting the countenance to establish the patient's constitution. The typical consultation concluded with the drawing up of elaborate prescriptions for laxatives. The physician who practised scientifically, by contrast, would take a systematic history of the present illness, perform a physical examination by pounding, listening and poking, consider all the possible diseases the patient might have on the basis of the signs and symptoms hitherto gathered (this is called the 'differential diagnosis'), then finally select the one disease most likely afflicting the patient by doing further examinations and laboratory tests (making the 'clinical' diagnosis). In this scientific practice, the clinical investigation as well as the differential diagnosis were historically quite new. It was a style that swept the traditional approach to primary care out the window.

The modern style of practice assumed that similar signs and symptoms of illness could be caused by a wide range of different disease mechanisms. Mechanism is a key word in modern medicine. It refers to the pathological processes leading to tissue changes in the body. We are, for example, dealing with a blue-ish, coughing patient who reports a history of blood-flecked sputum. The traditional doctor might conclude it was an excess of the humour phlegm. The scientifically oriented modern doctor approached the problem quite differently. He would have learned in medical school that vastly different mechanisms can cause this bedside ('clinical') picture. In pathology class, he would have studied slides of tuberculosis, pneumonia, and lung cancer, each with a different mechanism and producing its own unique changes in lung tissue, which were visible under the microscope.

The scientifically practising physician would proceed from this differential diagnosis to listen carefully to the chest, then take an X-ray (after 1896) or perform other tests that would pin down which of the three diseases was causing this patient's problems. At the end of the consultation the physician would be able to give the patient his or her prognosis, and determine a rational plan of treatment.

Traditional physicians had, of course, an instinct for prognosis, knowing generally what happened to patients who coughed up a lot of blood. But their therapeutics were based on humoral doctrines that totally lacked any kind of scientific basis. Thus, even if modern doctors could not cure their patients, at least an understanding of disease mechanisms and drug action *kept them from doing harm*. This ability to refrain from doing harm stands as one of the major acquisitions of primary care for the period from around 1840, when bloodletting began to go out of use, to 1935, when the first of the wonder drugs was introduced.

For modern doctors to draw up their differential diagnoses, a score of scientific advances had to occur. The science of microscopy and of different stains for making tissues visible under the microscope had to develop. The whole anatomical-clinical technique of identifying specific diseases had to be elaborated, in which researchers reason back and forth from autopsy findings to the patient's signs and symptoms before death. A germ theory of disease (see page 184) was required to put the understanding of fever on a scientific basis, the knowledge that specific kinds of infectious illnesses are caused by specific kinds of microbes. In other words, advances in many areas of background knowledge were required to transform medicine from being just an art to an art and a science.

How was all this science imported into primary care? The link between the doctor's scientific knowledge and the patient's subjective symptoms was the physical examination. To establish which disease mechanism was at work inside the body, the doctor would, in the first line, have to look at the patient's body, and touch and press him. The physical examination consisted of three innovations: palpating the patient's abdomen, percussing his chest, and listening – at first with one's ear against the major body cavities, later using a stethoscope – to the movement of blood, gas, and air within the limbs and major body cavities. All three innovations were first put into practice by the elite physicians of the Parisian teaching hospitals during the Napoleonic years (see page 173), then spread outwards to other centres of medicine in the years before 1850, finally diffusing into general practice in the second half of the nineteenth century.

Whereas traditional medical students memorized lists of herbal infusions and the kind of fevers for which each was appropriate, the modern medical student learned to observe the patient. Here is young Karl Stern, a resident physician in Frankfurt in the early 1930s, at the lectures of Professor Franz Volhard. Volhard, who himself had trained in the pathology department of a Berlin teaching hospital in the 1890s, was very much the image of the modern scientifically practising physician. Frequently, Stern said, Volhard would bring the patient in 'without any preliminary introduction'. 'The professor raised his hand in an imploring manner, glanced all over the audience, and then looked long and pensively at the patient. Presently there was a hush over the big room, and one could have heard a pin drop. The only thing one heard was the patient's breath. This silence went on for several minutes which seemed like half an hour.'

Suddenly, Stern continued, Volhard would call out, 'What do you see?' Again silence, because at first none of the medical students saw anything. Yet soon someone would call out, 'There is dyspnoea [shortness of breath]. The respiration is thirty-five per minute.' Volhard would remain silent, as if he had not heard. Someone else would say, 'Pallor around the area of the mouth' (a sign of lack of oxygen). Another would call, 'Club-shaped fingers', also an index that the lungs are poorly oxygenating the blood.

Jean-Martin Charcot (1825–93), the most eminent French physician of his day, was one of the new breed of specialist doctors. His early investigations were devoted to chronic diseases such as gout and arthritis, and the diseases of old age. Increasingly, however, he turned his active medical service at the Salpêtrière Hospital in Paris into an international centre for the investigation of neurological diseases.

One of the few dramatic successes achieved by medicine before the twentieth century was the prevention of smallpox. Inoculation, introduced in the early eighteenth century, was succeeded in the nineteenth century by the safer technique of vaccination, developed by Edward Jenner. The vaccination of children became compulsory in many countries. A doctor and his assistant run a visiting vaccination clinic in Germany, in this painting by Reinhard Zimmermann, 1857.

The students would be permitted to feel and touch only after having described what they had seen. 'It was quite extraordinary', Stern continued, 'to experience the varieties of tactile sensation.'

There was, quite aside from the world of sight, an entire world of touch which we had never perceived before. In feeling differences of radial pulse [at the wrist] you could train yourself to feel dozens of different waves with their characteristic peaks, blunt and sharp, steep and slanting, and the corresponding valleys. There were so many ways in which the margin of the liver [just below the right ribs] came up towards your palpating finger. There were extraordinary varieties of smell. There was not just pallor but there seemed to be hundreds of hues of yellow and gray.[17]

When these young physicians later entered primary care, everything they noted about the patient would be filtered through this riot of hues and sounds and touches.

The contrast between old and new could not be more striking. Young Arthur Hertzler in Kansas described traditionally oriented colleagues making a house call in the 1890s: 'The usual procedure for a doctor when he reached the patient's house was to greet the grandmother and aunts effusively and pat all the kids on the head before approaching the bedside. He greeted the patient with a grave look and a pleasant joke. He felt the pulse and inspected the tongue, and asked where it hurt. This done, he was ready to deliver an opinion and prescribe his pet remedy.'

Hertzler by contrast did as he had learned in medical school.

I examined my patients as well as I knew how. My puerile attempts at physical examination impressed my patients and annoyed my competitors … Word went out that the young doctor 'ain't very civil but he is thorough'. Only yesterday one of my old patients recalled that when I came to see her young son I 'stripped him all off and examined him all over'. Members of that family have been my patients for the intervening forty years, so impressed were they. Incidentally, it may be mentioned that in this case I discovered a pleurisy with effusion [an inflammation of the lining of the lungs producing serum] which had not been apparent to my tongue-inspecting colleague.[18]

A physician, probably Jean-Martin Charcot, listens to the internal reverberations of a patient being percussed – that is, having her ribcage tapped. Skilled physicians could learn much from the practice. Different pitches of sound indicated fluid on the chest and the condition of the lungs, especially important in an age when tuberculosis was common and deadly. Percussion of the chest was one of the new techniques used by scientifically practising doctors to make their differential diagnosis.

Being a country doctor at the turn of the nineteenth century did not necessarily mean being traditional: Hertzler was practising medicine based on science.

Something more than a lust for science lay behind these new clinical reflexes. As a result of the lax entry standards previously in effect, the medical profession had become quite overcrowded before the First World War. Being known as somebody who practised scientifically represented for young physicians a drawing card. So there was perhaps a public-relations tactic as well as a scientific motive in all this apparent meticulousness – the need to offer what the public demanded rather than what the practitioner deemed just. But, now, the public was demanding science.

Writing in 1924 with more than 50 years of medical practice under his belt, Daniel Cathell reflected how important this aura of science was in medical success. 'Working with the microscope and making analyses of the urine, sputum, blood, and other fluids as an aid to diagnosis, will not only bring fees and lead to valuable information regarding your patient's condition, but will also give you reputation and professional respect, by investing you, in the eyes of the public, with the benefits of being a very scientific man.'[19]

The ascendancy of science thus added a hands-on dimension to the doctor–patient relationship. The doctor now touched the patient, percussed, palpated, and listened. In addition to gathering important information for making a diagnosis, this physical contact also conveyed psychologically the impression of giving care, and fortified the psychological bond between physician and patient.

NEW MEDICATIONS

In the traditional doctor's medical bag, very little of the 'physic' had the power to do good. Of the hundreds of drugs listed in 1824 in the *Pharmacopoeia* of the Royal College of Physicians of London, only opium, dispensed as a deep-brownish 'tincture', or solution in alcohol, conferred much therapeutic benefit. Yet it lost much of its punch when taken orally (dissolved by stomach enzymes), and even though opium had been known in Europe since the sixteenth century to be effective against pain, a tincture of opium supplied little relief of severe pain. The college also proposed various forms of iron to its members, calling them useful, among other things, as a 'tonic'. Physicians did give iron for conditions that later would be diagnosed as iron-deficiency anaemia, but they did not do so systematically and 'chlorosis' – the term of the day for iron-deficiency anaemia – was not mentioned.

What other genuine good could the fellows of the Royal College of Physicians achieve in 1824 with drugs? It was very little. To say that they were able to relieve constipation is equivalent to saying that a shotgun may be used as a fly swatter: they purged ruthlessly with the many plant-based purgatives, such as aloes and senna, for every condition imaginable. In 1785, the Birmingham physician William Withering had disseminated within medicine the knowledge – already

Giving what the public wants

In one of Arthur Conan Doyle's short stories, 'A False Start' (1894), young 'Dr. Wilkinson' is just establishing his practice in town. He receives an unexpected call from the wealthy 'Sir John Millbank' to come and consult in the case of Sir John's bedridden wife, who apparently has some chest disease.

Sir John tells young Dr Wilkinson, 'And another thing. I won't have her thumped about all over the chest, or any hocus-pocus of the sort. She has bronchitis and asthma, and that's all. If you can cure it, well and good. But it only weakens her to have you tapping and listening; and it does no good, either.' (It comes out that the previous family doctor, 'Dr Mason', had never examined Sir John's wife.)

Dr Wilkinson is affronted at these peremptory instructions and picks up his hat to leave.

Sir John: 'Hullo, what's the matter now?'

Dr Wilkinson: 'It is not my habit to give opinions without examining my patient. I wonder that you should suggest such a course to a medical man. I wish you good day.'

Sir John rapidly backpedals, amazed at 'a young man who seemed to care nothing either for his wealth or title. His respect for [Wilkinson's] judgement increased amazingly'. Sir John consents to let Wilkinson examine his wife, and goes off to tell her.

Now two daughters, who have overheard the conversation, burst forth from their cover. 'Oh! well done, well done!', cries the taller daughter, clapping her hands.

'Don't let him bully you, doctor', says the other. 'Oh, it was so nice to hear you stand up to him. That's the way he does with poor Dr Mason. Dr Mason has never examined mamma yet. He always takes papa's word for everything.'

So impressed is Sir John with Wilkinson's careful physical examination that he dismisses Mason and makes Wilkinson the family doctor.[20] Sir John, his daughters, the entire entourage: all are wide-eyed at this new eruption of science in modern medicine, the physical examination.

---

long known in folk culture – that the foxglove plant was useful against certain forms of 'dropsy', or oedema caused by congestive heart failure (foxgloves contain digitalis). The college's *Pharmacopoeia* does mention a foxglove tea, or infusion, as a helpful diuretic, meaning a drug to stimulate the kidneys. This shows at least that they were in the right ballpark, since a strengthened heart causes the kidneys to start making urine. Yet medicine as a whole in the nineteenth century lost sight of digitalis as a cardiac drug, using it against tuberculosis and everything else, until London physicians James Mackenzie and Thomas Lewis reintroduced it before the First World War.

Therewith the list of genuinely useful drugs was at end. The physician practising before the middle of the nineteenth century had nothing against infectious disease, cancer, arthritis, diabetes, asthma, heart attacks, or vaginitis (inflammation of the vagina). The list of conditions he could not relieve (although he believed that he could) is much longer than those which he could. Arthur Hertzler, the Kansas frontier doctor, said in 1938 of his earlier colleagues, 'I can scarcely think of a single disease that the doctors actually cured during those early years … The possible exceptions were malaria and the itch [scabies]. Doctors knew how to relieve suffering, set bones, sew up cuts and open boils on small boys.'[21]

During the nineteenth century, some important new drugs became available, principally as a result of the growth of the organic chemical industry in Germany,

Cinchona, or Peruvian bark, became popular as a cure-all for fevers and tonic in the seventeenth century when it was introduced to Europe from South America. This drawing of the plant appears in a compendium of Aztec history and culture called the *Florentine Codex, c.* 1570. In reality, cinchona is effective only against malaria (quinine is one of its constituents) but this was not realized for some time. It tasted bitter, and its side-effects included vomiting and diarrhoea. The great demand for cinchona by Europeans during the period of colonial expansion had important consequences in promoting exploration and in developing new drugs.

490.

which synthesized new molecules from coal tar (benzene). By 1935, the list of useful drugs in the GP's bag would be much longer. In the area of pain relief, the nineteenth century saw the introduction of the alkaloids of opium (see page 258), which are much more concentrated than raw opium. After Alexander Wood made it known in 1855 that morphine could be administered with the hypodermic needle he had perfected, they could be injected directly into the blood stream, bypassing the stomach. The hypodermic syringe and the injectible opioids in the nineteenth-century medical bag became the subject of much mischief, for while they offered undoubted pain relief, they also were highly addictive. The old family doctors gave morphine at the drop of a hat, and tales are legion of patients whom these physicians casually addicted.

The aspirin family represented another innovation in pain relief (see page 261). Members of this family, all synthesized in the laboratory, cut pain effectively as well as reducing fever and inflammation. This is part of the larger story of the search for antifever drugs, or antipyretics. In the absence of a germ theory, earlier physicians had directed their attention to bringing down fever rather than to overcoming the underlying infection. Such efforts went back to experiments with quinine as a general febrifuge, not just an antimalarial drug. But quinine was ineffective against other fevers, and unbeloved among patients because of its bitter taste and side-effects.

Since its introduction in 1899, aspirin (acetylsalicylic acid) has been the most popular drug of all time. In the USA alone, some 10,000 to 20,000 tons of aspirin are used annually. If the members of the aspirin family had been consumed mainly over-the-counter, bought at the pharmacy without a prescription, they might not figure so prominently in the history of primary care. Yet many doctors themselves dispensed aspirin and its relatives, and wrote out prescriptions for them. By 1909, aspirin and the antipyretic phenacetin (another member of the acetanilid family) ranked among the ten items most prescribed by American physicians. The aspirin family had come to symbolize medicine's new therapeutic accomplishments.

An enduring problem in primary care is patients who cannot sleep, or are nervous, irritable, depressed, or agitated. The nineteenth-century German chemical industry had presents to offer them as well. In 1869, a foul-tasting hypnotic called chloral hydrate (made by adding water to chloral) came into medical use. Known popularly as a 'Mickey Finn', chloral hydrate was in reality a mild sleeping potion, one that starts to lose its efficacy after about the third night. (It has the potential for addiction, however, and 'chloral' addicts were a familiar sight in late-nineteenth -century private nervous clinics.)

In l888, a more powerful hypnotic called sulphonal came into medical use. Sulphonal was the first really popular drug of the Bayer Company's laboratories in Germany, and helped finance research on a further cascade of hypnotics. Bayer's final stroke in this area was to take barbituric acid, first synthesized in 1864, and add on several small hydrocarbon sidechains. The result, generically called barbital (barbitone in the UK), was marketed in l903 under the trade name Veronal. The barbiturates virtually put an end to all the earlier hypnotics except for chloral hydrate. A relative of barbital named phenobarbital was introduced in 1912 as Luminal, and has attained epic status in novels about psychoneurosis among the middle classes. Amytal, Seconal, Nembutal, and fifty or so other barbiturates followed later.

A detailed history of these sedatives and hypnotics would be more appropriate in a history of psychiatry were it not for the fact that general practitioners prescribed them so often. One Canadian family doctor, William Victor Johnston, wrote of the interwar years that Luminal, alongside aspirin, morphine, and digitalis, had been 'indispensable'. 'I bought Luminal tablets in five-thousand lots every few months', Johnston wrote, looking back on decades of practice.[22]

There were other advances, too – drugs such as amyl nitrite (Thomas Brunton discovered its usefulness in 1867) and nitroglycerine (William Murrell in 1879) to dilate the arteries of the heart in patients enduring anginal pain. These drugs tended to be administered more by specialists than by family doctors. What caused a sensation in primary care, a virtual revolution in the image of the physician, occurred in the realm of infectious diseases such as diphtheria.

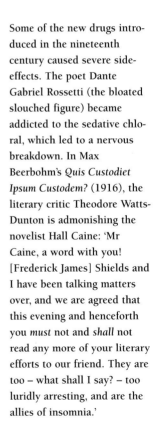

Some of the new drugs introduced in the nineteenth century caused severe side-effects. The poet Dante Gabriel Rossetti (the bloated slouched figure) became addicted to the sedative chloral, which led to a nervous breakdown. In Max Beerbohm's *Quis Custodiet Ipsum Custodem?* (1916), the literary critic Theodore Watts-Dunton is admonishing the novelist Hall Caine: 'Mr Caine, a word with you! [Frederick James] Shields and I have been talking matters over, and we are agreed that this evening and henceforth you *must* not and *shall* not read any more of your literary efforts to our friend. They are too – what shall I say? – too luridly arresting, and are the allies of insomnia.'

Of all the new drugs before 1935, that most to astonish the world was the antitoxin against diphtheria, developed in 1891 in Robert Koch's laboratory in Berlin. Emil Adolf von Behring and Shibasaburo Kitasato showed that the serum of a horse immunized against diphtheria (using techniques developed at the Pasteur Institute in Paris) could be used to immunize other horses. In 1892, the first commercial vaccines against diphtheria began to be produced. The introduction of the diphtheria antitoxin sharply upgraded the doctor's image in the eyes of the public. For the first time, medicine was truly capable of curing an infectious disease that threatened the children of every home in the nation.

Apart from the diphtheria antitoxin, however, it would be unwise to exaggerate the therapeutic accomplishments of the modern doctor before 1935. Syphilis was treatable with Salvarsan from 1910 (see page 264) but the reality of clinical practice reduced itself more to tonics and laxatives than to finely calibrated doses of Bayer's pharmaceutical products. In 1869, one observer described the scene at the casualty department of St Bartholomew's Hospital in London: '120 patients were seen by the physician and dismissed in an hour and ten minutes, or at the rate of 35 seconds each ... [The patients] were dismissed with a doubtful dose of physic, ordered almost at random, and poured out of a huge brown jug.'[23] Ten years later the medications dispensed at Bart's had scarcely become more sophisticated. 'They consist essentially,' said an anonymous contributor to *The Lancet*, 'of purgatives; a mixture of iron, sulphate of magnesia, and quassia [both laxatives], and cod-liver oil, fulfilling the two great indications of all therapeutics – elimination, and the supply of some elements to the blood.' The anonymous writer criticized Bart's for supplying medicine 'out of jugs, and patients seen at the rate of one a minute, for sixpence or a shilling'.[24]

What did the old-time US doctor around 1900 have in the saddlebags that he threw atop his horse as he made housecalls? 'In his case there are but few drugs', said Joseph Mathews, past-president of the American Medical Association in 1905, 'but he knows the quality of each one of them.' 'Calomel, opium, quinine, buchu [a diuretic to stimulate the kidneys], ipecac [an emetic; see page 254], and Dover's powder [a laxative; see page 255] constitute his armamentarium. He has never heard of many of the "new-fangled" remedies that are in the case of his young competitor, but he has managed to "get along" these many years without them'. Mathews felt that in time young physicians, too, would discover that all they really needed in their bags were drugs to make the patients defaecate and vomit.[25] Over a 12-month period in 1891–2 Americans consumed, among other drugs, 255,000 pounds (115,700 kg) of aloes (a laxative), 113,000 pounds (51,250 kg) of jalap (another laxative), 1,400,000 pounds (635,040 kg) of nux vomica (an emetic), and 13,000 pounds (5,900 kg) of 'calomel and other mercurial medicinal preparations'.[26] Thus medical therapeutics had clearly not experienced the same kind of scientific revolution as medical diagnostics.

Opposite: The causative bacillus of diphtheria was isolated in 1883 by Edwin Klebs. Seven years later, Emil Behring and Shibasaburo Kitasato developed the first diphtheria antitoxin. Horses were much used as experimental animals for producing the blood serum needed for the antitoxin. Watercolour by Fritz Gehrke, 1906.

The fight against diphtheria

It is difficult now to recall how awful epidemics of diphtheria once were, for the children caught up in them, for their grieving parents, and desperate doctors. One such epidemic from the 1890s was recalled by Thomas Shastid in the small Illinois town where he practised:

> Antitoxin had just been introduced, but, at least for us in that city, it did no good. Result: literally dozens of intubations and tracheotomies, especially the latter, because the former were ineffective. Night after night, sometimes for a week in succession, I would be called to get up and go to some residence, there to cut open some child's windpipe, therein to introduce a tube through which it might be able to breathe until it should be able, possibly, to throw off the terrible infection. Even then, not infrequently, the child died, because of the false membranes continuing to form — lower and lower, deeper and deeper, into the air-ways, until at length it had reached beyond the lowest extremity of our air-passing tube.

One night Shastid accompanied a colleague, nicknamed Misanthropus, whom everyone thought 'hard-boiled', to a home where a child lay ailing. To his horror, Shastid saw his colleague faltering, whining in a trembly voice, 'Of all my little — little — little patients I've loved this one the most'.

Shastid handed him the knife, pulled the skin tight over the child's trachea and picked up a retractor. The child stopped breathing. Shastid cried, 'Quick, Doctor, quick. Your patient'll be dead'.

Misanthropus 'leaned over with the knife as if to make an incision, attempted to cut — but his hand vibrated, shook, went all wobbling around everywhere'.

'Cut!', Shastid shouted, 'Cut!'

Misanthropus again tried to use the knife, pressing it so deeply into the child's neck that Shastid thought the blade must be back at the neck bone. Misanthropus had inadvertently used the back edge of the blade. He turned and handed the knife to Shastid.

'I took it', Shastid said later, 'and, I think (I am not boasting), performed an excellent operation. Yet, next morning, the child was dead'.[27]

Consider the relief that diffused among both doctors and patients after the antitoxin had become available. Alfred Schofield, a physician with an upper-middle-class practice in London, described the first case of diphtheria he encountered after the antitoxin had arrived, 'obtained from certain horses kept near Harrow for the purpose'.

> I found the boy very ill, the whole back of his throat being like white velvet. I had never used the new remedy before, but determined to try it to save the boy's life. I injected a small quantity under the skin of the stomach and watched the throat. I can only compare the marvellous result to the disappearance of snow beneath a hot sun. After the second dose every trace of the membrane disappeared, and the boy soon recovered.[28]

TECHNOLOGY AND PRIMARY CARE

When 'Dr Stark Munro', one of Arthur Conan Doyle's fictional characters, set up medical practice in the 1890s, he had little with him by way of equipment. 'In my box were a stethoscope, several medical books, a second pair of boots, two suits of clothes, my linen and my toilet things.'[29] Was that really all that one needed for the practice of medicine in those days? One must distinguish between innovations that remain the monopoly of a small group of specialists, and those that diffuse widely among general practitioners.

The panoply of new technology in primary care that emerged in the late nineteenth century (see page 140) was reassuring to the patients, and extended the range of medical diagnosis far beyond what the simple techniques of physical examination permitted. One US study between the two world wars found, for example, that of 100 cases of heart disease seen in general practice sixty-five were chronic cases requiring no new visits for a diagnosis and, in thirty-five, the general practitioner should require no more than a single visit of 30 minutes to make the diagnosis. 'For 30 cases, this is sufficient; 2 need an additional visit of 20 minutes; the remainder are referred to a specialist after the first visit to the general practitioner.'[30]

The study was focused on medical economics, but it assumed that a general practitioner would be able competently to determine what the heart was doing in a single surgery visit of half an hour. By contrast the great English heart specialist James Mackenzie had complained just a decade previously about the 'utmost confusion prevailing as to the significance of the signs detected in the heart'.[31]

SCEPTICSM AND THE PATIENT-AS-A-PERSON MOVEMENT

The combination of scientifically trained physicians thinking systematically about the mechanisms of disease, together with the persistence of tides of laxatives dispensed from big brown jugs, made it inevitable that doctors would become sceptical about the possibilities of drug treatment in general. This scepticism was called therapeutic nihilism. In the second half of the nineteenth century the nihilists ruled the roost in academic medicine, teaching generations of medical students, quite correctly, that the decoctions and infusions then available in the formulary were either useless or harmful, that physicians could do relatively little to cure disease (although they could relieve suffering with opium), and, by implication, that the real function of medicine was to accumulate scientific information about the human body rather than to heal.

Therapeutic nihilism had begun in the big European medical centres in the 1840s. The term itself is associated with the Viennese academic Joseph Dietl, a pupil of the famous physician Josef Škoda. Dietl wrote in 1841: 'Medicine as a natural science cannot have the task of inventing panaceas and discovering miracle cures that banish death, but instead of discovering the conditions under which people become ill, recover, and perish, in a word, of deepening a doctrine of the

Opposite: *Diphtheria*, attributed to a follower of Goya, 1802–12. Diphtheria, a highly contagious bacterial infection whose symptoms include a moderate fever, general malaise, sore throat, and a hard cough, was often fatal to children. It spread widely in the eighteenth century There were also epidemics during the nineteenth century until the development of the antitoxin and improved methods of treatment. In the twentieth century, programmes of mass immunization have greatly reduced the incidence of the disease worldwide but epidemics still occasionally occur, as recently in the former Soviet Union.

Innovations in primary care

The second half of the nineteenth century saw several innovations, among them the microscope, the thermometer, the X-ray, the stethoscope, and the electrocardiograph.

The microscope

The microscope reached university medicine in the 1840s, and was central in diagnosing the true cause of death from tissue taken at autopsy. But the typical family doctor would not have this objective, and used the microscope instead to study specimens. For example, it was highly useful for studying blood samples taken from patients to determine if they were anaemic and to judge from the size and shape of the red blood cells the kind of anaemia. One could also look at urine specimens under the microscope for evidence of pus to see if, say, an infection of the urinary tract were causing that deep pelvic pain. Or one could try to find the bacteria of pneumonia, tuberculosis, or bronchitis in samples of sputum. Also, a microscope 'looked good' in one's office.

Snickered Daniel Cathell in 1882 of the microscope and similar equipment, 'If, at your office and elsewhere, you make use of instruments of precision ... they will not only assist you in diagnosis, etc., but will also aid you greatly in curing people by heightening their confidence in you and enlisting their co-operation'.[33]

The thermometer

It was the Berlin physician Ludwig Traube who introduced the thermometer into clinical medicine around 1850. Indeed, it was Traube who introduced to Germany the whole modern investigation of the patient.

Above: The Russian zoologist Elie Metchnikoff with a microscope. In the late nineteenth century, his microscopic studies led to the modern science of immunology. Right: An early X-ray (*c.* 1897) of an arthritic hand.

The thermometer was brought into the New York Hospital in 1865. Thomas Clifford Allbutt, the distinguished Leeds physician who later became the Regius Professor of Medicine at Cambridge, initiated its use in England in 1867.

By the 1880s the thermometer had become part of the scientific doctor's medical bag because of its obvious utility in measuring fever. It also had a gratifying psychological effect on patients. William Macartney, as a house doctor (intern) at Bellevue Hospital in the late 1880s in New York, remembered being one day in the midst of a surgical operation when called to the women's ward. 'I was supposed to give immediate first aid to every accident case, so I rushed to the bedside and, finding that she probably had merely a broken arm, I put a thermometer in this old Irish lady's armpit and told her I would be back soon. On my return, she said with a grateful smile, "Shure, Doctor, that did me a wor-rld of good".'[34]

The X-ray

In 1895, the Würzburg physicist Wilhelm Röntgen discovered that by passing a high voltage through a vacuum tube (perfected by the English scientist William Crookes), he could generate electromagnetic vibrations capable of penetrating human flesh and leaving an imprint on a photographic plate on the other side. On 22 December 1895, he used these 'Röntgen rays' to make a photograph of the bones of his wife's hand; the picture became one of the century's most potent images. It was instantly apparent that these 'X-rays'could be used diagnostically. By March 1896 doctors in, for example, Chicago were excitedly discussing X-ray plates showing 'bones of the hand and the leg and a few coins and keys in a pocketbook'.[35]

The X-ray helped greatly in areas where physical diagnosis produced confusion. Was there was a percussion note of dullness in the chest? What unwelcome object was in that region to dampen the normal high note caused by the hollowness of the lungs? With the X-ray it could be determined if the pathology were an aneurysm (or bulging) of the aorta — a typical late consequence of syphilis, a tumour, or tuberculosis. All of these diseases create areas of dullness, but the X-ray would show exactly what was at fault.

Burton Wood, in charge of the outpatient department at a London hospital for chest diseases, remembered what a nightmare the early diagnosis of tuberculosis had once been using the techniques of physical examination (quickness of diagnosis was thought important in order to send the patient to a spa or sanatorium before the disease had spread):

> The unmusical were bewildered by dissertations on the varying quality of tones that might be elicited. In auscultation we were taught to take note of the slightest differences in breath sounds. Slight weakening of inspiration at one apex [top of lung] or a roughening of the breath sounds or a catchy quality might all be significant of disease.

They had once taken skin pencils 'to mark the limits of resonance, and closed eyes during percussion were calculated to impress the patient'. Now all of that was over. 'Radiology supplies more direct evidence. It enables us, in common phrase, "to see for ourselves"'.[36]

In orthopaedics, for problems like fractures, the X-ray opened a new world. 'A badly set limb or an unnecessary or bungled amputation injures our whole profession', said Cathell in 1924. 'And the limb or stump may be held up in court in a suit for damages.' 'Unless you are an idiot, X-ray them all.'[37] By the 1950s almost half of American general practitioners — far fewer in Britain — had an X-ray machine on hand in their offices.

The sphygmomanometer

A knowledge of the blood pressure is useful as a measurement of the work the heart has to do: the higher the arterial resistance against the blood being pumped out of the heart, the tireder the heart gets. In 1896, the Italian physician Scipione Riva-Rocci invented a simple device for measuring blood pressure — a rubber bag that went around the arm, which was then filled with air in order to block the circulation in the brachial artery and determine at what pressure the blood was passing through.

In 1905, the Russian Nikolai Korotkoff added the refinement of having the doctor listen with a stethoscope at the pit of the elbow for the noises made by the blood when its circulation is cut off (these noises indicate the systolic pressure, or highest force at which the heart can expel the blood) and when the sound terminates as the blood resumes circulating (the diastolic, or resting pressure of the heart). Around the time of the First World War clinicians were not sensitive to hypertension, or high blood pressure. But patients and doctors hung upon the idea that one's blood pressure might be too low, and surgeons as well wanted to know their patients' blood pressures during operations. Quite quickly, therefore, the measurement of blood pressure became standard in primary care. In 1912, for example, doctors at the Massachusetts General Hospital in Boston started noting the blood pressure of their patients on admission. By the 1920s it was customary for British and American general practitioners to have in their offices the instruments required for measuring blood pressure.

The electrocardiograph

Determining what the heart is doing is the toughest of all assignments in bedside medicine, for the clues are so few and so difficult to interpret. A wave of electrical current crosses the heart from the right side to the left every time it beats. In certain kinds of heart disease, such as when a heart attack has damaged the heart muscle, the passage of this current is interrupted. Both doctors and patients have a keen interest in knowing about the extent of such damage. The electrocardiograph (ECG, or EKG using the German initials of the term) makes possible this measurement.

In 1901, a Dutch physiologist named Willem Einthoven hitched up a galvanometer (for measuring current) to a device that projected a record of its readings onto a photographic plate, thus creating an image of the heart wave. This device required the patient to place hands and feet in four buckets of water (see page 200) and was at first quite complicated to operate, although of great usefulness to specialists. By the 1930s, however, an American general practitioner might reasonably expect to acquire an ECG — 'for example, a 'Sandorn Cardiette' — and by the 1950s almost half of all general practitioners in the USA had one in their surgeries.

human condition that is based scientifically upon the study of nature, physics and chemistry.'[32] Thus the task of medicine was to be not healing at all, but research into scientific mechanisms. Bernhard Naunyn, who later became a professor of internal medicine in Germany, remembered of his professors in Berlin in the 1860s: 'They knew that the healing part of medicine rested upon the discipline's scientific basis, and that the physician's compulsion to cure [*Drang zum Heilen*] had to be reigned in.'[38]

In the USA, therapeutic nihilism surfaced as praise of 'nature's healing ways', or the *vis medicatrix naturae*, and a rejection of the classic heroic therapies of bleeding and purging. In 1844, Harvard's Jacob Bigelow cautioned medical students against 'always thinking that you must make your patients worse before they can be better. I believe that much of the medical imposition of the present day is sustained in places where practice has previously been over-heroic, and because mankind are gratified to find that they and their families can get well without the lancet, the vomit, and the blister, indiscriminately applied'.[39]

Another Harvard professor in the mid-nineteenth century, Oliver Wendell Holmes, would rescue only opium, wine, and anaesthesia from the formulary. The rest of it could be sunk to the bottom of the sea. 'The best proof of it is, that no families take so little medicine as those of doctors.'[40] By the 1890s this kind of dubiety about heroic therapy had gathered enough steam to plough up not just bleeding and purging but virtually the entire traditional pharmacopoeia. William Osler, Canadian-born professor of medicine at Johns Hopkins University and one of the most influential physicians in the English-speaking world, limited himself in his 1892 textbook to a handful of drugs and said that for many diseases there was no treatment at all. For example, for malignant scarlet fever, 'The disease cannot be cut short. In the presence of the severer forms we are still too often helpless.'[41]

But family doctors do not want to be helpless. In primary care, the doctrine of therapeutic nihilism was anathema because physicians enjoy the feeling of helping and because patients crave a prescription at the end of the consultation. It was entirely unacceptable that patients should be sent away with the news that medicine was powerless in their case. Kansas doctor Arthur Hertzler summed up the position of the general practitioner around the turn of the century,

> In some cases I knew, even in the beginning, that my efforts would be futile in the matter of rendering service to anyone … Often I knew before I touched harness that the trips would be useless … Of course, one left some medicine in case of a recurrence of the trouble; this was largely the bunk, but someone had to pay for the axle grease and just plain advice never was productive of revenue unless fortified by a few pills. It was about as important as the deacon's 'Amen' during the preacher's sermons – it did no harm and it was an evidence of good faith.[42]

So what was the family doctor to do? His medicines were mainly 'the bunk' and he realized that in scientific terms either the patient would recover spontaneously from the infectious illness or he would not. Organically based medicine could do little save yield a diagnosis and prognosis. But the patients craved help.

In this logical dilemma was born the patient-as-a-person movement, a doctrine that would run through primary care from the l880s until the Second World War. The patient could not be helped with medicines, although these would be given anyway, but with the psychological support of the doctor. In seeing the patient as 'a person' and not just as 'a case of disease' the physician was able to approach him in an understanding and sympathetic manner that was *in and of itself therapeutic*. Here was born the reputation of the 'old-time GP' as being someone willing to sit and listen to his patients, to give them time to tell their stories, and advise them patiently about how to cope with their problems. It was not that the old-time doc was necessarily a more sensitive and humane individual than his predecessors or his successors, merely that he was therapeutically desperate and realized that he had nothing to give them except such psychological benefits as inherently resided in the consultation.

The patient-as-a-person movement originated within the commanding heights of medical science in Europe, but among physicians, whose particular bent was healing, rather than anatomical pathology. In Vienna, Hermann Nothnagel, professor of medicine after 1882, embodied the new philosophy. As he said in his l882 inaugural lecture, 'I repeat once again, medicine is about treating sick people and not diseases'.[43] Nothnagel was well known for his views about 'being a friend to the patient', and fought for their best interests, even at the cost of harsh words with the family doctor. He emphasized to the house staff at the Vienna General Hospital the importance of history-taking in the consultation – a key theme in the movement as a whole because in taking a long and careful history the doctor has the chance to establish an emotional rapport with the patient.

Nothnagel was fond of quoting a saying from an earlier prince of German medicine, Christoph Wilhelm Hufeland, to the effect that, 'Only a truly moral person can become a physician in the truest sense of the term'. (Interestingly, it was the nihilist Josef Škoda who had turned the whole world of romantic medicine that Hufeland embodied upside down.) Nothnagel's good nature did indeed shine through: he was unfavourably known among the generally anti-Semitic Viennese medical faculty as being philo-Semitic. Nothnagel, who had a huge consulting practice in the Vienna hotels, prescribed great quantities of the useless medications of the time, but established close rapport with his patients and was much loved by them.

Among the significant professors of medicine in Germany was Adolf Kussmaul. Towards l880 at Strasbourg, Kussmaul admonished the medical students. A young American physician, who was sitting in, recalled his words: 'the physician examines and treats the "patient" and not the "case". It was this insistence on the human and the humane side of medicine that made the deepest impression on me', wrote New York neurologist Barney Sachs many years later.[44]

In advocating 'Nature's healing ways', some late-nineteenth-century doctors were rejecting the classic therapies of bleeding and purging. Many came to believe that most medicines were 'bunk'. From a German guide to domestic medicine by Anna Fischer-Dückelmann (1903).

Noted American physicians also kept up a drumfire of support for seeing the patient as a person, which was not incompatible with a scientific disbelief in drugs. Most notably, William Osler embodied these humanistic values, teaching the medical students on rounds at Johns Hopkins University that, 'The good physician treats the disease but the great physician treats the patient who has the disease'.[45] One of his young students, Clarence B. Farrar who later became a psychiatrist, noted: 'Osler was instinctively practising psychotherapy without ever having studied it.'[46]

Another Osler student who went on to become a Hopkins clinician, developing all the while a successful private practice, was Lewellys Barker. Why has your practice been so successful, Dr Barker? 'I am of the opinion that to make patients like him, a doctor must himself have a real liking for people; he must be interested in *them* as well as in their *diseases*.'[47] In 1939, George Canby Robinson, another Osler student, wrote a book entitled *The Patient as a Person*, deploring that 'scientific satisfaction' was replacing 'human satisfaction' in medicine and urging the 'treatment of the patient as a whole'.[48]

Physicians in primary care found one aspect of the patient-as-a-person movement of particular interest: the utility of this approach in treating patients whose symptoms were 'functional' or 'psychosomatic' – in other words, symptoms that had arisen in the absence of any organic lesion but were defined by the patient as organic in nature. Such symptoms constituted – and constitute today – a huge amount of what was seen in primary care: a third or more of all patients. Here the patient-as-a-person movement had stellar advice to offer. As Francis Weld Peabody, the professor of internal medicine at Harvard University, volunteered in 1927, 'The successful diagnosis and treatment of these patients ... depends almost wholly on the establishment of that intimate personal contact between physician and patient which forms the basis of private practice. Without this, it is quite impossible for the physician to get an idea of the problems and troubles that lie behind so many functional disorders'.[49]

Harvard even started a course in 1941 on the 'Treatment of patients as persons'. Writing in 1936, William Houston, a professor of medicine in Georgia, commented that this kind of psychological sensitivity, was what distinguished the doctor from the veterinarian: 'All that part of a doctor's work that rises above the veterinary level, that part in which the personality of the doctor is the therapeutic agent and the personality of the patient is the object acted upon, may properly be called "psychological treatment".' But the psychology consisted in spending lots of time with patients and talking to them, and having some 'awareness of what [one] is about'.[50]

There is no doubt that this message was picked up by physicians in primary care. Daniel Cathell, in the 1924 edition of his famous doctors' guide, said 'It is often very satisfying to the sick to be allowed to tell, in their own way, whatever they deem important for you to know. Give a fair, courteous hearing, and, even though Mrs Chatterbox, Mr Borum, and Mrs Lengthy's statements are tedious, do not abruptly cut them short, but endure and listen with respectful attention, even though you are ready to drop exhausted.'[51] In Guy de Maupassant's novel *Mont-Oriol* (1887) about spa life, the newly arrived 'Docteur Black' draws the custom of all the wealthy elderly ladies at the spa. Why was this successful? Among other things, 'He heard their stories out without interruption, taking notes of all their observations, of all their questions, of all their wishes. Every day he would increase or decrease the dosage of water drunk by his patients, which gave them complete confidence in the care he was taking of them'.[52]

Hermann Nothnagel was probably wrong that to be successful in medicine a physician had to be a good person. Dr Black and countless other physicians doubtlessly used the show of concern as a marketing tactic in primary care. But why not? It was a tactic of great therapeutic effectiveness that responded to the patient's desire to be cared for, in the face of diseases that could not be cured.

SHIFTING THE SITE OF PRIMARY CARE

In 1950, after finishing a study of Britain's National Health Service, Joseph Collings announced that the day of the horse-and-buggy doctor was gone: 'It is absurd to try to recapture the 19th-century concept of the benign old doctor in his frock coat and silk hat sitting through the night, awaiting the pneumonia crisis or the delayed arrival of the first-born.'[53] Two things were killing off this old-style family doctor – a shift in the locus of medical practice from general practitioner to specialist, and a shift in the physical site of primary care from the patient's home to the doctor's surgery and the hospital outpatient department.

The rise of specialism at the end of the nineteenth century was in part pushed by public demand, in part pulled by medical supply. To specialists even more than to general practitioners clung the mantle of science, a powerful attraction for a public with implicit confidence in the wonders of progress. 'The inexorable public', mocked Walter Rivington in 1879, a surgeon at the London Hospital, 'will not believe in a man who is good all round. With the public a physician who can treat the liver is not good for the stomach, certainly not for the kidneys. The heart has no connexion with the lungs, and all the organs of the body are totally independent of one another.' Rivington spoke of patients who would 'come up from the country, and consult four or five separate practitioners – one for his general state, one for his ear, another for his chest, and another for his throat … The force of subdivision of the human body can no further go.'[54] Rivington mirrored the traditional distaste of British doctors for specialism.

But physicians followed the internal logic of their own interests to specialism, not just the fancy of the public. Subjects such as ophthalmic surgery did indeed possess demanding cores of knowledge that could not be mastered while staying abreast of the information needed for general practice. 'The line of skirmishers advancing into the No Man's Land of fresh knowledge is always radiating outwards, and breaking up into smaller groups', said Wilmot Herringham, himself a London physician, in 1920. 'First there is a continual invention of fresh instruments of precise observation or treatment' that called for specialized skill. He cited the laryngoscope and the urethral catheter. Then came inventions that called for specialized knowledge, such as the electrocardiograph.[55] All these specialists had something to offer the general practitioner in their function as consultants (giving opinions or doing procedures) but not – at this point – taking the family doctor's patients away.

The 1870s saw the flourishing of societies devoted to specialized knowledge on the East coast of the USA. New York City had, for example, a dermatological society, an obstetrical society, and a forensic-medicine society by the 1870s. London saw in the 1880s the formation of six specialty societies, including dental surgery, ophthamology, dermatology, gynaecology, neurology, and ear-nose-and-throat surgery. London's Harley Street, which had three doctors in 1840, had acquired ninety-seven by 1890, becoming the centre of gravity of London's consultant and specialty practice.

Now at this point an interesting divergence between the UK and the USA occurred. In Britain, family doctors retained an important share of primary care whereas, in the USA, they became a vanishing breed. In Britain, a fairly strict line had already been drawn by the turn of the century between primary care in the hands of general practitioners and specialist care in hospitals, for GPs lost the right to attend patients in hospital. As one writer commented, 'the demarcation of responsibilities between the urban GP and consultant was to take place at the gates of the city hospital'.[56] This cut GPs off from hospital science and hospital care, but preserved them as a group because a letter from a family doctor was

The medical profession grew enormously in the nineteenth century and for the first time prominent members began to meet in congresses. Their presence was readily immortalized by the new invention of photography. This is the 1881 International Medical Congress in London. International cooperation was, however, dashed by international rivalries, in medicine as in politics, in the era leading up to the First World War.

essential for referral to a hospital outpatient department or to a consultant. The National Health Insurance Act of 1911 then safeguarded the GP's survival by creating a system of 'panel doctors' in which GPs were paid to take on state-insured workers. By 1939 there were some 2,800 full-time consultants and specialists and 18,000 general practitioners in Britain. Among the 43,000 physicians in the UK in 1980, 65 per cent were still GPs.

In the USA, by contrast, general practitioners began disappearing around 1900, the result of the pressure of the specialists from above and the hospital outpatient departments from below. By the mid-1920s perhaps a quarter of the population of the largest cities was receiving its medical care in clinics and outpatient departments. In 1928, of some 152,000 physicians in the USA, 27 per cent had either limited themselves entirely to a specialty or were interested in one. By 1942 only 49 per cent of all doctors were GPs. The American public flocked to the specialists, shunning the 'old-time family doctor'. Daniel Cathell commented in 1924: 'Today a specialist wisely located in any large city must be but an ordinary man, not to get considerable business. While a general practitioner in a large city must be an extraordinary man to get much or any good, desirable business at all.'[57]

This drift away from general practice continued inexorably in the following decades in the USA. By 1989, of 469,000 physicians in active patient care, only 12 per cent were in general and family practice. Within the specialty practices, the great bulk of care was primary care. Several medical specialities were surveyed in 1977: only 3.5 per cent of all patient visits in internal medicine were referrals, the others were walk-ins; in obstetrics and gynaecology, only 4.4 per cent were referrals, in ophthamology 7.7 per cent, and so on. In no medical specialty were more than 13 per cent of the patients referred (urology), meaning that these doctors were giving primary care to most of their patients.

In a second change in locus, medical practice shifted from the patient's home to the doctor's surgery. Although the figure of the kindly old doc making housecalls retains its nostalgic appeal, one forgets easily how tough this work was on the physicians themselves, especially the arduousness of night calls, when a note that simply said 'come at once' could mean anything from a headache to a ruptured appendix.

Bernhard Naunyn recalled from the time of his general practice in the late 1860s in Berlin being hauled from bed in the wee hours three nights in a row. On the first night he had to climb up the stairs of some tenement in Kreuzberg to the bedside of a 'healthy looking young lad who was sleeping'. Naunyn woke him up. The boy looked about a bit dazed. 'So you see', said the father, 'that's the way he looked before too.' Naunyn assured the father that nothing was wrong with the boy and went home.

Medical practitioners took great pride in their instruments, and elaborate anaesthetists' bags and midwifery cases were offered for sale. Before the late nineteenth century, however, the importance of proper sterilization was not appreciated, and so instrument cases could be veritable deathtraps, harbouring lethal bacteria. In this advertisement from 1913, it is still assumed that the doctor will be going around in a horse-drawn carriage.

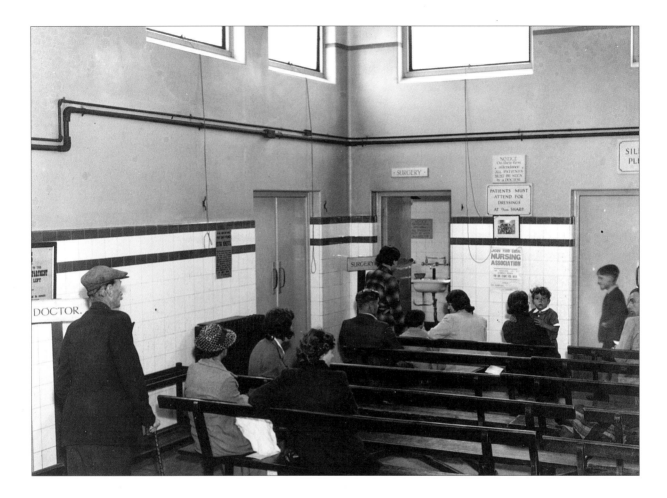

This hospital outpatient waiting-room on the eve of the Second World War indicates the strengths and weaknesses of public medicine as it emerged in Britain in the early to mid-twentieth century. On the one hand, is the scrupulous cleanliness of the tiled walls; on the other, the institutional officiousness of the 'silence' notice and the bleakness of the atmosphere. Patients were being reduced to medicine fodder.

On the second night at 3 a.m., there was another, similar occurrence, 'completely unfounded anxiety on the part of a worried mother'. 'When on the third night I was supposed to go out again between three and four, because the child was said to have "internal fits" I didn't go at once. I said I'd come as soon as I was up. Of course I couldn't then go back to sleep. I thought about the sick child, and soon I did get up, and went over there, and I found the child dead.'[58]

The maddening thing about housecalls, therefore, was that one could not tell which were emergencies: all summonses had to be answered. Then there was the sheer exhaustion of being on the road in a horse and buggy or on horseback, and spending the night on top of tables in the waiting rooms of railway stations.

Wasn't there a better way? The telephone made it possible for the physician to establish whether an emergency existed before going out. Motor transport, of course, let the doctor get about more easily on house calls but, more important, it permitted the patient to come to the doctor, or to the hospital emergency department. The first rudimentary telephone exchange on record, built in 1877, connected the Capital Avenue Drugstore in Hartford, Connecticut, with twenty-one local doctors.

House calls in winter

William Macartney, a general practitioner in Fort Covington, New York in the l890s and after, remembered what it was like to make house calls in the winter.

> On many a wintry night I got lost when there were no tracks, or the tracks were drifted over and the blizzard blotted out all landmarks. Occasionally I would have to tie my horse to a near-by fence, cover him with a big buffalo-robe and continue my journey on snowshoes. I recall such a night when my pony, exhausted by long battling with the drifts, fell, and was unable to rise. I covered her carefully with robes and my fur coat, and started through a sugar-wood for the nearest farm-house.

After himself collapsing in the deep snow and the bitter wind, Macartney was 'all in'. Then by chance 'the farmhouse door opened and two men came out on the way to the barn. I yelled, and the wind being favorable, they heard me, came with their lantern and dug me out'. Macartney warmed up in the farmhouse a bit, went back with the men to rescue his pony, and continued on his way.

When Macartney reached farm patients who were surgical emergencies, he would operate on the kitchen table. He carried with him a 50 per cent solution of mercuric chloride in glycerine and his instruments, and would use clean linen tablecloths for gauze material that the neighbours brought over. 'Thus equipped', Macartney 'opened abdomens, operated on hernias, mostly strangulated [a piece of the gut trapped in the groin], appendix cases and similar acute conditions.'[59]

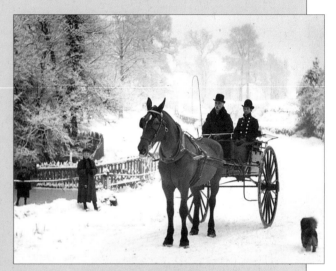

The horse-and-buggy doctor was a familiar and reassuring sight until the coming of the motor car speeded up the doctor's rounds early in the twentieth century.

Motorcars first became available in the l890s, and physicians were among the earliest customers for them. Ecstatic doctors talked of making housecalls in 'half the time', and increased their business as well by broadening their range. By l928, one small-town doctor in New Hampshire, USA, was covering 30,000–35,000 miles a year. 'With a single exception, it is five years since I have driven a horse', Ralph Tuttle wrote. 'This increased facility of transportation not only helps the doctor get to his patients but makes it possible to take the patients to a hospital'.[60] It had even become possible for a physician 'to keep office hours'. There was one more consequence. Because it was now possible for patients to get about easily, doctors stopped settling in rural areas in the USA. In 1926, physicians polled in 283 counties reported that in l00 of those counties no new medical graduate had settled within the previous 10 years. Cars had stimulated the urbanization of medical practice and the denuding of the countryside.

Urban medical practice itself became increasingly office- and hospital-based. Although in the USA as a whole in the late 1920s 50 per cent of all medical calls took place at home, big cities saw somewhat less home visiting. In 1929, in Philadelphia, only 39 per cent of the average GP's 64 hours a week was spent on housecalls. (Of the 50 hours that full-specialists put in a week, only 12 per cent were spent doing housecalls.) In the early 1950s, in 'Regionville' – an anonymous community selected for research – of 1,318 illnesses treated by doctors, only 22 per cent were seen at the patient's home, 71 per cent in the doctor's surgery (and the others in a variety of settings). By 1990, only 2 per cent of all physician contacts in the USA took place in the patient's home, 60 per cent in the surgery, and 14 per cent in a hospital outpatient department.

In Britain, home visiting remained more intact, doubtlessly because the National Health Service, enacted in England and Wales in 1946 and coming into being on 5 July 1948, had fortified the position of the general practitioner. According to one survey, as late as 1977, 19 per cent of all patient contact still took place in the form of home visits.

THE CHANGING NATURE OF THE CONSULTATION

In primary care during the twentieth century, serious infectious disease has become much less common, at least in the Western world; the subjective sensations of illness on the other hand have become more frequent, but they are cared for less intensively. These are the major changes over the past hundred years in patterns of help-seeking and care-giving.

The dominance of fever in general practice lasted right up to the years between the world wars. Describing in 1927 his own practice in Leeds, England, over a period of several years, Stanley Sykes put influenza as the commonest complaint with 335 cases: six of his patients had died of it. Then came acute bronchitis, tonsilitis, measles, whooping cough, and impetigo (a bacterial skin infection). Each of these, all major infectious illnesses, had occurred fifty or more times. Of Dr Sykes's thirty-two tuberculosis patients, ten had died. Pneumonia on his list (twenty-four patients with twelve deaths) beat cancer (twenty-three patients with twelve deaths). Only thirty-nine of his patients had heart disease, twenty of whom died. Dr Sykes was still seeing patients with typhoid fever, rheumatic fever, and erysipelas (a streptococcal infection causing redness and swelling under the skin).[61]

This picture of disease in general practice in the developed world would soon change radically. The major infections would fall away – a result of improvements in public health (such as more effective quarantining), of apparently spontaneous changes in the virulence of some infectious agents (such as the organisms causing scarlet fever and tuberculosis), and, finally, of improved therapy (such as the introduction of the sulpha drugs in 1935). A practice like Stanley Sykes's soon became a thing of the past. One British family doctor, Keith Hodgkin, wrote in 1963: 'Tuberculosis, meningitis, polio ... rheumatic fever, chilblains [reddening of fingers and toes from mild frostbite] and lobar pneumonia continue to decline and are disappearing from practice in Western countries.'[62]

In a report published in 1963 it was noted that the average general practitioner in the developed world 'might wait eight years to see a case of rheumatic fever in a child under the age of fifteen; sixty years to see a case of typhoid or paratyphoid fever; and as long as 400 years to see a case of diphtheria'.[63] Replacing the former major infectious illnesses in Western countries have come diseases related to modern lifestyles – lung cancer and coronary artery disease. Because upper respiratory infections – coughs and colds – also count as infectious illnesses, it is difficult to make the claim that infectious illness as a whole has declined. Yet the conclusion is justified that among serious medical problems in the Western world, the major infectious diseases of the past have given way to chronic degenerative diseases today, such as cancer, heart disease, and arthritis.

In spite of the decline of acute infectious illness, the population seems to be feeling worse than better. Systematic door-to-door surveys of the USA in 1928–31 and again in 1981 make it possible to compare rates of illness, or the sense of wellbeing, of the population over this 50-year period. The annual number of self-reported illnesses per hundred population rose from 82 in 1928–31 to 212 in 1981, a 158 per cent increase. This increase was not the result of a rise in chronic illness, for among children aged 5–14 (an age group generally not subjected to chronic disease) the rate of reported illness rose by 233 per cent. The explanation of this striking rise in the subjective sensation of illness, at a time when major infectious disease in the developed world has declined, may be that individuals as a whole have become more sensitive to bodily symptoms and more inclined to seek help for physical sensations that earlier generations would have dismissed as trivial.

With this increase in the perception of illness, there has been an increase in medical helpseeking. In the USA, in 1928–31, the average person visited the doctor only 2.9 times a year; by 1964, this had risen to 4.6 times a year, and to 5.5 times in 1990. In Britain, in 1975, the average person had three NHS consultations a year; by 1990, this had risen to five.

But these rising global rates of consultation do not necessarily mean that each individual illness is intensively seen. In the years before 1940, doctors would see an ill patient quite often. How many home calls were necessary for a typical illness? An American survey done in 1928–31 found that for a cold, the doctor would consult 2.4 times (either at home or the surgery), for a reportable communicable disease, 3.6 times, and for a digestive disease 6.2 times. On the whole, 3.6 home calls would be necessary for a typical illness.

In England, patients expected the doctor to visit often. It was, explained Stanley Sykes, so easy for the family doctor to get backlogged. Of a hundred patients on your visiting list, 'You see perhaps fifteen on the first day. The arrears accumulate with alarming rapidity, and the inevitable result is that indignant messages or relatives are arriving every day demanding to know why the doctor hasn't been. It is futile to explain that you are busy. To a sick man there is only one patient in the universe, and that is himself.'[64] This adds up to an extraordinary intensity of care in illness.

Although we do not have comparable statistics on the intensity of treatment today, people sometimes lack the feeling that their woes are being looked after. The much higher annual rates of consultation today, combined with the decline in acute infectious illness, suggests that patients of today consult more regularly over the course of the year, in a kind of ongoing anxiety about wellness, rather than demanding the doctor's presence at the bedside on the odd occasion when they are genuinely ill.

But even if today's patient did lie febrile, he or she would probably see the doctor only in the surgery or in the hospital emergency department, and not at home. Physicians have many techniques for keeping the patient at bay, including unlisted phone numbers, answering services, and nurse-receptionists who have their own notions of the hierarchy of urgency in medical diagnosis. Hence, as one observer said, 'There is a longing on the part of patients for that old doctor – one always available, ever kindly, modest in fees, and inspiring in manner'.[65]

PRIMARY CARE AND MEDICINE TODAY

A cartoon in *The Spectator* in 1990 captured the mood of the post-modern patient. The wife, who has just hung up the phone, informs the bedridden husband, 'The doctor doesn't visit any more. He says why don't you drop in when you're feeling better?'

In February 1935, a German biochemist, Gerhard Domagk wrote an article in a German medical journal on the subject of a brick-red sulphonamide dye called 'Prontosil Rubrum' that combated staphylococcal and streptococcal infections (page 269). At last, a medication had been found that was effective against many different bacterial killers. Prontosil and its relatives became known as the 'sulpha' drugs, and their appearance marked the beginning of the post-modern period of medicine. The discovery of prontosil represented a turning of the page. For the first time in history medicine could really heal diseases that were common and affected large numbers of the population – the many fevers and bacterial infections of the past. They became known as the 'wonder drugs': the long list of sulpha drugs introduced after 1935 and then penicillin and the many antibiotics used for the first time on the civilian population after the Second World War. They gave to medicine enormous new therapeutic power.

The antibiotics were just the beginning. In the explosion of biochemical and pharmacological research that followed the Second World War, drugs were discovered that relieved arthritis, that fought cancer, that reduced high blood pressure, and that dissolved clots in blocked coronary arteries. These drugs caused a transformation not just of clinical medicine, but of doctors' attitudes towards patients, and towards the consultation. The introduction of these drugs and the investigation of the biochemical mechanisms that lie behind their success represented the beginning of medicine's post-modern period. If the modern period had been characterized by the doctor's ability to diagnose disease scientifically while being therapeutically powerless against it, the post-modern period was characterized by the ability to triumph over the classic killers of humankind and to relieve suffering on a scale hitherto undreamt.

A basic theme in the history of primary care has been the necessity of giving the patients what they want. The irony of post-modern medicine is that, although doctors have become therapeutically far more awesome than ever before, they have ceased giving the patients what they want. Effective against disease at an organic level, doctors have often found it no longer necessary to enlist the psychological benefits of the doctor–patient relationship in bolstering the patient through an illness. The whole patient-as-a-person movement fell into desuetude after 1950, replaced by a new generation of physicians filled with an overweening therapeutic self-confidence. The aspects of the doctor–patient relationship to which patients had once thrilled, such as the physician's show of interest in the history-taking or the laying on of hands in the physical exam, became downplayed in favour of using the resources of diagnostic imaging and of laboratory tests in the diagnosis of disease. It was not that physicians became somehow more inhumane, merely that the previous display of apparent humanity had now become therapeutically unnecessary.

Thus post-modern medicine has become haunted by a growing dissatisfaction among patients with primary care. The sympathetic old doc, always willing to turn an apparently attentive ear, has become a totemic figure in tirades against the impersonality of the health-care system. Grateful as patients have been for the new drugs, they have become increasingly resentful of those who prescribe them, hurling showers of malpractice suits against physicians perceived as remote and arrogant. Alternative medicine, with its confidence in the therapeutic benefits of stroking the soles of the feet or getting those poisons out of there with colonic irrigation, has undergone a rebirth.

This failure to supply what is psychologically required to gratify the patient has thus produced a supreme irony. At the very moment that science has conferred success over much of the vast range of disease that plagues humanity, the crown of victory has been snatched from the physician's head. An adversarial note has entered the doctor–patient relationship, and it has become, rightly or wrongly, increasingly anachronistic to claim of a post-modern doctor what the patients of an old family doctor in Chicago once said to him, with a hug about the neck: 'Oh, you dear, good man, how we all love you!' [66]

<table>
<tr><td>CHAPTER 5</td><td></td></tr>
</table>

CHAPTER 5   *Medical Science*

Roy Porter

In medieval times, the educated physicians of the Islamic East and the Christian West practised medicine on the basis of the teachings of the Ancient Greeks. By the late Middle Ages, however, there was growing dissatisfaction with certain deeply entrenched doctrines, and the new intellectual ferment we call the Renaissance – the quest to purify old doctrines and discover new truths – encouraged fresh biomedical inquiry. During the Renaissance, medicine was put on a surer footing, particularly once the Scientific Revolution brought glowing success to the mechanical sciences, physics, and chemistry.

LAYING THE ANATOMICAL FOUNDATIONS

Of fundamental importance in enhancing the standing of medicine was the pursuit of systematic human anatomy. Doctors in ancient Athens had treated the human body as sacred, and honoured it by refraining from cutting up dead bodies. In spite of their many contributions, therefore, Hippocratic and the later Galenic medicine were anatomically weak. Analogous views about the sanctity of the body (the belief that it belonged to God not man) later led the Roman Catholic Church to voice some opposition to dissecting the dead. Common people also felt deep misgivings. Grass-roots hostility to dissection made itself felt in Britain even as late as the passing of the Anatomy Act in 1832. This was not surprising, given the notorious activities of William Burke and William Hare and other 'resurrection men'. In Edinburgh, Burke and Hare murdered the subjects they then sold for research to the medical school.

A sound anatomical and physiological basis is to us essential to scientific medicine, but it could develop only out of systematic dissection. Ecclesiastical opposition to dissection slowly melted away in medieval times. During the Black Death in the mid-fourteenth century, the Papacy sanctioned postmortems to search the cause of the pestilence, but it was not until 1537 that Pope Clement VII finally accepted the teaching of anatomy by dissection. From the fourteenth century, however, dissections grew more common, especially in Italy, which was then the centre of scientific inquiry (see page 75). Early anatomical demonstrations were public occasions, almost spectacles, for the purpose not of research but instruction – they allowed the professor to parade his proficiency. Dressed in long robes he would sit in a high chair reading out relevant passages from the works of Galen, while his assistant pointed to the organs alluded to and a dissector did the knifework. Early in the sixteenth century Leonardo da Vinci produced some 750 anatomical drawings. These were done in a purely private capacity, perhaps in secret, and made no impact at all on medical progress.

The real breakthrough came with the work of Andreas Vesalius. Born in 1514 the son of a Brussels pharmacist, Vesalius studied in Paris, Louvain, and Padua,

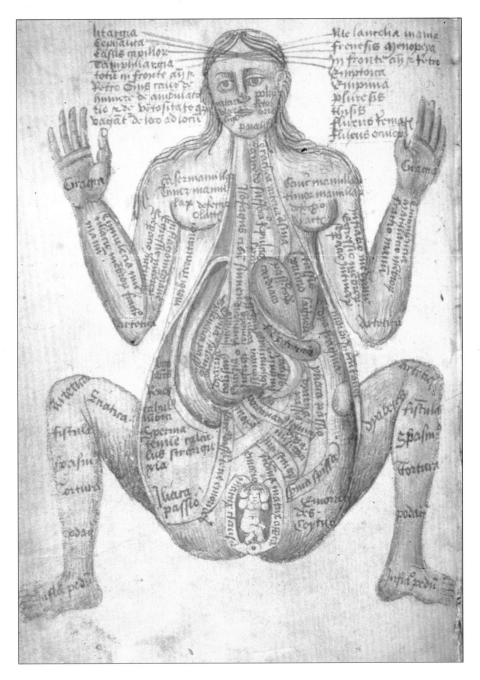

Before the invention and spread of printing from the mid-fifteenth century, anatomical illustrations were relatively rare and lacked the precision and standardization that reproduction techniques made possible – and, of course, the anatomical expertise that came with Renaissance dissections. Here the female body is laid bare. The apparent visual crudity of this and similar late-medieval anatomical images is not due to the absence of artists skilled in representing reality. In the Later Middle Ages, illustrations served not to depict what was before the artist's eye but to represent general truths in visual form. Squatting figures, depicted frontally and with legs astride, were used to show disease, wounds, and the influence of the zodiac on parts of the body. Realism was irrelevant: the aim was to reinforce the verbal message, to indicate the standard conclusions of learned physic. These images were evidently successful for they survived into the age of print, woundmen in particular being used in books of sixteenth-century surgery. They presented the body as a teaching-aid, neatly labelled and connected to the macrocosm.

where he took his medical degree in 1537, becoming at once a professor there; later, he became court physician to the Holy Roman Emperor Charles V and to Philip II of Spain. In 1543, he published his masterwork, *De Humani Corporis Fabrica* (On the Structure of the Human Body). In the exquisitely illustrated text, printed in Basel, Vesalius praised observation and challenged Galenic teachings on various points, recognizing that Galen's beliefs rested on knowledge of animals rather than humans. He criticized other doctors for describing the *plexus reticu-*

Andreas Vesalius was the first Renaissance anatomist systematically to test the teachings of the Ancient Greeks against the visual evidence of personal dissection. His massive *De Humani Corporis Fabrica* (1543) was brilliantly and profusely illustrated. Produced by the press of Joannes Oporinus, it is one of the jewels of Renaissance printing as well as a turning point in the medical view of the structure of the human body. Vesalius tested Galen by reference to the human body. The *Fabrica* gained immensely by the contributions of the artist, John Stephen of Kalkar in Germany, who provided the text with naturalistic yet technically precise drawings that showed the dissected body in life-like poses.

laris because they had seen it in Galen's writings but never actually in a human body. He chided himself for once believing in Galen and the writings of other anatomists.

Vesalius's great contribution lay in creating a new atmosphere of inquiry and in setting anatomical study on solid foundations of observed fact. Although his work contained no startling discoveries, it induced a shift in intellectual strategy. After Vesalius, appeals to ancient authority lost their unquestioned validity, and his successors were compelled to stress precision and personal, and first-hand observation. Vesalius's work was quickly honoured: Ambroise Paré, the leading surgeon of the day, used it for the anatomical section of his classic work on surgery, published in 1564 (see page 206).

Vesalius presented exact descriptions and illustrations of the skeleton and muscles, the nervous system, the viscera, and the blood vessels. His followers developed his techniques in greater depth and detail. In 1561, his student and successor as professor of anatomy at Padua, Gabrielle Falloppio (Fallopius), published a volume of anatomical observations that elucidated and corrected aspects of his work. Falloppio's findings included structures in the human skull and ear, and research into the female genitalia. He coined the term vagina, described the clitoris, and was the first to delineate the tubes leading from the ovary to the uterus. Ironically, however, he failed to grasp the function of what became known as the Fallopian tubes; only two centuries later was it recognized that eggs were formed in the ovaries, passing down those tubes to the uterus. Early anatomy thus outran physiology.

By the close of the sixteenth century, Vesalian anatomy had become the golden method for anatomical investigations. Another Italian pioneer, Bartolommeo Eustachio, discovered the Eustachian tube (from the throat to the middle ear) and the Eustachian valve of the heart; he also examined the kidneys and explored the anatomy of the teeth. In 1603, Falloppio's successor at Padua, Girolamo Fabrizio (Fabricius ab Acquapendente), published a study of the veins that contained the first descriptions of their valves; this was to prove an inspiration to the English physician William Harvey. Slightly later, Gasparo Aselli of Padua drew attention to the lacteal vessels of the mesentery and identified their function as carrying chyle from food. This led to further studies of the stomach; Franz de le Boë (Franciscus Sylvius) of Leiden was later able to outline a chemical theory of digestion. Work also proceeded on the structure of the kidney, while Regnier de Graaf, a Dutch physician, was able to provide by 1670 a high-quality description of the reproductive system, discovering the Graafian vesicles of the female ovary.

Thus the work of Vesalius lent impetus to explorations of the organs of the body, although it must be said that Renaissance researches generally had a better grasp of structure than function. A climate of opinion had, however, been created in which anatomy became the foundation of medical science.

WILLIAM HARVEY AND THE NEW SCIENCE

The growing prestige of anatomical knowledge began to change the orientation of study of the body and its disorders. The humoral theories of Hippocrates and his followers had viewed health and disease in terms of overall fluid balance. This was challenged in the Renaissance by a new concern with precise bodily mechanisms.

From earliest times, blood had been viewed as a life-giving fluid, perhaps the most significant of the four humours (see page 58): it was recognized to nourish the body, although when disordered it was the cause of inflammation and fever. Galen's theory of the production and motion of blood long held sway. He believed that the veins that carried blood originated in the liver (the arteries stemmed from the heart). Blood was concocted (literally 'cooked') in the liver; it then migrated outwards on a kind of tidal motion through the veins into organs, where it carried nourishment and was consumed. The part of the blood proceeding from the liver to the right ventricle of the heart divided into two streams. The former passed along the pulmonary artery to the lungs, the latter traversed the heart through 'interseptal pores' into the left ventricle, where it mingled with air (*pneuma*), became heated, and proceeded from the left ventricle to the aorta, to the lungs and the periphery. The linkage of arteries with veins permitted some *pneuma* to enter the veins, while the arteries received some blood.

Galen's characterization of the blood system carried authority for fifteen hundred years. By 1500, however, his teachings were beginning to be questioned. Michael Servetus, a Spanish theologian and physician, offered a hypothesis about a 'smaller circulation' through the lungs, and implied that blood could not (Galen notwithstanding) flow through the septum of the heart but must find its way across the lungs from the right to the left side of the heart. In 1559, Servetus's hints about the pulmonary circulation of the blood were reiterated by the Italian anatomist, Realdo Colombo. In his *De Re Anatomia* Colombo showed, against Galen, that there were no openings in the heart's dividing wall between its auricles and ventricles. Colombo's theory became widely known, but in the short term it did not produce any serious threat to Galen's doctrines. In his 1603 treatise, Girolamo Fabrizio described venous valves but drew no inferences regarding the operations of the blood system. That was left to William Harvey.

Harvey's revolutionary work was not universally accepted. Parisian physicians, notoriously conservative, remained loyal for some time to Galenic teachings, and Harvey supposedly complained that his medical practice 'fell off mightily' after he published *De Motu Cordis* in 1628

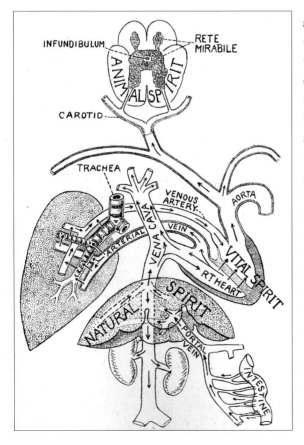

Galen's physiological scheme, as interpreted in 1946 by the medical historian Charles Singer.

The revolutionary ideas of William Harvey

William Harvey was born in Folkestone, Kent, the eldest of seven sons in the family of a yeoman farmer. He went to school in Canterbury, proceeding to study medicine at Caius College, Cambridge. Graduating in 1597, he moved to Padua, working under Girolamo Fabrizio. In 1602, he set up in practice in London as a physician and was elected a Fellow of the Royal College of Physicians in 1607. Two years later he was appointed physician to St Bartholomew's Hospital, and in 1615 he was Lumleian lecturer at the College of Physicians.

While studying under Fabrizio from 1600 to 1602, Harvey pursued investigations into the operations of the heart, which allowed him to write as early as 1603: 'the movement of the blood occurs constantly in a circular manner and is the result of the beating of the heart'.[1] These new ideas he finally published in Frankfurt in 1628 under the title *Exercitatio Anatomica de Motu Cordis et Sanguinis in Animalibus* (An Anatomical Disquisition Concerning the Motion of the Heart and the Blood in Animals).

Harvey developed his revolutionary theory of blood circulation by painstaking observation and cautious reasoning from such phenomena as the one-way system of valves. He made no use of microscopes – these had only recently been introduced – and he followed what might be called an old-fashioned Aristotelian approach to the philosophy of Nature, emphasizing the perfection of circular motion when formulating and vindicating his theory that blood circulates round the body. Harvey approved of Aristotle's teleological perception of the body's operations – that the body's structures must be designed to fulfil the particular functions they perform. Yet, he insisted, when he compared the old Galenic doctrines about the heart and blood with the actual structures, he found many problems and paradoxes. If, as Galen maintained, the pulmonary veins were destined 'for the conveyance of air', why, queried Harvey, did they have the same structure as blood vessels? Such questions excited Harvey's inquisitiveness.

In *De Motu Cordis*, tellingly dedicated to King Charles I, Harvey set forth his radically new theory, asserting that the heart was a pump that effected the circulation of the blood around the body. 'The heart of animals is the foundation of their life', he maintained:

> the sovereign of everything within them, the sum of their microcosm, that upon which all the growth depends, from which all power proceeds. The King, in like manner, is the foundation of his kingdom; the sun of the world around him, the heart of the republic, the fountain whence all power, all grace doth flow . . . Almost all things human are done after human examples, and many things in a king are after the pattern of the heart. The knowledge of his heart, therefore, will not be useless to a Prince, as embracing a kind of Divine example of his functions, – and it has still been usual with men to compare small things with great. Here . . . you may at once contemplate the prime mover in the body of man, and the emblem of your own sovereign power.[2]

There was a certain irony in this view. Harvey extolled the heart ('the sovereign of everything'), yet reduced it to a piece of machinery, a mere pump, just another part in the corporeal engineering.

The veins of the forearm, in Harvey's *De Mortu Cordis*. Harvey could not see the minute connections – the capillaries – between the arteries and veins, but he showed that a connection must exist. He ligated an arm tightly so that the arterial blood could flow between the ligature down the arm. He then loosened the ligature so that arterial blood flowed down the arm, but the ligature remained tight enough to stop venous blood from moving up above the ligature. When the ligature had been tight, the veins below the ligature appeared normal, but with it loosened they became swollen, indicating that blood had moved down the arteries and then back up the arm inside the veins. At the extremities, therefore, there had to be connections for the blood to travel from the arteries to the veins.

A folio from Marcello Malpighi's *Opera Omnia* (1686), showing microscopic views of the lung and its network of capillaries. The development of the microscope in the seventeenth century opened major new opportunities for physiological research, involving, for example, the discovery of red blood cells. The disclosure of capillaries showed for the first time the pathways of the blood from the arteries to veins and hence gave visual proof of William Harvey's theory of the circulation of the blood.

because patients, too, were suspicious of new-fangled teachings. Nevertheless, Harvey's inspiration spurred and guided further physiological inquiry. A clutch of younger English researchers continued his work on the heart, lungs, and respiration.

One was Thomas Willis, who became a founder member of London's Royal Society (1662) and Sedleian Professor of Natural Philosophy at Oxford, and was also a fashionable London physician. Willis pioneered study of the anatomy of the brain, and of diseases of the nervous system and muscles, discovering the 'circle of Willis' in the brain. The most brilliant of the English Harveians, however, was Richard Lower. Born into an old Cornish family, he studied at Oxford and followed Willis to London. He collaborated with the mechanical philosopher Robert Hooke in a series of experiments, exploring how the lungs changed dark-red venous blood into bright-red arterial blood, and publishing his findings in *Tractatus de Corde* (Treatise on the Heart) in 1669. Lower earned a certain immortality by conducting at the Royal Society the first blood-transfusion experiments, transferring blood from dog to dog, and from person to person.

Physicians met scientists (or 'natural philosophers' as they were then called) at such venues as the Royal Society and exchanged ideas and techniques. Physicians felt there was all to gain from making their doctrines more 'scientific'. A new aid was the microscope, developed by Antoni van Leeuwenhoek in the Netherlands and taken up by Robert Hooke. Another lay in the startling contemporary advances in natural philosophy in general, above all in the physical sciences. The mechanical philosophy promoted by René Descartes, Robert Boyle, Hooke, and others presented the idea of the machine (with its levers, cogs, pulleys, and so forth) as the model for the body. Building on Harvey, many suggested a hydraulic understanding of its pipes, vessels, and tubes. Fashionable philosophers now rejected the old humoral theories as nothing but verbal flimflam, lacking any basis in material reality.

The mechanical philosophy stimulated new research programmes. In Italy, Marcello Malpighi conducted a remarkable series of microscopic studies of the structure of the liver, skin, lungs, spleen, glands, and brain, many of which were published in early numbers of the *Philosophical Transactions* of the Royal Society. Giovanni Borelli of Pisa and other 'iatrophysicists' (doctors convinced that the laws of physics offered the key to the body's operations) studied muscle behaviour, gland secretions, respiration, heart action, and neural responses. Working in Rome under the sponsorship of Sweden's Queen Christina, Borelli's main contribution was a treatise, *De Motu Animalium* (On Animal Motion), published in 1680–1. He made remarkable observations on birds in flight, fish swimming, muscular contraction, the mechanics of breathing, and a host of similar subjects, and attempted, more boldly than any before him, to comprehend body functions primarily in terms of the laws of physics.

Exploring what made the body machine work, Borelli postulated the presence of a 'contractile element' in the muscles; their operation was triggered by processes similar to chemical fermentation. He viewed respiration as a purely mechanical process that drove air through the lungs into the bloodstream. Familiar with the air-pump experiments conducted by Otto von Guericke and Robert Boyle, in which small animals expired in 'rarified' air (that is, a vacuum), he maintained that 'aerated blood' included elements vital to life. Air possessed, he said, a life-sustaining function because it served as a vehicle for 'elastic particles' that entered the blood to impart internal motion to it. In Borelli's highly innovative work, physics and chemistry together promised to unravel the secrets of life.

Seventeenth-century anatomists treated the body as a machine, activated by devices such as pulleys and levers, and understandable in terms of geometry, statics, and dynamics. Perhaps the fullest attempt to give a quantitive description of the body was made by a disciple of Galileo, Giovanni Alfonso Borelli, who was also an astronomer and mathematician. In his *De Motu Animalium* of 1680–1, from which this demonstration of the leg joints is taken, he calculated the force exerted by the pull of different muscles, and analysed in geometrical terms how human muscles act when used in walking and running.

Another innovative attempt to analyse the body in scientific terms lay in iatrochemistry. Whereas iatrophysics read the human frame through the laws of physics, iatrochemists applied chemical analysis. Repudiating the humours as archaic and fanciful, certain investigators looked back to the chemical theories of the sixteenth-century Swiss iconoclast, Paracelsus dismissed by some as a quack but respected by many as a major medical reformer. Paracelsus harked back to the simplicity of Hippocrates, learned from folk medicine, and believed in the power of nature to cure the body and heal the mind (see page 248).

Devotees of Paracelsus also drew on the opinions of his Netherlandish follower, Johannes (Jean) Baptiste van Helmont. Van Helmont rejected Paracelsus's notion of a single *archeus* (or indwelling spirit), developing instead the idea that each organ has its own specific *blas* (spirit) regulating it. His concept of 'spirit' was not mystical but material and chemical. He held all vital processes to be chemical, each being due to the action of a particular ferment or gas. These ferments were imperceptible spirits capable of converting food into living flesh. Transformative processes occurred throughout the body, but particularly in the stomach, liver, and heart. Van Helmont deemed body heat a by-product of chemical fermentations, arguing that the whole system was governed by a soul situated in the pit of the stomach. Chemistry, broadly understood, was thus the key to life. Views like these were radical. Gui Patin, leader of the ultra-orthodox medical faculty in Paris, denounced van Helmont as a 'mad Flemish scoundrel'.

One of van Helmont's chief followers was Franciscus Sylvius. A supporter of William Harvey who taught at Leiden, Sylvius emphasized the salience of blood

circulation for general physiology. He disparaged van Helmont's ideas as too eso-
teric, seeking to substitute for his gases and ferments notions of bodily processes
that combined chemical analysis with circulation theory. Even more than van Helmont, Sylvius concentrated on digestion, arguing that this fermentive process
occurred in the mouth, in the heart – where the digestive fire was kept burning by
chemical reactions – and in the blood, moving outwards to the bones, tendons,
and the flesh.

By 1700, in other words, advances in gross anatomy – and, after William Harvey, in physiology also – had created the dream of a scientific understanding of the
body's structures and functions, drawing on and matching those of the new and
highly prestigious mechanics and mathematics. Scientific medicine during the
following century fulfilled certain of these goals, but also saw them frustrated.

THEORIES OF LIFE IN THE AGE OF ENLIGHTENMENT

During the eighteenth century, the Age of Enlightenment, research into general
anatomy – bones, joints, muscles, fibres, and so on – continued along lines developed by Andreas Vesalius and his followers. Demonstrating supreme artistic skill
and capitalizing on improvements in printing, many splendid anatomical atlases
were published, including folios such as the *Osteographia* (1733) of the London
surgeon-anatomist William Cheselden.

Careful investigation into individual organs continued, spurred by the fascination shown by Marcello Malpighi and other exponents of the 'new science' in bellows, syringes, pipes, valves, and the similar contrivances. Anatomists struggled
to lay bare the form/function relationship of minute (sometimes microscopical)
structures, in the light of images of the organism as a system of vessels, tubes, and
fluids. The laws of mechanics thus underwrote anatomical inquiry.

The Dutch anatomist Herman Boerhaave, the greatest medical teacher of his
times (see page 124), proposed that physical systems operating throughout the
body comprised an integrated, balanced whole in which pressures and liquid
flows were equalized and everything found its own level. Spurning the earlier
'clockwork' models of René Descartes as too crude, Boerhaave treated the body as
a plumbing network of pipes and vessels, containing, channelling, and controlling
body fluids. Health was explained by the movement of fluids in the vascular system; sickness was largely explained in terms of its obstruction or stagnation. The
old humoral emphasis on balance had thus been preserved but translated into
mechanical and hydrostatic terms.

Yet the fascination felt by Boerhaave and others in the mechanics of the body
does not mean that medicine had become dogmatically reductionist or materialist. The presence of a soul in human beings could be taken for granted, but (Boerhaave judiciously maintained) inquiry into the essence of life or the immaterial
soul was irrelevant to the nitty-gritty of medicine, whose business lay in the investigation of tangible physiological and pathological structures and processes. Con-

siderations of the soul, in Boerhaave's opinion, were best left to priests and metaphysicians: medicine should study secondary causes not primary causes, the 'how', not the 'why' and 'wherefore'.

Certain aspects of Newton's natural philosophy, however, encouraged investigators to dismiss narrowly mechanistic views of the body and to pose wider questions about the properties of life. That meant reopening old debates over historic subjects, such as the doctrine of the soul. Highly significant was the work of the German chemist and physician Georg Ernst Stahl.

The founder of the distinguished Prussian medical school at the University of Halle in 1693, Stahl advanced classic anti-mechanistic arguments. Purposive human actions could not, he maintained, be wholly explained in terms of mechanical chain-reactions – like a stack of dominoes toppling over or balls cannoning round a billiard table. Wholes were greater than the sum of their parts. he claimed. Purposive human activity presupposed the presence of a soul, understood as a constantly intervening, presiding power, the very quintessence of the organism. More than a Cartesian 'ghost in the machine' (present but essentially separate), Stahl's *anima* (soul) was the ever-active agent of consciousness and physiological regulation, and a body-guard against sickness. For disease, in his view, was a disturbance of vital functions provoked by maladies of the soul. The body,

strictly speaking, was guided by an immortal spirit. Because the soul acted directly at bottom – that is, without need for the mediation of the *archæi* (ferments) of van Helmont or any other physical intermediaries – neither gross anatomy nor chemistry had much explanatory power: to fathom the operations of the body required understanding the soul and life itself.

Friedrich Hoffmann, Stahl's younger colleague at Halle, looked rather more favourably upon the new mechanical theories of the body. 'Medicine', he pronounced, 'is the art of properly utilizing physico-mechanical principles, in order to conserve the health of man or to restore it if lost.'[3]

Experimental researches into living bodies in the eighteenth century continually raised the question: is the living organism essentially a machine, or something different? Certain discoveries revealed the phenomenal powers possessed by living beings, not least a wonderful capacity to regenerate themselves in a manner unlike clocks or pumps. In 1712, the French naturalist René Réaumur demonstrated the ability of the claws and scales of lobsters to grow again after being severed. In the 1740s, the Swiss investigator Abraham Trembley divided polyps or hydras, and found that complete new individuals grew; he got a third generation by cutting up the latter. There was obviously more to life than the mechanists suspected.

During the eighteenth century, the movement towards elaborate, accurate, and beautiful anatomical atlases, begun with Vesalius in the Renaissance, reached its peak. William Cheselden's *Osteographia* (1733), from which this drawing of the torso is taken, was one of the finest of such works. It provided a full illustration of his masterpiece, *Anatomy of the Human Body* (1713). Cheselden taught anatomy and performed surgery at St Thomas's Hospital, London, specializing in the removal of bladder stones.

Mechanistic views of the body

The soaring prestige of the physical sciences stimulated the urge to measure the operations of the body machine. The great pioneer was the Italian Santorio Santorio, who settled in Venice in 1599 after 14 years as physician to the King of Poland and moved to Padua as professor of theoretical medicine in 1611. Santorio carried out an elaborate series of calculations of his own weight, food intake, and excreta, in particular so as to quantify weight loss through insensible perspiration. A friend of Galileo, he invented instruments to gauge humidity and temperature, and a pendulum for measuring the pulse rate. Early in the eighteenth century, Gabriel Daniel Fahrenheit, a German man of science, improved the reliability and accuracy of the alcohol thermometer and, in 1714, invented the mercury thermometer and the temperature scale still associated with his name. Around the same time, an Englishman, John Floyer, developed a watch for quantifying the pulse.

The most daring physiological experimentalist of the early eighteenth century was, however, an Anglican clergyman, Stephen Hales, vicar of Teddington in Middlesex. He devised 'haemodynamic' experiments to calibrate blood circulation, expounded in gory detail in his *Statical Essays* (1731–3). He gauged the force of the blood by inserting long brass tubes into the jugular vein and carotid artery of living horses, observing that the arterial pressure (measured in terms of column height) was far greater than the venous. Through his quantifying experiments with blood pressure, heart capacity, and blood-flow velocity, the Revd Hales made notable headway in circulation physiology. A dauntless animal experimenter, the clergyman also followed up Descartes' interest in reflex action by decapitating frogs and then exciting their reflexes by pricking the skin.

A portrait of Stephen Hales published in 1800. Vivisection experiments like those of Hales did not lack critics in the eighteenth century. By 1758, the normally tough-minded Samuel Johnson was deploring the fact that animal experiments were 'being published every day with ostentation' by doctors who 'extend the arts of torture'.

Experimentation led to new opinions regarding the character of vitality – and, by implication, the relations between body and mind, body, and soul. The premier figure in these debates was a Swiss polymath, Albrecht von Haller, who produced a pathbreaking text, the *Elementa Physiologiae Corporis Humani* (Elements of the Physiology of the Human Body) in 1757–66. Building on Boerhaave's concern with the fibres, Haller's finest contribution was his laboratory demonstration of the hypothesis proposed by Francis Glisson in the mid-seventeenth century that irritability (also known as contractility) was a property inherent in muscular fibres, whereas sensibility (feeling) was the exclusive attribute of nervous fibres.

Haller thus established the fundamental division of fibres according to their reactive properties. The sensibility of nervous fibres lay in their responsiveness to painful stimuli; the irritability of muscle fibres was their property of contracting in reaction to stimuli. Haller thereby advanced a physical explanation – something William Harvey had lacked – of why the heart pulsated: it was the most 'irritable' organ in the body. Composed of layers of muscular fibres, it was stimulated by the inflowing of blood, responding with systolic contractions.

On the basis of experimental procedures used on animals and humans, Haller's theories thus differentiated organ structures according to their fibre composition, ascribing to them intrinsic sensitivities independent of any transcendental, religious soul. Like Newton when faced with the phenomenon of gravity, Haller believed that the causes of such vital forces were beyond knowing – if not completely unknowable, at least unknown. It was sufficient, in true Newtonian fashion, to study effects and the laws of those effects. Haller's concepts of irritability and sensibility achieved widespread acclaim and formed the basis for further neurophysiological investigation.

A Scottish school of 'animal economy' (the contemporary phrase for physiology) also arose, centred on the impressive new Edinburgh University medical school, founded in 1726. Like Haller, Robert Whytt, a pupil of Alexander Monro *primus*, explored nervous activity, but Whytt contested Haller's doctrine of the inherent irritability of the fibres. In *On the Vital and Other Involuntary Motions of Animals* (1751), he argued that the reflex involved 'an unconscious sentient principle . . . residing in the brain and spinal cord', although he denied that his teaching entailed any undercover reintroduction of the *anima* of Stahl or the Christian soul. Whytt's view that body processes involved insensible purposive activities may be seen as an early attempt to grapple with the problem of what Sigmund Freud would later call the unconscious.

One who built on Haller's concept of irritability as a property of fibres was William Cullen, professor of medicine at the University of Edinburgh and, at the time, the most influential medical teacher in the English-speaking world. Born in 1710, Cullen taught chemistry in Glasgow before moving to Edinburgh to teach chemistry, materia medica, and medicine. He was the leading light of the Edinburgh Medical School during its golden age, publishing the best-selling nosologically arranged *First Lines of the Practice of Physic* (1778–9).

Cullen interpreted life itself as a function of nervous power and emphasized the importance of the nervous system in disease causation, coining the word 'neurosis' to describe nervous diseases. His one-time follower but later foe, John Brown, a larger-than-life figure who radicalized Scottish medicine (his followers were called Brunonians) but died an alcoholic, was to go further than Haller by reducing all questions of health and disease to variations around the mean of irritability. In place of Haller's concept of irritability, however, Brown substituted the idea that fibres were 'excitable'. Animation was hence to be understood as the

Among the finest anatomical atlases of the time was Albrecht von Haller's *Icones Anatomicæ* (1743–56), from which this plate of the facial arteries is taken. For the Swiss-born Haller, anatomy and physiology were insepara-bly linked: they formed a sin-gle science of 'living anatomy' – *anatomia animata*. Much of his physiological research was done by dissection, injection, or extirpation. He specialized in explorations of the nervous system.

product of external stimuli acting on an organized body: life was a 'forced condition'. Sickness, he ruled, was distur-bance of the proper functioning of excitement, and dis-eases were to be treated as 'sthenic' or 'asthenic', depending on whether the body was over- or underexcited.

In France, graduates of the distinguished University of Montpellier – more go-ahead than Paris – led the vitality debate. Francois Boissier de Sauvages denied that mecha-nism on the Boerhaave model could explain the origin and continuation of motion in the body. Rather like Haller, he maintained that anatomy made little sense on its own; what was needed was physiological study of the structure of a living (not a dissected) body, endowed with a soul. Later Montpellier teachers such as Théophile de Bordeu adopted a more materialist stance, stressing the inherent vitality of living bodies rather than the operation of an implanted soul.

Comparable researches were pursued in London. John Hunter, who was Scottish-born but had trained in the dis-secting-rooms of his brother William (see page 222), proposed a 'life-principle' to account for properties distin-guishing living organisms from inanimate matter: the life-force was in the blood. Thus philosophies of the 'machine of life' characteristic of the age of Descartes gave way to the more dynamic idea of 'vital properties' or vitalism. It is no acci-dent that the very term 'biology' was coined around 1800, by, amongst others, Gottfried Reinhold Treviranus, a professor at Bremen, and the French naturalist and trailblazing evolutionist Jean-Baptiste Lamarck.

Debates about the nature of life were not conducted simply by armchair philosophers. They were advanced by particular researches into human and ani-mal bodies: conjectures were put to the test. The processes of digestion, for exam-ple, earlier raised by Johannes van Helmont and Franciscus Sylvius, were subjected to sophisticated experimentation. Was digestion performed by some internal vital force, by the chemical action of gastric acids, or by the mechanical activities of churning, mincing, and pulverizing by the stomach muscles? The digestion debate had rumbled on since the Greeks, but eighteenth-century inquiries were characterized by striking experimental ingenuity, pioneered by René Réaumur. Having trained a pet kite to swallow and regurgitate porous food-filled tubes, Réaumur demonstrated the powers of gastric juices, and showed that meat is more fully digested in the stomach than are starchy foods.

As studies of digestion suggest, medicine fruitfully interacted with chemistry. A Scottish chemist, Joseph Black, formulated the idea of latent heat and identified 'fixed air' or what came to be known, in the new chemical nomenclature, as car-

The spark of life

With the development of condensers and the Leiden jar, electricity made great strides and became a fashionable object of experimental display in the eighteenth century. Guinea-pigs, animal and human, were routinely 'electrified' out of curiosity and mildly sadistic amusement.

Experimental electrophysiology — the application of currents to nerve and muscle preparations — was pioneered by Luigi Galvani. In *De Viribus Electricitatis in Motu Musculari* (On Electrical Powers in the Movement of Muscles) of 1792, the Italian anatomist described animal experiments in which he suspended the legs of dead frogs by copper wire from an iron balcony. When twitching followed, he concluded that electricity was involved and connected to the life force. His experiments were extended by Alessandro Volta, professor at Pavia, whose *Letters on Animal Electricity* appeared in 1792. Volta showed that a muscle could be made to contract by electric stimuli.

The connexions between life and electricity implied by such experiments proved immensely suggestive for later neurophysiology. They were also to provide the inspiration for science-fiction fantasies such as Mary Shelley's *Franken-stein* (1818), whose theme was the artificial creation of life through physicochemical experimentation and the dangers attending such power.

bon dioxide. Major advances followed in understanding respiration. Black had noted that the 'fixed air' given off by quicklime and alkalis was also present in expired air; while non-toxic, it was physiologically incapable of being breathed. It was the French chemist Antoine-Laurent Lavoisier who best explained the passage of gases in the lungs. He showed that the air inhaled was converted into Black's 'fixed air', whereas the nitrogen ('azote') remained unchanged. Respiration was, Lavoisier believed, the analogue within the living body to combustion in the external world; both needed oxygen, both produced carbon dioxide and water. Lavoisier thus established that oxygen was indispensable for the human body,

Many experimenters in the late eighteenth century believed that gases were the secret of life and that the new chemistry would lay bare their mysteries. The greatest chemist of the time was the Frenchman Antoine-Laurent Lavoisier, who is credited with the discovery of oxygen in 1775. This drawing of Lavoisier's laboratory was done by Mme. Lavoisier around 1785 (the colouring was added later). She included herself in the group, seated at a desk on the right.

showing that, when engaged in physical activities, the body consumed greater quantities of oxygen than when at rest. Alongside chemistry, advances in other physical sciences, such as electricity, also promised medical payoffs.

THE ORIGINS OF CLINICAL SCIENCE

Anatomy and physiology thus forged ahead in the eighteenth century, and the new-found faith in science probed the laws of life. But the relations between basic biological knowledge and medical practice remained opaque, and few scientific breakthroughs had direct payoffs for the mastery of disease. Many eminent physicians recorded their opinions on disease. William Heberden, who trained in Cambridge and practised in London, developed an impressive grasp, in the Hippocratic manner, of the characteristic disease syndromes. Heeding the advice of the great seventeenth-century clinician Thomas Sydenham, that clinical symptoms should be described with the same minuteness and accuracy observed by a painter in painting a portrait, Heberden emphasized the importance of distinguishing symptoms that were 'particular and constant' from those due to extraneous causes such as ageing. The fruit of 60 years' conscientious bedside notetaking, his *Commentaries* (1802) debunked hoary errors (for instance, the supposed prophylactic qualities of gout) and offered shrewd diagnostic and prognostic counsel.

Certain new clinical skills emerged. In his *Inventum Novum* (New Discovery) of 1761, Leopold Auenbrugger, physician-in-chief to the Hospital of the Holy Trinity at Vienna, advocated the technique of percussion of the chest. An innkeeper's son, Auenbrugger had been familiar since childhood with the trick of striking casks to test how full they were. Switching from barrels to patients, he noted that when tapped with a finger's end, a healthy subject's chest sounded like a cloth-covered drum; by contrast, a muffled sound, or one of unusually high pitch, indicated pulmonary disease, especially tuberculosis.

In general, eighteenth-century physicians rested content with the traditional diagnostic uses of the 'five senses'; they would feel the pulse, sniff for gangrene, taste urine, listen for breathing irregularities, and attend to skin and eye colour – looking out for the *facies Hippocratica*, the cast on the face of a dying person. These time-honoured methods were almost exclusively qualitative. Thus, what standardly counted in 'pulse lore' was not the number of beats per minute (as later), but their strength, firmness, rhythm, and 'feel'. Some attention was given to urine samples, but the historic art of urine-gazing (uroscopy) was now repudiated as the trick of the quackish 'pisse prophet': serious chemical analysis of urine had barely begun. Qualitative judgements dominated, and the good diagnostician was he who could size up a patient by acuity and experience.

CONCEPTS OF DISEASE

The good clinician thus knew his patients, but he also knew his diseases. Eighteenth-century practitioners trod in the footsteps of Thomas Sydenham and

Sex and gender

Before the nineteenth century, precisely how fertilization took place, and the respective roles played by the male and female, was rather fruitlessly debated. Aided in part by microscopical studies, so-called animalculist or *emboîte-ment* theories had risen to prominence in the seventeenth century. These contended that the new individual was already completely developed (in miniature) first in the seminal fluid and then in the womb from the moment of conception. William Harvey, on the other hand, had lent his authority to a separate theory, ovism or epigenesis, attributing a key role to the female egg in generation, and showing, through experiments on deer kindly donated by Charles I, the gradual and successive appearance of vital parts in the developing foetus.

This 'preformationism' versus 'epigenesis' dispute bubbled on well into the eighteenth century, buoyed up by wider questions of theology (*emboîtement* could be seen as predestinarian) and gender politics (Harvey's ovism dignified the female role). The most refined embryological study came from Caspar Friedrich Wolff of Berlin. His *Theoria Generationis* (Theory of Generation) of 1759 supported Harvey's epigenetic opinions by providing experimental evidence of the gradual evolution of the foetal parts. No organs were present in the egg, organs became differentiated step-by-step, rather than being preformed and merely swelling in bulk, like a balloon being blown up, in the fertilized egg.

Wolff's work looked forward to that of the great nineteenth-century embryologists such as Karl Ernst von Baer, who discovered the mammalian egg (ovum) in the ovary, explicated the nature of ovulation, and formulated the 'biogenetic law' that in embryonic development general characters appear before special ones. In the nineteenth century, embryology became one of the fundamental building-blocks of biology, since it explained development itself.

In the modern age, Cupid possessed not only a bow and arrow but cannons too, but the result was the same: instant babies everywhere. Sex remained an inflammatory and explosive topic.

ultimately of Hippocrates, amassing comprehensive empirical case records, especially of epidemic disorders. Sydenham was much admired in England. 'The English Hippocrates' had served as captain of horse for the Parliamentarian army in the Civil War. In 1647, he went to Oxford and from 1655 practised in London. A friend of Robert Boyle and John Locke, he stressed observation rather than theory in clinical medicine, and instructed physicians to distinguish specific diseases and find specific remedies. He was a keen student of epidemic diseases, which he believed were caused by atmospheric properties (he called it the 'epidemic constitution') that determined which kind of acute disease would be prevalent at any season.

Following Sydenham's teachings, a Plymouth doctor, John Huxham, published extensive findings about disease profiles in his *On Fevers* (1750); and a Chester practitioner, John Haygarth, undertook analysis of smallpox and typhus epidemics. John Fothergill, a Yorkshireman and a Quaker who built up a lucrative London practice, was another avid follower of Sydenham. In *Observations of the*

Weather and Diseases of London (1751–4), Fothergill gave a valuable description of diphtheria ('epidemic' sore throat), which was then growing more common especially among the urban poor. His friend and fellow Quaker, John Coakley Lettsom, was the driving-force behind the clinical investigations pioneered by the Medical Society of London, founded in 1778. Such medical gatherings, developing also in the provinces, collected clinical data and exchanged news. The birth of medical journalism also helped pool experience and spread information.

Systematic epidemiological and pathological research programmes did not develop until the nineteenth century; yet many valuable observations on diseases were made before 1800. In 1776, Matthew Dobson demonstrated that the sweetness of the urine in diabetes was due to sugar; in 1786, Lettsom published a fine account of alcoholism; Thomas Beddoes and others conducted investigations into tuberculosis, which was already becoming the great 'white plague' of urban Europe. But no decisive breakthroughs followed in disease theory. Questions as to true causation (*vera causa*) remained highly controversial. Many kinds of sickness were still attributed to personal factors – poor stock or physical endowment, neglect of hygiene, overindulgence, and bad lifestyle. This 'constitutional' or physiological concept of disease, buttressed by traditional humoralism, made excellent sense of the uneven and unpredictable scatter of sickness: with infections and fevers, some individuals were afflicted, some were not, even within a single household. It also drew attention to personal moral responsibility and pointed to strategies of disease containment through self-help. This personalization of illness had attractions and pitfalls that are still debated today.

Theories that disease spread essentially by contagion were also in circulation. These had much common experience in their favour. Certain disorders, such as syphilis, were manifestly transmitted person-to-person. Smallpox inoculation, introduced in the eighteenth century (see page 39), offered proof of contagiousness. But contagion hypotheses had their difficulties as well: if diseases were contagious, why didn't everyone catch them?

Such misgivings explain the popularity of long-entrenched miasmatic thinking – the conviction that sickness typically spread not by personal contact but through emanations given off by the environment. After all, everyone knew that some locations were healthier, or more dangerous, than others. With intermitting fevers like 'ague' (malaria), it was common knowledge that those living close to marshes and creeks were especially susceptible. Low and spotted fevers (typhus) were recognized as infecting populations in the overcrowded slum quarters of great towns, just as they also struck occupants of gaols, barracks, ships, and workhouses. It was thus plausible to suggest that disease lay in poisonous atmospheric exhalations, given off by putrefying carcases, food and faeces, waterlogged soil, rotting vegetable remains, and other filth in the surroundings. Bad environments, the argument ran, generated bad air (signalled by stenches), which, in turn, triggered disease. Late in the century, reformers directed attention to the 'septic'

Opposite: *Der Arzt* by Gerard Dou (1653). The old-style physician had almost no diagnostic technology at his disposal, nor did he conduct full, hands-on physical examinations as we know them but worked on the basis of his senses: sight, touch (of the wrist for the pulse), hearing, smell, and taste (sampling urine, for example, for the sweetness symptomatic of diabetes). Galenic medicine largely diagnosed illness on the basis of fluids passing from the body, hence the primacy of the inspection of urine. From the seventeenth century, with the decline of Galenism and the rise of medical science, uroscopy declined; but artists still liked to identify the doctor by his urine flask, especially if there was some satirical inention in mind. Urine-gazing became the mark of the quack.

diseases – gangrene, septicaemia, diphtheria, erysipelas, and puerperal fever – especially rampant in slum quarters and in ramshackle gaols and hospitals. The Hôtel Dieu in Paris had an atrocious reputation as a hotbed of fevers.

Disease theory greatly benefited from the rise of pathological anatomy. The trail was blazed by the illustrious Italian, Giovanni Battista Morgagni, professor of anatomy at Padua, who built on earlier postmortem studies by Johann Wepfer and Théophile Bonet. In 1761, when close to the age of eighty, Morgagni published his great work *De Sedibus et Causis Morborum* (On the Sites and Causes of Disease), which surveyed the findings of some 700 autopsies he had carried out. It quickly became famous, being translated into English in 1769 and German in 1774.

It was Morgagni's aim to show that diseases were located in specific organs, that disease symptoms tallied with anatomical lesions, and that pathological organ changes were responsible for disease manifestations. He gave lucid accounts of many disease conditions, being the first to delineate syphilitic tumours of the brain and tuberculosis of the kidney. He grasped that where only one side of the body is stricken with paralysis, the lesion lies on the opposite side of the brain. His explorations of the female genitals, of the glands of the trachea, and of the male urethra also broke new ground.

Others continued his work. In 1793, Matthew Baillie, a Scot and a nephew of William Hunter practising in London, published his *Morbid Anatomy*. Illustrated with superb copperplates by William Clift (they depicted, among other things, the emphysema of Samuel Johnson's lungs) Baillie's work was more of a textbook than Morgagni's, describing in succession the morbid appearances of each organ.

Before the discovery of microbial pathogens late in the nineteenth century, the prime source of disease was believed to be miasma – poisonous gases given of by unhealthy environments. These included stagnant waters, as well as overcrowded slums and rotting animal and vegetable materials.

He was the first to give a clear idea of cirrhosis of the liver, and in his second edition he developed the idea of 'rheumatism of the heart' (rheumatic fever).

Pathology was to yield an abundant harvest in early nineteenth-century medicine, thanks to the publication in 1800 of the *Traité des Membranes* by François Xavier Bichat, who focused particularly on the histological changes produced by disease. Morgagni's pathology had concentrated on organs, Bichat shifted the focus. The more one will observe diseases and open cadavers, he declared, the more one will be convinced of the necessity of considering local diseases not from the aspect of the complex organs but from that of the individual tissues.

Born in Thoirette in the French Jura, Bichat studied at Lyon and Paris, where he settled in 1793 at the height of the Terror. From 1797 he taught medicine, working at the Hôtel Dieu. His greatest contribution was his perception that the diverse organs of the body contain particular tissues or what he called 'membranes'; he described twenty-one, including connective, muscle, and nerve tissue. Performing his researches with great fervour – he undertook more than 600 post mortems – Bichat formed a bridge between the morbid anatomy of Morgagni and the later cell pathology of Rudolf Virchow.

A nineteenth-century drawing of a tumour in the gallbladder.

MEDICINE BECOMES SCIENTIFIC

The seventeenth century had launched the New Science; the Enlightenment propagandized on its behalf. But it was the nineteenth century that was the true age of science, with the state and universities promoting and funding it systematically. For the first time, it became essential for any ambitious doctor to acquire a scientific training. Shortly after 1800, medical science was revolutionized by a clutch of French professors, whose work was shaped by the opportunities created by the French Revolution for physicians to use big public hospitals for research. Among physicians, they acquired a heroic status, not unlike Napoleon himself. Perhaps the most distinguished was René-Théophile-Hyacinthe Laënnec, a pupil of François Bichat. In 1814, he became physician to the Salpêtrière Hospital and two years later chief physician to the Hôpital Necker. In 1816, Laënnec invented the stethoscope. Here is how he described his discovery:

> In 1816 I was consulted by a young woman presenting general symptoms of disease of the heart. Owing to her stoutness little information could be gathered by application of the hand and percussion. The patient's age and sex did not permit me to resort to the kind of examination I have just described (direct application of the ear to the chest). I recalled a well-known acoustic phenomenon: namely, if you place your ear against one end of a wooden beam the scratch of a pin at the other extremity is distinctly audible. It occurred to me that this physical property might serve a useful purpose in the case with which I was then dealing. Taking a sheet of paper I rolled it into a very tight roll, one end of which I placed on the precordial region, whilst I put my ear to the other. I was both surprised

The early nineteenth century brought the invention of some of the diagnostic technology familiar today, notably the stethoscope, invented by René Laënnec. Above: three early monaural stethoscopes based on Laënnec's design.

Right: Laënnec at the Necker Hospital in Paris, where he introduced the stethoscope (after a painting by Chartran in the Sorbonne, 1816). Laënnec diagnosed a multiplicity of pulmonary conditions with the help of his new invention: bronchitis, pneumonia, and, above all, pulmonary tuberculosis (phthisis or consumption). From then on, physicians could listen directly to the body, bypassing the story told by the patient.

and gratified at being able to hear the beating of the heart with much greater clearness and distinctness than I had ever before by direct application of my ear.

I saw at once that this means might become a useful method for studying, not only the beating of the heart, but likewise all movements capable of producing sound in the thoracic vacity, and that consquently it might serve for the investigation of respiration, the voice, rales and possibly even the movements of liquid effused into the pleural cavity or pericardium.[4]

By experiment, his instrument became a simple wooden cylinder about 23 centimetres (9 inches) long that could be unscrewed for carrying in the pocket. It was monaural (only later, in 1852, were two earpieces added – by the American George P. Cammann – for binaural sound). The stethoscope was the most important diagnostic innovation before the discovery of X-rays in the 1890s.

On the basis of his knowledge of the different normal and abnormal breath sounds, Laënnec diagnosed a multiplicity of pulmonary ailments: bronchitis, pneumonia, and, above all, pulmonary tuberculosis (phthisis or consumption). His oustanding publication, *Traité de l'Auscultation médiate* (1819), included clinical and pathological descriptions of many chest diseases. Ironically, Laënnec himself died of tuberculosis.

Laënnec's investigations paralleled those of his colleague, Gaspard Laurent Bayle, who in 1810 published a classic monograph on phthisis, on the basis of more than 900 dissections. Bayle's outlook was different from Laënnec's. He was more interested in taxonomy, and distinguished six distinct types of pulmonary phthisis. Laënnec had no interest in classification; rather, his ability to hear and interpret breath sounds made him primarily interested in the course of the diseases he examined. Like other contemporary French hospital physicians, he was accused of showing greater concern for diagnosis than for therapy – but this stemmed not from indifference to the sick but from a deep awareness of therapeutic limitations. Translations of Laënnec's book spread the technique of stethoscopy, as did the foreign students drawn to Paris. A man with a stethoscope draped round his neck became the prime nineteenth-century image of medicine: the instrument had the word science written on it.

Laënnec remains the one famous name amongst the generation of post-1800 French physicians who insisted that medicine must become a science and who believed that scientific diagnosis formed its pith and marrow. At the time, however, the most illustrious was Pierre Louis, whose writings set out the key agenda of the new 'hospital medicine'. Graduating in Paris in 1813, Louis spent 7 years practising in Russia. On returning home, he plunged into the wards of the *Pitié* hospital and published the results of his experiences in a massive book on tuberculosis (1825), followed 4 years later by another on fever.

Louis' *Essay on Clinical Instruction* (1834) set the standards for French hospital medicine. He highlighted not only bedside diagnosis but also systematic investi-

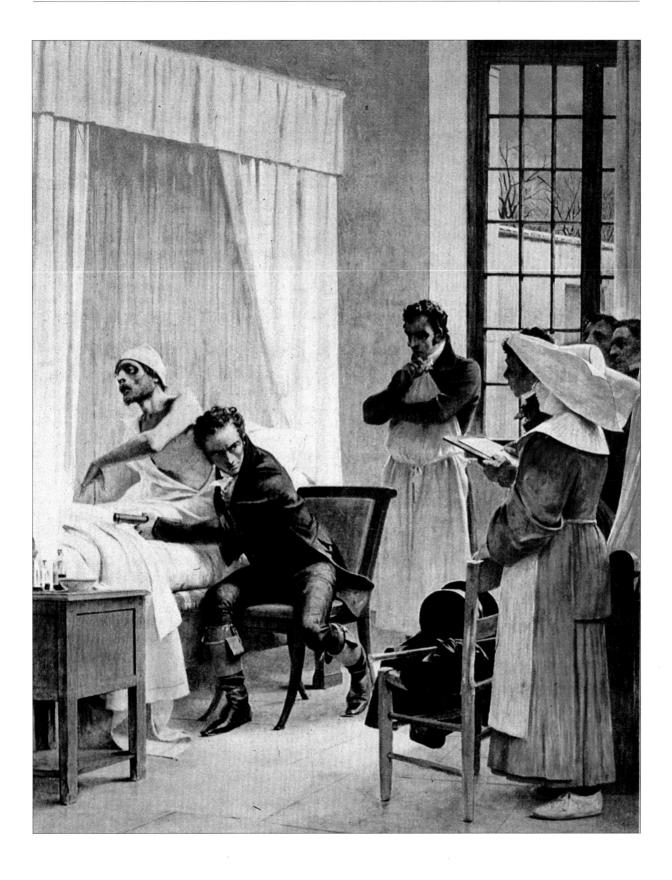

gation into the patient's circumstances, history, and general health. He deemed the value of the patient's *symptoms* (that is, what the patient felt and reported) secondary, stressing the far more significant *signs* (that is, what the doctor's examination ascertained). On the basis of such signs, the lesions of the pertinent organs could be determined, and they were the most definite guides to identifying diseases, devising therapies and making prognoses. For Louis, clinical medicine was an observational rather than an experimental science. It was learned at the bedside and in the morgue by recording and interpreting facts. Medical training lay in instructing students in the techniques of interpreting the sights, sounds, feel, and smell of disease: it was an education of the senses. Clinical judgement lay in astute explication of what the senses perceived.

Louis was, furthermore, a passionate advocate of numerical methods – the culmination of an outlook that had begun in the Enlightenment. Louis' mathematics were little more than simple arithmetic – quantitative categorizations of symptoms, lesions, and diseases, and (most significantly) application of numerical methods to test his therapies. To some degree, Louis sought to use medical arithmetic to discredit existing therapeutic practices: he was thus a pioneer of clinical trials. Only through the collection of myriad instances, he stressed, could doctors hope to formulate general laws.

Overall, the leading lights among French hospital doctors were more confident about diagnosis than cure, although Laënnec highlighted the Hippocratic concept of the healing power of nature – the power of the body to restore itself to health. But in the French school, therapeutics remained subordinate to pathological anatomy and diagnosis. The meticulousness with which Laënnec, Louis, Bayle, and others delineated disease reinforced the nosological concept that diseases were discrete entities, real things. The move from reliance upon symptoms (which were variable and subjective) to constant and objective lesions (the sign) supported their idea that diseased states were fundamentally different from normal ones.

The 'Paris school' was not a single cohesive philosophy of medical investigation. Nevertheless, there was something distinguished about Paris medicine; and during the first half of the nineteenth century students from Europe and North America flocked to France. Young men who studied in Paris returned home to fly the flag for French medicine. Disciples in London, Geneva, Vienna, Philadelphia, Dublin, and Edinburgh followed the French in emphasizing physical diagnosis and pathological correlation. They often also took back with them knowledge and skills in basic sciences such as chemistry and microscopy. Several leading English stethoscopists, including Thomas Hodgkin (of Hodgkin's disease), learned the technique directly from Laënnec himself.

Imitating the French example, medical education everywhere grew more systematic, more scientific. Stimulated by teachers who had studied in Paris, medical teaching in London expanded: by 1841, St George's Hospital had 200 pupils, St Bartholomew's 300. There were hundreds of students in other London hospital schools as well, and from the 1830s London also boasted a teaching university, with two colleges, University and King's, each with medical faculties and purpose-built hospitals.

London become a major centre of scientific medicine. Amongst the most eminent investigators was Thomas Addison, who became the leading medical teacher and diagnostician at Guy's Hospital where he collaborated with Richard Bright and identified Addison's disease (insufficiency of the suprarenal capsules) and Addison's anaemia (pernicious anaemia). Bright for his part was a member of the staff at Guy's Hospital from 1820. His *Reports of Medical Cases* (1827–31) contain his description of kidney disease (Bright's disease), with its associated dropsy and protein in the urine.

Vienna also grew in eminence. The University of Vienna had well-established traditions: the old medical school had bedside teaching on the model espoused by Herman Boerhaave in the early eighteenth century, but decay had set in towards 1800. However, new teaching was introduced by the Paris-inspired Carl von Rokitanski, who made pathological anatomy compulsory. The age's most obsessive dissector (supposedly performing some 60,000 autopsies in all), Rokitanski had a superb mastery of anatomy and pathological science, and left notable studies of congenital malformations and reports of numerous conditions, including pneumonia, peptic ulcer, and valvular heart disease.

In the USA, by contrast, high-quality medical schools and clinical investigations developed more slowly. In its *laissez-faire*, business-dominated atmosphere, many schools were blatantly commercial, inadequately staffed, and offered cut-price degrees (see page 127).

Pierre-Charles-Alexandre Louis (1787–1872), one of the most distinguished French clinicians, pathological anatomists, and statisticians of the nineteenth century.

MEDICINE IN THE LABORATORY

Influenced by the Paris school, hospitals became the key sites for medical science. Remarkable advances also started taking place in the laboratory. By 1850, laboratories were transforming physiology and pathology and beginning to make their mark on medical education. Laboratories were not new – they had grown up with seventeenth-century science – nor was experimental medicine; the Revd Stephen Hales, for instance, conducted experiments on blood circulation in the early eighteenth century (see page 164). Nevertheless, nineteenth-century practitioners of organic chemistry, microscopy, and physiology rightly believed they were giving birth to a new enterprise, based on the laboratory and its stress on vivisection. The hospital was a place to observe, the laboratory to experiment.

Science went from strength to strength in the nineteenth century, winning greater public funds and a place in the sun. German universities, in particular, became associated with the research ethos. Justus von Liebig's Institute of Chemistry at the University of Giessen established the mould for German laboratory science. Liebig studied chemistry at Bonn and Erlangen before spending 2 years in Paris, gaining laboratory experience. In 1824, at the tender age of twenty-one, he was appointed professor of chemistry at Giessen, where his institute became a magnet, attracting students seeking practical instruction in qualitative analysis. It proved a huge success, being enlarged to house more students and research facilities before the University of Munich lured him away in 1852 with an offer he could not refuse.

Liebig's goal was to subject living beings to strictly quantified chemical analysis. By measuring what went in (food, oxygen, and water) and what came out (urea, various acids and salts, water, and carbon dioxide in the excretions and exhalations), vital information would be discovered about the chemical processes occurring within. Liebig thought of the body in terms of chemical systems. Respiration brought oxygen into the body, where it mixed with starches to liberate energy, carbon dioxide, and water. Nitrogenous matter was absorbed into muscle and comparable tissues; when it was broken down, urine was the final product, together with phosphates and assorted chemical by-products.

Becoming the age's great breeder of chemists, Liebig encouraged his students to undertake chemical analyses on such animal tissues as muscle and liver, or on blood, sweat, tears, urine, and other fluids. They attempted measurement of the relationship in living organisms between food and oxygen consumption and energy production. In short, Liebig's school launched energetic investigation of nutrition and metabolism, developing what was later to be called biochemistry.

Liebig's career proved crucial. He trained scores of students in research methods and organized systematized laboratory research. He emphasized the cardinal importance of physicochemical thinking in understanding biological processes, developing the reductionist ambition of applying the physical sciences to living organisms. As early as 1828 his lifelong friend, Friedrich Wöhler (from 1836 pro-

The German chemist Justus von Liebig in his laboratory at the University of Geissen. After Wilhelm Trautschold, *c.* 1840.

fessor of chemistry at Göttingen), synthesized the organic substance urea from inorganic substrates: this served as a persuasive proof that no categorical barrier separated 'vital' compounds found in living beings from ordinary chemicals. Such findings gave impetus to the programme known as scientific materialism, whose adherents were engaged in a militant repudiation of the speculative, idealistic philosophy (*Naturphilosophie*) that, in the musings of Goethe and others had achieved much prestige in German culture in the Romantic era. Liebig and his followers were sober experimentalists scornful of mystical and poetic aspirations to understand the Meaning of Life.

The enshrinement of physiology as a high-status experimental discipline was a key feature of nineteenth-century medical science. Johannes Müller was its trailblazer. Born in Coblenz, Müller became professor of physiology and anatomy at Bonn and from 1833 at Berlin. Gifted at neurophysiological research, Müller's enormous two-volume *Handbuch der Physiologie des Menschen* (1833–40) was fundamental to the progress of the discipline. He was above all an inspiring teacher, and his students – Theodor Schwann, Hermann von Helmholtz, Emil du Bois-Reymond, Ernst Brücke, Jacob Henle, Rudolf Virchow, and many others – became trendsetters in scientific and medical research.

Four promising young physiologists associated with Müller – Helmholtz, du Bois-Reymond, Karl Ludwig and Brücke – published a manifesto in 1847 proclaiming that physiology's goal was to explain all vital phenomena in terms of physicochemical laws. Before he turned to physics in the 1870s, Helmholtz devoted himself to central physiological problems, including measurement of animal heat and the velocity of nerve conduction, and investigation of sight and hearing. He invented the ophthalmoscope, aiding work on vision. Ludwig for his part did pioneer research on glandular secretions, notably the manufacture of urine by kidneys. Du Bois-Reymond, professor of physiology in Berlin, was mainly immersed in electrophysiology, studying muscles and nerves. Brücke went to Vienna, where his concerns spanned physiological chemistry, histology, and neuromuscular physiology. Tough-mindedly committed to scientific naturalism, Brücke became one of Sigmund Freud's teachers and heroes.

The thrust of the experimental physiology carried out by such field-leaders was, in Ludwig's words, to understand functions 'from the elementary conditions inherent in the organism itself'.[5] It required the use of experimental animals and drew on new instruments to record data. In 1847, Ludwig introduced the technological device that epitomized physiological research: the kymograph – the machine designed to trace body alterations onto a line on a graph. Growing technological sophistication was central to modern medical science. There were other developments in instrumentation. The design of the microscope was greatly improved, correcting distortion and so enabling histology to create a bridge between anatomy and physiology. Learn to see microscopically, Rudolf Virchow insisted, summing up the message that Müller taught all his pupils.

Microscopy was intimately linked with the new study of cells, in 1838 begun by another of Müller's pupils, Theodor Schwann. Schwann discovered the enzyme pepsin in the stomach, investigated muscle contraction, and demonstrated the role of microorganisms in putrefaction. But he is chiefly remembered for extending the cell theory, previously applied to plants, to animal tissues. His model was reductionist: cells, he believed, were the fundamental units of zoological and botanical activity. Incorporating a nucleus and an outer membrane, they could be formed (in a manner he compared to crystals growing within solutions) out of a formless organic matrix that he called the blastema.

Schwann's views were modified by Rudolf Virchow, professor of pathological anatomy at Würzburg (1849) and later Berlin (1856). His microscopical work carried profound biological significance. In his *Cellularpathologie* (1858), he disputed Schwann's notion of the blastema, and developed the maxim: *omnis cellula e cellula* (all cells from cells). If François Bichat's *Traité des Membranes* (1800) put tissues on the map, Virchow's treatise did the same for cells: it established a new, productive unit for making inferences about function and disease. Virchow's

Rudolf Virchow, photographed in his study, was probably the most distinguished German pathologist of his age, and is regarded as the founder of cellular pathology. He contributed to the study of tumours, leukaemia, hygiene, and sanitation. He was a politician as well as a scientist, and, as a Liberal member of the German Parliament from 1880 to 1893, he strenuously opposed the policies of Bismarck.

hypothesis had special pertinence for such biological events as fertilization and for pathophysiological ones, such as the source of the pus cell in inflammation. Diseases arise (he argued) from abnormal changes within cells; such abnormal cells multiply through division. Virchow thus regarded the study of cells as basic to the understanding of cancer, on which he lavished great attention, describing leukaemia for the first time. His view of disease was essentially an internal one, and he proved distrustful of the bacteriology of Louis Pasteur (see page 184), which he regarded as rather shallow. German laboratories attracted students from all over Europe and North America. In the 1830s, the migration was a trickle: chemists went to Justus von Liebig in Giessen and microscopists to Johannes Müller in Berlin. Half a century later, it had become a deluge, with medical students flocking to complete their education in the German-speaking universities.

French hospital medicine in its heyday had not relied on laboratory-based inquiries, although foreign medical students sometimes gained instruction in microscopy as well as experience in hospital wards and morgues. France gradually slipped behind Germany because it failed to create the new laboratories necessary for physiological research. Nevertheless, France continued to produce eminent researchers. For example, François Magendie, professor of anatomy at the Collège de France (1831), made important studies of nerve physiology, the veins, and the physiology of food. His real distinction lay in helping to launch the career of Claude Bernard.

Born near Villefranche, Bernard failed as a dramatist and so studied medicine at Paris, in 1841 becoming Magendie's assistant at the Collège de France. Thereafter, all was success, including chairs at the Sorbonne and the Museum of Natural History, a seat in the Senate, and the presidency of the French Academy. Bernard's brilliance lay in his superb operative techniques and the simplicity of his experiments. His earliest researches were on the action of the secretions of the alimentary canal, pancreatic juice, and the connection between the liver and nervous system. Later researches were, for example, on changes of temperature of the blood, levels of oxygen in arterial and in venous blood, and the opium alkaloids. He reached major physiological findings: the role of the liver in synthesizing glycogen and in keeping blood-glucose levels within a healthy range; the digestive functions of the secretions of the pancreas; the vasodilator nerves and their role in regulating the flow of blood in blood vessels; and the effects on muscles of carbon monoxide and curare (the South American arrow poison; see page 257).

Claude Bernard carrying out an experiment. His greatest contribution to physiological theory was the notion that life requires a constant internal environment. Combining experimental skill with a partiality for theory, he was notably innovative and one of the great masters of productive research.

The Four Doctors by John Singer Sargent (1905). Seated in the Welch Medical Library at Johns Hopkins University Medical School are members of the first clinical faculty: (from left to right) William Henry Welch, professor of pathology and dean; William Stewart Halsted, professor of surgery; William Osler, professor of medicine; and Howard Kelly, professor of gynaecology. When the medical school was opened in 1893, the emphasis was on advanced teaching and research. The early professors, some of whom were educated in Germany, began the tradition of excellence in clinical science for which the USA has been distinguished in the twentieth century.

Bernard's most famous book, *Introduction à la Médecine expérimentale* (1865), was a systematic exposition of the experimental method for biomedical sciences. Traditional hospital medicine, Bernard maintained, had two key limitations. As an observational science, it was purely passive, akin to natural history. The progress of physiology required the active observation of the experimentalist under controlled conditions. At the sickbed, there were too many imponderables to allow precise understanding. Moreover, he argued (contradicting Pierre Louis, René Laënnec, and their school), the pathological lesion itself was not the origin but the end point of disease. Pathophysiological knowledge could be fulfilled only in the laboratory, and only through use of laboratory animals in controlled environments. No pathology without physiology, he insisted. The interplay of physiology, pathology, and pharmacology constituted for him the foundations of experimental medicine, and each had to be a laboratory science.

Yet Bernard was no crass materialist or physical reductionist. Animals and human beings, he maintained, were not automata at the mercy of the external environment. And the reason for this was because higher organisms did not live solely in the exterior environment; they actively created their own internal environment, the *internal milieu*, the home of live communities of cells. Numerous physiological mechanisms, mediated through fluids such as blood and lymph, were devoted to balancing concentrations of sugar, salt, and oxygen in the blood and tissue fluids; it was their job to preserve a uniform body temperature in relation to the fluctuations of variable external ones. It was through these mechanisms – later to be called 'homeostasis' by the Harvard physiologist Walter Bradford Cannon – that higher organisms achieved a degree of autonomy within the more fundamental determinism of the natural order.

Scientific medicine developed later in Britain and the USA, owing profound debts to developments in France and Germany. By the 1880s, droves of Americans were studying biology and medicine in German-speaking universities: there were perhaps 15,000 between 1850 and the First World War, mostly in Vienna, Göttingen, Berlin, and Heidelberg. They primarily went for clinical instruction, but some, like the pathologist William Henry Welch, homed in on the laboratories. It was Welch who introduced the Germanic spirit into American experimental medicine, building his career at the most Germanic of American universities, Johns Hopkins in Baltimore, Maryland. The Johns Hopkins Hospital opened its doors to patients in 1889, although the medical school – unusual in admitting women – was delayed for a further four years because of a shortage of funds. The emphasis was on advanced teaching

The Russian physiologist and psychologist Ivan Petrovitch Pavlov with co-researchers carrying out a demonstration on a dog of his theory of 'conditioned' or acquired reflexes. One of his experiments involved studying the secretion of juices by the stomach in response to stimuli, such as the sound of a tinkling bell that the dog associated with food. His studies attracted worldwide praise and in 1904 he received one of the first Nobel Prizes for physiology or medicine. In Victorian times, experiments on dogs were so criticized by the British public that the government was forced to pass the Cruelty to Animals Act in 1876. This required experimenters on animals to be licensed and to operate under strict conditions.

and research. British medical students also went in droves to Germany, but institutions in Britain supporting medical research remained small all through the Victorian age – British medicine was mainly practical and geared to private practice. Research achieved little status in the universities, and there was hardly any state support. Moreover, the British situation was not helped by public hostility to vivisection to a degree not experienced elsewhere.

The antivivisection campaign grew vocal at the 1874 Norwich meeting of the British Medical Association after a demonstration by a French physiologist – he injected alcohol into two dogs – made headline news. A summons for wanton cruelty was issued. Although unsuccessful, the prosecution put animal experimentation on the political agenda, leading to the setting up of a Royal Commission to examine experimental medicine. The resultant 1876 Cruelty to Animals Act was a compromise that satisfied neither antivivisectionists nor the science lobby. It permitted medically trained investigators to conduct vivisection experiments under licence and strictly stipulated conditions. No other nation passed legislation regulating animal experimentation before the twentieth century.

Neither the 1876 Act nor the activities of the antivivisectionists prevented British physiology from increasing its international status in the decades before the First World War. Working first in London and then in Edinburgh, Edward Schafer (later Sharpey-Schafer) achieved fame for his researches on muscular contraction. Around the same time, Michael Foster and his pupils John Newport Langley and Walter Holbrook Gaskell created a research school in Cambridge that produced a number of future Nobel Laureates and boosted Cambridge's reputation as Britain's most enterprising medical school. Foster set himself the problem

The germ theory of disease

The complexity of the interplay of science and medicine is indicated by the fact that the most illustrious of all investigators, Louis Pasteur, was not even a physician, but a chemistry graduate of the Ecole Normale Supérieure, the main science school in Paris. Born a tanner's son from the Jura Mountains near the Swiss border, Pasteur trained as a chemist, becoming a professor in Strasbourg, Lille, and then Paris. His interest in microorganisms was triggered by analysing the activity of certain chemicals, especially the tartrates, and this led to a growing fascination with fermentation. Puzzles regarding wine- and beer-making drew him to microorganisms such as yeast.

Pasteur devised experiments to disprove the old notion of spontaneous generation. He showed that all grubs arose from minute insect-laid eggs and organisms pervading the atmosphere, invisible to the naked eye. He conducted extensive experimentation on fermentation and the role of microorganisms in phenomena such as the souring of milk and the fermentation of sugar into alcohol. He developed a method for eliminating microbes from milk – 'pasteurization'. The heating of milk to a prescribed temperature ensured that milk would cease to be a source of the spread of tuberculosis and typhoid.

The diseases that first led to Pasteur's germ theory were those of silkworms, and he went on to explore the role of microorganisms in the diseases of cattle, pigs, poultry, and, finally, human beings. Research on chicken cholera, swine erysipelas, and anthrax led to new 'vaccines', the term he coined to honour Edward Jenner. Pasteur showed the worth of his anthrax vaccine in a sensational experiment. On 28 April 1881, he injected twenty-four sheep with his new vaccine. This was repeated 3 weeks later. A further fortnight later, this group, and a control group of unvaccinated animals, were implanted with virulent anthrax bacilli. When the animals were inspected again on 2 June all the vaccinated animals were healthy, whereas all the unvaccinated ones were dead or dying. Pasteur's crowning achievement, the rabies vaccine, developed in 1885, was for a disease, like anthrax, common to animals and human beings.

Dismissing traditional notions of miasmata and chemical poisons, Pasteur championed the germ theory of disease. A superb microscopist, he identified streptococci and staphylococci and waved the banner for bacteriology as a science. He was, nevertheless, less successful in providing convincing proof for his new ideas than his younger German contemporary, Robert Koch, whose meticulous demonstrations won assent for the bacterial theory of disease causation once and for all.

Trained by Friedrich Wöhler in Göttingen and rising to become Professor of Public Health in Berlin, Koch published a paper, 'The etiology of traumatic infectious diseases' in 1879 that proved a milestone in scientific method, confirming the germ theory of disease. It set out to differentiate between diverse bacteria, connect specific bacteria with specific indications, and so settle whether bacteria were the consequences of infections or (as Koch insisted) their causes.

---

of determining whether the heartbeat was muscular or neurological in nature; and his Cambridge protégés in due course broadened out this question to explore the anatomy and physiology of the autonomic nervous system, the chemical transmission of nerve impulses, and the control of reflexes and movement.

TROPICAL MEDICINE IN THE ERA OF IMPERIALISM

During the nineteenth century medicine grew international, indeed global: the Red Cross was established by the Geneva Convention of 1864, and international medical congresses were inaugurated in 1867 in Paris. The specialism of tropical medicine emerging from the 1870s reflects the spirit of the era of imperialism, when the great powers battled to settle the less 'civilized' parts of the globe. Scientists became embroiled in an uneasy mix of competition and cooperation.

To meet these questions, he adumbrated a series of principles later known as Koch's Postulates. These held that to prove a particular bacterium produced a specific condition, four requirements must be satisfied:

- the specific organism must be proven to be present in every instance of the infectious disease;
- the organism must be capable of being cultivated in pure culture;
- inoculating an experimental animal with the culture would reproduce the disease; and
- the organisms could be recovered from the inoculated animal and grown again in a pure culture.

These have proved valuable criteria for confirming the demonstration of particular bacterial causes for specific diseases. The germ theory of disease was thereby refined into a bacterial explanation of disease causation.

Koch's greatest discoveries were the bacillae that caused tuberculosis (1882) and cholera (1883). He also made useful technical innovations, notably the use of solid cultures for growing bacteria. Perceiving the need to isolate specific bacterial strains, Pasteur had used artificial cultivation in broths, but Koch showed up the distortions such liquid media created. Searching for solid media, he eventually chose to solidify the standard 'nutrient broth' by adding gelatin to develop a universal medium.

Koch's achievements were enormous, and his students and rivals used his methods to discover the causal microbes for typhoid, diphtheria, pneumonia, gonorrhoea, undulant fever, meningitis, leprosy, tetanus, plague, syphilis, whooping cough, and staphylococcal and streptococcal infections. Through its new attention to living pathogens, bacteriology went a long way to solving the old problem of disease aetiology. In the process it opened up questions of susceptibility and immunity.

Pasteur in his laboratory. He used rabbits to develop his rabies vaccine.

Imperial expansion had long been thwarted by diseases such as malaria (from the Italian *mala aria*, bad air) that remained troublesome around the Mediterranean and continued to thwart colonial endeavours in Asia, Africa, and Latin America; and generations of experience had taught that the tropics were the white man's grave. Yet the relations between climate, disease, and victims had long been a puzzle. Some 'tropical' diseases, such as sleeping sickness and schistosomiasis, primarily affected natives. Others, like malaria, afflicted Europeans too. And from the 1830s, cholera had moved beyond its traditional home in the Indian subcontinent, circling the globe in great pandemics (see page 41). Malaria remained. Plague had never disappeared from Asia and the Near East; as late as the 1890s an outbreak in China inaugurated a pandemic that spread catastrophically to India and beyond; in 1900, the USA itself was hit by an epidemic in San Francisco.

The German physician and medical bacteriologist Robert Koch (centre, facing camera) in Africa, studying the tsetse fly. The fly transmits sleeping sickness or African trypanosomiasis, a serious disease in sub-Saharan Africa. Koch made many outstanding discoveries on disease-causing pathogens. He received a Nobel Prize in 1905 for his work on tuberculosis.

Each of the diseases just mentioned was 'tropical' in the sense that it was more frequent in hot climates; and certain diseases – for example, schistosomiasis in the Nile Valley – seemed to be restricted almost exclusively to hot climates and the native inhabitants. Not surprisingly, traditional explanations of diseases of hot climates had drawn on the general framework of miasmatic environmentalism: heat produced severe fevers and tendencies to putrescence. But new explanations emerged in the last quarter of the nineteenth century; their pioneer was Patrick Manson.

A Scot, Manson had gone to the Far East in 1866 as a Customs Medical Officer. During a dozen years in Amoy (now Xiamen) off the south-east China coast, he studied elephantiasis, the chronic disfiguring disease that through blockage of lymph flow leads to massive swelling of the genitalia and limbs. He was also able to demonstrate that it was caused by a parasite – a nematode worm called *Filaria* or *Wuchereria* – spread through mosquito bites. This was the first disease shown to be transmitted by an insect vector. Returning to London in 1890, he became the

British soldiers cleaning plague houses in Hong Kong in the 1890s. The third great pandemic of bubonic plague spread through much of the world in the late nineteenth century. In 1894, the infection reached the S. Chinese coast in Guangdong Province, appearing in the ports of Guangzhou, Hong Kong, and Beihai. It later spread from Asia to San Francisco. In the absence of a cure or a vaccine then, strict hygienic measures were the only relief.

leading consultant on tropical diseases, in 1899 helping to found the London School of Tropical Medicine. His *Tropical Diseases* (1898) delineated the new specialism, emphasizing that entomology, helminthology, and parasitology were the keys to understanding diseases exclusive to tropical climates.

Building a reputation as a scientific parasitologist, Manson stamped his vision on the emergent specialism, not just in Britain but also throughout Europe and the Americas. Assimilating but going beyond bacteriology, his work led to the spotlighting of a new class of parasitic organisms as the precipitants of tropical diseases: schistosomiasis was found to be produced by the trematode worms *Bilharzia*; tropical dysentery was caused by an amoeba; sleeping sickness by a trypanosome protozoan; and malaria by another sort of protozoan, *Plasmodium*.

Other diseases were mastered, in theory if not in practice, by extending the new parasitological model. The Spanish-American War in Central America led to shocking mortality from yellow fever and hence to the foundation in 1900 of a US Army Yellow Fever Commission. A local Havana doctor, Carlos Finlay, was

The puzzle of malaria

The puzzle of malaria was unravelled by Ronald Ross, whose career Patrick Manson helped launch. The son of an army officer, Ross studied medicine at St Bartholomew's Hospital in London and entered the Indian Medical Service. In 1894, Manson informed him of his belief that malaria was transmitted through mosquito bites; Ross returned to India determined to examine this hypothesis.

Repeating and thereby confirming earlier work by the French microbiologist Charles Laveran, he discovered the malaria parasite *Plasmodium* (a protozoan slightly smaller than a bacterium) in the stomachs of *Anopheles* mosquitoes that had bitten malaria sufferers. Ross then showed that the mosquito was a necessary vector in malaria transmission; in addition, he elucidated the relationship between the *Plasmodium* life cycle and disease.

Independently, the Italian Giovanni Grassi related malaria to the *Anopheles* mosquito and demonstrated that this mosquito itself first became infected by feeding off the blood of a person with the *Plasmodium* parasite in the bloodstream. In 1901, Ross was awarded a Nobel Prize for his account of the life cycle of the malaria parasite.

Here is Ross in his laboratory in Secunderabad on 20 August 1897 — the anniversary of which he always called Mosquito Day:

At about 1 p.m. I determined to sacrifice the seventh *Anopheles*... of the batch fed on the 16th, Mosquito 38, although my eyesight was already fatigued. Only one more of the batch remained.

The dissection was excellent, and I went carefully through the tissues, now so familiar to me, searching every micron with the same passion and care as one would search some vast ruined palace for a little hidden treasure. Nothing. No, these new mosquitoes also were going to be a failure: there was something wrong with the theory. But the stomach tissues still remained to be examined — lying there, empty and flaccid, before me on the glass slide, a great white expanse of cells like a great courtyard of flagstones, each of which must be scrutinized — half an hour's labour at least. I was tired, and what was the use? I must have examined the stomachs of a thousand mosquitoes by this time. But the Angel of Fate fortunately laid his hand on my head; and I had scarcely commenced the search again when I saw a clear and almost perfectly circular outline before me of about 12 microns in diameter. The outline was much too sharp, the cell too small to be an ordinary stomach-cell of a mosquito. I looked a little further. Here was another, and another exactly similar cell.

The afternoon was very hot and overcast; and I remember opening the diaphragm of the sub-stage condenser of the microscope to admit more light and then changing the focus. *In each of these cells there was a cluster of small granules, black as jet* and exactly like the black pigment granules of the *Plasmodium* crescents. As with that pigment, the granules numbered about twelve to sixteen in each cell and became blacker and more visible when more light was admitted through the diaphragm. I laughed, and shouted for the Hospital Assistant — he was away having his siesta. 'No, no,' I said; 'Dame Nature, you are a sorceress, but you don't trick me so easily. The malarial pigment cannot get into the walls of the mosquito's stomach; the flagella have no pigment; you are playing another trick upon me!' I counted twelve of the cells, all of the same size and appearance and all containing exactly the same granules. Then I made rough drawings of nine of the cells on page 107 of my notebook, scribbled my notes, sealed my specimen, went home to tea (about 3 p.m.), and slept solidly for an hour...

When I awoke with mind refreshed my first thought was: Eureka! the problem is solved![6]

Ronald Ross and Mrs. Ross outside the laboratory of the hospital in Calcutta, where Ross's theory on the mosquito transmission of malaria was completed in 1898.

already championing a mosquito-borne theory of yellow fever, based on experiments in which healthy volunteers were bitten by mosquitoes that had fed on yellow-fever victims: they then typically fell sick. The Yellow Fever Commission enlisted the help of Finlay and the Chief Sanitary Officer in Havana, the American military doctor, Colonel William Gorgas, and, building on the work of the British parasitologist Ronald Ross and Giovanni Grassi, it followed up Finlay's mosquito hypothesis, subjecting healthy volunteers under supervised conditions to mosquitoes that had previously bitten yellow-fever patients. This time a different species of mosquito, *Aedes aegypti*, proved to be responsible. Laboratory and field studies led Gorgas to inaugurate a successful mosquito-eradication programme in Havana.

A similar scheme followed in the Panama Canal Zone. The French had begun to construct the Panama Canal, but they had abandoned the enterprise because losses from yellow fever had been exorbitant. Through draining marshes, oiling ponds over, and reducing stagnant water in townships, the number of mosquitoes was reduced, with significant decline in the incidence of mosquito-borne diseases. The construction of the canal then went ahead between 1904 and 1914 – a dramatic vindication of the potential of medical science in the tropics.

TWENTIETH-CENTURY BREAKTHROUGHS

Building on the developments of the nineteenth century, the past hundred years have brought unparalleled developments in biology, chemistry, and physiology and the opening up of new specialities within medical science. It would be quite impossible even to list here all the main twentieth-century breakthroughs in medical science, but a few fields and salient advances may be outlined.

The microbiological research promoted by Louis Pasteur and Robert Koch led to the creation around 1900 of immunology. The word 'immunity' – exemption from a particular disease – was popularized as researchers grew more familiar with the enigmatic relations of infection and resistance. Fascinated by the nutritional requirements of microorganisms, Pasteur had suggested a nutritional dimension to the resistance of a host and the attenuation of a parasite: the microorganism lost its power to infect because it could not longer flourish and reproduce.

Pasteur was more concerned with vaccine production than with the theoretical reasons why vaccines protected (or immunized). In 1884, however, a Russian zoologist, Elie Metchnikoff (see page 140), observed in the water flea (*Daphnia*) a phenomenon he termed phagocytosis (cell-eating), subsequently developing his observations into a comprehensive cellular view of resistance. Metchnikoff saw amoeba-like cells in these lower organisms apparently ingesting foreign substances like vegetable matter. He deduced that these amoeba-like cells in *Daphnia* might be comparable to the pus cells visible in higher creatures. Microscopic examination of animals infected with various pathogens, including the anthrax bacillus, showed white blood cells assaulting and appearing to digest the disease

Overleaf: Testing Carlos Finlay's theory that healthy people succumbed to yellow fever if bitten by mosquitoes that had previously fed on yellow-fever victims. The theory was confirmed in 1900 in Havana through the use of volunteers by the US Army Commission on Yellow fever headed by Major Walter Reed. This knowledge made it possible later to eradicate the disease by destroying the insect carriers. With Finlay and Reed in Dean Cornwell's reconstruction of one of the US Army's experiments in Cuba are American physicians Jesse Lazear and James Carroll. Carroll volunteered to be bitten by an infected mosquito and in 1900 was the first experimental case of yellow fever – presumably the victim in the painting. He survived the mosquito bite but Lazear died from the disease in 1900.

germs. Metchnikoff likened white blood cells to an army that was 'fighting infection'. Extrapolating from these hypotheses, Metchnikoff subsequently turned into a scientific guru, expounding striking beliefs on diet, constipation, ageing, and humanity's biological future. He became noted for his advocacy of eating yoghurt, arguing that the bacilli used in producing it inhibited the bacteria in the gut that caused harmful putrefactive by-products.

Metchnikoff's cellular theory of immunity gained prominence within the French scientific community; in an era of tense scientific rivalry, German researchers proposed chemical theories. Robert Koch's scepticism about the immunological significance of phagocytosis carried great weight in Germany, and two of his younger colleagues, Emil Adolf von Behring and Paul Ehrlich, argued that immunological warfare was waged less by the white blood cells than in the blood serum. Their chemical hypothesis had important factors in its favour. It was known that the cell-free serum of immunized creatures could destroy lethal bacteria, and that protection could be transmitted via serum from animal to animal: this implied there was more to immunity than the operation of white blood cells alone. Moreover, two of Pasteur's own pupils, Emile Roux and Alexandre Yersin, showed in 1888 that cultures of diphtheria bacilli were toxic even when the cells themselves had

been filtered out. This seemed to suggest that it was not necessarily the bacterial cell itself that bred disease but rather some chemical toxin the cell manufactured.

On the strength of these observations serum therapy was developed. Working with a Japanese associate, Shibasaburo Kitasato, Behring claimed in 1890 that the whole blood or serum of an animal, rendered immune to tetanus or diphtheria by injecting the relevant toxin, could treat another creature exposed to an otherwise fatal dose of the bacilli. Serum therapy had some genuine triumphs, but it never proved a wonder cure – not least because epidemic diseases such as diphtheria were notoriously variable in their virulence. Nevertheless, serum therapies grew in popularity after 1890, and antitoxins were prepared for diseases other than tetanus and diphtheria, including pneumonia, plague, and cholera. Many, however, remained convinced of the superior protective possibilities of vaccines. Vaccines developed from the treated organisms of plague and cholera were introduced around 1900 by the Russian-born bacteriologist, Waldemar Haffkine.

From the 1880s Ehrlich had been exploring the physiological and pharmacological properties of various dyes (see page 264), demonstrating, for example, the affinity of the newly discovered malaria parasite for methylene blue. Applying the

The anthrax bacillus, from a paper published by Robert Koch in 1877. Koch built on the work of the French investigator Casimir-Joseph Davaine, who first identified the bacterium in the blood of sheep dying from anthrax. Koch elucidated the life history of the microorganism and its mode of infection, and showed that anthrax spores can survive for many years in soil.

stereochemical ideas of Emil Fischer and other organic chemists, Ehrlich devised a 'side-chain' notion to explain how antigens and antibodies interacted. His formulation was essentially a chemical interpretation of immunity, part of a molecular vision of reality that included the possibility of pharmacological 'magic bullets', the ultimate aim of chemotherapy. Ideas of immunity linked in various ways with the study of the relations between nutrition and health. Nutrition studies had various traditions on which to draw. Back in the eighteenth century, the problem of scurvy aboard ship had led to conjectures connecting diet and disease and to the first clinical trials by the Scottish doctor James Lind (see page 256).

The researches of Justus von Liebig in Germany helped put the organic chemistry of digestion and nourishment on a sound footing. Liebig's pupils explored the creation of energy out of food and launched the idea of dietary balance. Notable work was done by German physiologist Wilhelm Kühne, a professor at Heidelberg from 1871, who introduced the term 'enzyme' to describe organic substances that activate chemical changes. There was a long tradition of explaining sickness in terms of absolute lack of food. Around 1900, however, a new concept was emerging: the idea of deficiency disease – the notion that a healthy diet required certain very specific chemical components. Crucial were the investigations of Christiaan Eijkman into beriberi in the Dutch East Indies. The first to produce a dietary deficiency disease experimentally (in chickens and pigeons), Eijkman proposed the concept of 'essential food factors', or roughly what would later be called vitamins. He demonstrated that the substance (now known as vitamin B_1) that gives protection against beriberi was contained in the husks of grains of rice – precisely the element removed when rice is polished. Through clinical studies on prisoners in Java, he determined that unpolished rice would cure the disorder.

Eijkman's researches were paralleled by the Cambridge biochemist Frederick Gowland Hopkins, who similarly discovered that very small amounts of certain substances found in food (his name for them was 'accessory food factors') were requisite for the body to utilize protein and energy for growth. An American physiologist, Elmer Verner McCollum, showed that certain fats contained an essential ingredient for normal growth: this provided the basic research for the understanding of what became known as vitamins A and D. In 1928, Albert von Szent-Györgyi isolated vitamin C from the adrenal glands, and it became recognized that that was the element in lemon juice that acted as an antiscorbutic. The idea of deficiency disease proved highly fruitful. In 1914, Joseph Goldberger of the US Public Health Service concluded that pellagra, with its classic pot-bellied symptoms, was not an infectious disorder but was rather caused by poor nutrition. Goldberger was able to relieve pellagra sufferers in the southern States by feeding them protein-rich foods. By the 1930s the pellagra-preventing factor was proved to be nicotinic acid (niacin), part of the B vitamin complex.

Study of nutrition could broadly be seen as part of the programme of research into the 'internal environment' launched by Claude Bernard. So, too, was another new specialty – endocrinology or the investigation of internal secretions. Its key concept was that of the hormone, which arose out of the energetic research programme in proteins and enzymes pursued at University College London, by William Bayliss and Ernest Starling. In 1902, an intestinal substance called secretin that activates the pancreas to liberate digestive fluids was the first specifically to be named a hormone (from the Greek: I excite or arouse). It opened up a new field: the study of the chemical messengers travelling from particular organs (ductless or endocrine glands) to other parts of the body in the bloodstream.

The relations between the thyroid gland, goitre (an enlargement of the gland), and cretinism (defective functioning of the gland) were early established, and surgical procedures followed (their mixed success is examined on page 232). The pancreas, ovaries, testes, and the adrenals were all recognized to be endocrine glands, like the thyroid. Researchers sought to ascertain precisely what metabolic processes they controlled, and which diseases followed from their imbalances. Once it was discovered that the pancreas releases into the circulation a material contributing to the control of the blood sugar it became clear that diabetes was a hormone-deficiency disease. With a view to treating diabetes, a race followed to extract the active substance (called 'insuline' by Edward Sharpey-Schafer) produced by the 'islets of Langerhans' in the pancreas.

Attention was also given to the pituitary gland, which was recognized to secrete growth hormone. In his *The Pituitary Body and its Disorders* (1912), an American surgeon, Harvey Cushing, showed that its abnormal functioning produced obesity (he described the sufferer as a tomato head on a potato body with four matches as limbs). As with thyroidism, surgery was used to remove the adrenal gland or the pituitary tumour. Further endocrinological researches led to the isolation of the female sex hormone, oestrone. By the 1930s the family of the oestrogens had been elucidated, as had the male sex hormone, testosterone. Twenty years later, on the basis of these discoveries, an oral contraceptive for women was developed (see page 267).

Some of the most fundamental advances in the biomedical sciences have arisen with the progress of neurology. Their potential significance for medical practice is still imperfectly understood. From René Descartes onwards, the importance of the nervous system for the regulation of behaviour was acutely recognized, but speculation long outran experimentation.

Experimental neurophysiology made great strides during the nineteenth century. The series of major studies stretching from Charles Bell (after whom Bell's palsy is named) to Charles Sherrington cannot be described here. Sherrington's book, *The Integrative Action of the Nervous System* (1906), which is often called the 'Bible of neurology', clearly established that the operation of the brain cells involved two neurones with a barrier between one cell and the next, enabling the impulse to pass with differing degrees of ease (the synapse). What remained a

A laboratory at the Liverpool School of Tropical Medicine in 1899. The first dean of the school and Holt Professor of Pathology, Rubert (later Sir Rubert) Boyce, is shown on the right, examining a blood-film. On his left is Charles Scott (later Sir Charles) Sherrington, then Holt Professor of Physiology. In the left foreground is Surgeon Major (later Sir Ronald) Ross, first lecturer in tropical diseases in the school. Sherrington, dubbed the father of modern neurophysiology, left Liverpool in 1913 to become Waynflete Professor of Physiology at Oxford. His book *The Integrative Action of the Nervous System* (1906) is a classic of neurology. He shared a Nobel Prize for medicine with Lord Adrian in 1932. Grisaille by W.T. Maud.

subject of passionate debate was how the nerve currents, identified in the work of David Ferrier, Sherrington, and others, were transmitted from nerve to nerve, across synapses, to their targets. Evidence began to accumulate that chemical as well as electrical processes were at work. The English physiologist and pharmacologist, Henry Hallett Dale, found a substance in 1914 in ergot (a fungus), which he called acetylcholine. This affected muscle response at certain nerve junctions. In 1929, Dale isolated acetylcholine from the spleens of freshly killed horses, and showed it was secreted at nerve endings after electric stimulation of motor nerve fibres. Acetylcholine was thus the chemical agent through which the nerves worked on the muscles. This was the first neurotransmitter to be identified.

Meanwhile in 1921, the German physiologist, Otto Loewi, was investigating the chemical basis of the muscular actions of the heart. He was to record that

> In the night of Easter Saturday, 1921, I awoke, and jotted down a few notes on a tiny slip of paper. Then I fell asleep again. It occurred to me at six o'clock in the morning, that during the night I had written down something most important, but I was unable to decipher the scrawl. That Sunday was the most desperate day in my whole scientific life. During the night, however, I woke again, and I remembered what it was. This time I did not take any risk; I got up immediately, went to the laboratory, made the experiment on the frog's heart . . . and at five o'clock the chemical transmission of nerve impulses was conclusively proved.[7]

Loewi's experiments showed that the heart, when stimulated, secreted a substance directly responsible for certain muscular actions: this was the enzyme cholinesterase, a chemical inhibitor that interrupted the acetylcholine stimulator and produced the nerve impulse pattern.

Further work brought to light numerous other chemical agents that were found at work in the nervous system. At Harvard University, Walter Cannon identified the stimulative role of adrenaline, and this led to a classification of nerves according to their transmitter substances. More research provided evidence of monamines in the central nervous system, including noradrenaline, dopamine, and serotonin.

The transmitter–inhibitor pattern thus became known, stimulating fresh work on controlling or correcting basic problems in brain function. For instance, the action of tetanus and botulism on the nervous system could for the first time be explained. Parkinson's disease, a degenerative nervous condition identified in the nineteenth century, was considered largely untreatable until it was associated with chemical transmission in the nervous system. In the late 1960s, however, it was discovered that the adrenergic side could be stimulated with L-dopa, a drug that enhances dopamine in the central nervous system and acts on the precursor of noradrenaline, presumed to be the transmitter substance. Every further development in the understanding of neurotransmission and the chemicals involved therein opens new prospects for the control and cure of neurological disorders.

One other dimension of modern science and its medical applications that must be mentioned here is genetics. The establishment of Darwin's theory of evolution by natural selection inevitably gave prominence to the component of inheritance in human development. But Darwin himself lacked a satisfactory theory of inheritance, and specious concepts of degenerationism and eugenics (see page 326) achieved great and sometimes lethal consequence before modern genetics became soundly established from the 1930s.

Valuable advances were achieved, early in the twentieth century, in demonstrating the hereditary component of metabolic disorders. Archibald Edward Garrod, a physician at St Bartholomew's Hospital in London, investigated what he first called *Inborn Errors of Metabolism* (1909), using as a model for this concept alkaptonuria, an inherited metabolic disorder in which an acid is excreted in quantities in the urine. The real breakthrough came when the infant subdiscipline of molecular biology paved the way for the elucidation of the double-helical structure of DNA in 1953 by Francis Crick and James Watson, working at the Medical Research Council's laboratory in Cambridge. The cracking of the genetic code has in turn led to the Human Genome Project, set up in 1986 with the goal of mapping all human genetic material (see page 347). Opinion remains divided as to whether this project will reveal that more diseases than conventionally thought have a genetic basis. Many believe that the next enormous medical breakthroughs will lie in the field of genetic engineering. In the meantime, a combination of clinical studies and laboratory research has firmly established the genetic component in disorders such as cystic fibrosis and Huntington's chorea (see page 345). The latter was shown to run in families as long ago as 1872 by the American physician, George Huntington.

CLINICAL SCIENCE IN THE TWENTIETH CENTURY

It is clear that the scientific pursuit of medical knowledge has undergone structural shifts during the past hundred years. Early nineteenth-century French medical science developed in the hospital, and German medical science pioneered the laboratory. New sites have emerged in more recent times to create and sustain clinical science. In some cases, this has meant special units set up by philanthropic trusts or by government. A key initiative in encouraging clinical research in the USA was the foundation in 1904 of the Rockefeller Institute for Medical Research in New York. Although the institute was at first entirely devoted to basic scientific studies, from the start the intention was to set up a small hospital alongside it, to be devoted to research in the clinic. The hospital was opened in 1910.

A vital influence on clinical research in the USA was Abraham Flexner's report on medical education, published in 1910. Flexner, educationalist brother of Simon Flexner, the first director of the Rockefeller Institute, drew attention to the parlous situation of many medical schools. An enthusiastic supporter of the German model then developing at Johns Hopkins in Baltimore, Flexner considered that there were only five US institutions that could be regarded as true centres of medical research – Harvard and Johns Hopkins, and the universities of Pennsylvania, Chicago, and Michigan. Soon after the publication of the Flexner report, the Rockefeller Foundation made funds available to Johns Hopkins for the establishment of full-time chairs in clinical subjects. This innovation spread throughout the USA, so that by the mid-1920s there were twenty institutions that could match the best in Europe. The system received a further boost with the foundation in 1948 of the National Institutes of Health. Research grants were awarded to clinical departments, which grew enormously.

Since the First World War, American clinical research has been notable both for quantity and for quality. The award of Nobel Prizes may be taken as some index. No British clinical research worker has won a Nobel Prize since Sir Ronald Ross, who won it in 1902 for the discovery of the role of the mosquito in the transmission of malaria (see page 188). Nevertheless, numerous British individuals have made internationally recognized contributions to clinical research in the twentieth century, among them James Mackenzie, who pioneered the use of the polygraph for recording the pulse and its relationship to cardiovascular disease. His work was particularly important in distinguishing atrial fibrillation and in treating this common condition with digitalis. His *Diseases of the Heart* (1908) summarized his vast experience, although he never properly appreciated the possibilities of the electrocardiograph, then being taken up by the more technologically minded Thomas Lewis.

Thomas Lewis has been dubbed the architect of British clinical research. Born in Cardiff, Lewis went in 1902 to University College Hospital (London), where he remained as student, teacher, and consultant until his death. He was the first completely to master the use of the electrocardiogram. Through animal experiments he was able to correlate the various electrical waves recorded by an electrocardiograph with the sequence of events during a contraction of the heart, which enabled him to use the instrument as a diagnostic tool when the heart had disturbances of its rhythm, damage to its valves, or changes due to high blood pressure, arteriosclerosis, and other conditions. In later life, Lewis turned his attention to the physiology of cutaneous blood vessels and the

Alice Ruhdé, assistant pharmacologist at John J. Abel's laboratory at Johns Hopkins University Medical School, c. 1915. Abel, Johns Hopkins first professor of pharmacology and the 'father of American pharmacology', believed firmly in the importance of chemistry for medicine. He was one of the first to isolate the adrenal hormone adrenaline (in 1897). In 1914, he showed that blood contains amino acids, by dialysis through a cellophane tube, and this work paved the way towards dialysis in the treatment of kidney disease. In 1925, insulin was crystallized in his laboratory and shown to be a protein.

Nobel Prizewinners in physiology or medicine

Date	Name	Country	Subject
1901	Emil A. von Behring	Germany	Serum therapy
1902	Ronald Ross	GB	Malaria
1903	Niels R. Finsen	Denmark	Treatment with light radiation
1904	Ivan P. Pavlov	Russia	Physiology of digestion
1905	Robert Koch	Germany	Tuberculosis
1906	Camillo Golgi	Italy	Structure of the nervous system
	Santiago Ramón y Cajal	Spain	
1907	Charles L. A. Laveran	France	Role of protozoans in causing disease
1908	Elie Metchnikoff	Russia	Immunity
	Paul Ehrlich	Germany	
1909	Emil T. Kocher	Switzerland	Thyroid gland
1910	Albrecht Kossel	Germany	Proteins
1911	Allvar Gullstrand	Sweden	Dioptrics of the eye
1912	Alexis Carrel	France	Structure of blood vessels
1913	Charles R. Richet	France	Anaphylaxis (abnormal reactions to antigens)
1914	Robert Bárány	Austria	Balancing apparatus of the inner ear
1915	–		
1916	–		
1917	–		
1918	–		
1919	Jules Bordet	Belgium	Immunity
1920	Schack A. S. Krogh	Denmark	Regulation of the motor mechanism of capillaries
1921	–		
1922	Archibald V. Hill	GB	Production of heat in muscle contraction
	Otto F. Meyerhof	Germany	Relationship of oxygen consumption and metabolism of lactic acid in muscles
1923	Frederick G. Banting	Canada	Discovery of insulin
	John J. R. MacLeod	Canada	
1924	Willem Einthoven	Netherlands	Electrocardiogram
1925	–		
1926	Johannes A. G. Fibiger	Denmark	*Spiroptera* carcinoma
1927	Julius Wagner-Jauregg	Austria	Treatment of general paralysis by infection with malaria
1928	Charles J. H. Nicolle	France	The louse as the vector of typhus
1929	Christiaan Eijkman	Netherlands	Dietary-deficiency diseases
	Frederick G. Hopkins	GB	Accessory food factors
1930	Karl Landsteiner	Austria	Human blood groups
1931	Otto H. Warburg	Germany	Cellular respiration
1932	Charles S. Sherrington	GB	Function of neurones
	Edgar D. Adrian	GB	
1933	Thomas H. Morgan	USA	Role of chromosomes in heredity

Date	Name	Country	Subject
1934	George Hoyt Whipple	USA	Liver treatment of pernicious anaemia
	George R. Minot	USA	
	William P. Murphy	USA	
1935	Hans Spemann	Germany	Mechanics of embryonic development
1936	Henry H. Dale	GB	Chemical transmission of nerve impulses
	Otto Loewi	Austria	
1937	Albert Szent-Györgyi	Hungary	Isolation of vitamin C
1938	Corneille J.F. Heymans	Belgium	Sinus and aortic mechanisms that regulate respiration
1939	Gerhard Domagk	Germany	Antibacterial effects of the sulphonamide prontosil
1940	–		
1941	–		
1942	–		
1943	C. P. Henrik Dam	Denmark	Discovery of vitamin K
	Edward A. Doisy	USA	Chemical nature of vitamin K
1944	Joseph Erlanger	USA	Functions of single nerve fibres
	Herbert S. Gasser	USA	
1945	Alexander Fleming	GB	Discovery of penicillin
	Ernst B. Chain	GB	
	Howard W. Florey	GB	
1946	Hermann J. Muller	USA	Use of X-rays to induce genetic mutations
1947	Carl F. Cori	USA	Carbohydrate metabolism
	Gerty T. Cori	USA	
	Bernado A. Houssay	Argentina	Role of pituitary hormones in sugar metabolism
1948	Paul H. Müller	Switzerland	Development of the insecticide DDT
1949	Walter R. Hess	Switzerland	Functional mapping of the brain
	António Egas Moniz	Portugal	Leucotomy for the relief of schizophrenia
1950	Edward C. Kendall	USA	Hormones of the adrenal cortex
	Tadeus Reichstein	Switzerland	
	Philip S. Hench	USA	
1951	Max Theiler	S. Africa	Yellow fever and the vaccine for it
1952	Selman A. Waksman	USA	Streptomycin
1953	Hans A. Krebs	GB	Citric acid cycle
	Fritz A. Lipmann	USA	Molecular structure of coenzyme A
1954	John F. Enders	USA	Cultivation of polio virus
	Thomas H. Weller	USA	
	Frederick C. Robbins	USA	
1955	Alex Hugo T. Theorell	Sweden	Oxidation enzymes
1956	André-Frédéric Cournand	USA	Heart catherization
	Werner Forssmann	Germany	
	Dickinson W. Richards	USA	

Nobel Prizewinners in physiology or medicine

Year	Name	Country	Description
1957	Daniel Bovet	Italy	Antihistamine drugs and muscle relaxants
1958	George W. Beadle	USA	How mutations affect genetic reactions
	Edward L. Tatum	USA	
	Joshua Lederberg	USA	Genetic recombination
1959	Severo Ochoa	USA	Biological synthesis of ribonucleic and deoxyribonucleic acids
	Arthur Kornberg	USA	
1960	Frank Macfarlane Burnet	Australia	Acquired immunological tolerance
	Peter B. Medawar	GB	
1961	Georg von Békésy	USA	Analysis and transmission of sound by the human ear
1962	Francis H. Crick	GB	Structure of nucleic acids
	James D. Watson	USA	
	Maurice H. F. Wilkins	GB	
1963	John C. Eccles	Australia	Biophysics of nerve transmission
	Alan L. Hodgkin	GB	
	Andrew F. Huxley	GB	
1964	Konrad E. Bloch	USA	Cholesterol and fatty acid metabolism
	Feodor Lynen	Germany	
1965	François Jacob	France	Control of gene action
	André Lwoff	France	
	Jacques Monod	France	
1966	Francis Peyton Rous	USA	Tumour-inducing viruses
	Charles B. Huggins	USA	Hormonal treatment of prostatic cancer
1967	Ragnar Granit	Sweden	Primary physiological and chemical processes in the eye
	Haldan K. Hartline	USA	
	George Wald	USA	
1968	Robert W. Holley	USA	The genetic code and its function in protein synthesis
	Har Gobind Khorana	USA	
	Marshall W. Nirenberg	USA	
1969	Max Delbrück	USA	Gene replication and viral genetics
	Alfred D. Hershey	USA	
	Salvador E. Luria	USA	
1970	Bernard Katz	GB	Release of neurotransmitters at nerve terminals
	Ulf von Euler	Sweden	
	Julius Axelrod	USA	
1971	Earl W. Sutherland, Jr	USA	Hormone action
1972	Gerald M. Edelman	USA	Chemical structure of antibodies
	Rodney R. Porter	GB	
1973	Karl von Frisch	Germany	Individual and social behaviour patterns
	Konrad Lorenz	Austria	
	Nikolaas Tinbergen	GB	
1974	Albert Claude	Belgium	Structural and functional organization of the cell
	Christian de Duve	Belgium	
	George E. Palade	USA	
1975	David Baltimore	USA	Interaction of tumour viruses and the genetic material of cells
	Renato Dulbecco	USA	
	Howard M. Temin	USA	
1976	Baruch S. Blumberg	USA	Origin and dissemination of infectious disease
	D. Carleton Gajdusek	USA	
1977	Roger Guillemin	USA	Peptide-hormone production by the hypothalamus
	Andrew V. Schally	USA	
	Rosalyn S. Yalow	USA	Radioimmunoassay of peptide hormones
1978	Werner Arber	Switzerland	Restriction enzymes and problems of molecular genetics
	Daniel Nathans	USA	
	Hamilton O. Smith	USA	
1979	Alan M. Cormack	USA	Computer-assisted tomography (CAT)
	Godfrey N. Hounsfield	GB	
1980	Baruj Benacerraf	USA	Genetically determined structures on the cell surface that regulate the immunological response
	Jean Dausset	France	
	George D. Snell	USA	
1981	Roger W. Sperry	USA	Functional specialization of the cerebral hemispheres
	David H. Hubel	USA	Information-processing in the visual system
	Torsten Wiesel	Sweden	
1982	Sune K. Bergström	Sweden	Prostaglandins and related biologically active substances
	Bengt I. Samuelsson	Sweden	
	John R. Vane	GB	
1983	Barbara McClintock	USA	Mobile genetic elements
1984	Niels K. Jerne	Denmark	Specificity in the development and control of the immune response
	Georges J. F. Köhler	Germany	
	César Milstein	GB	
1985	Michael S. Brown	USA	Regulation of cholesterol metabolism
	Joseph L. Goldstein	USA	
1986	Stanley Cohen	USA	Growth factors
	Rita Levi-Montalcini	Italy	
1987	Susumu Tonegawa	Japan	Genetic principles for the generation of antibody diversity
1988	James W. Black	GB	The design of new drugs
	Gertrude B. Elion	USA	
	George H. Hitchings	USA	
1989	J. Michael Bishop	USA	Cellular origin of retroviral oncogenes
	Harold E. Varmus	USA	
1990	Joseph E. Murray	USA	Organ and cell transplantation
	E. Donnall Thomas	USA	
1991	Erwin Neher	Germany	Function of single ion channels in cells
	Bert Sakmann		
1992	Edwin Krebs	USA	Reversible protein phosphorylation as a biological regulatory mechanism
	Edmund H. Fischer	USA	
1993	Richard Roberts	GB	Split genes
	Phillip Sharp	USA	
1994	Alfred Gilman	USA	G proteins
	Martin Rodbell	USA	
1995	Edward Lewis	USA	Genetic control of embryonic growth
	Christiane Nüsslein-Volhard	Germany	
	Eric F. Wieschaus	USA	

Sir Thomas Lewis's electrocardiograph, a device for recording the electrical activity of the heart, 1912. Notice the buckets of water. Lewis was the first physician completely to master the electrocardiogram, which the Dutch physiologist Willem Einthoven had introduced in 1901 (see page 141).

mechanisms of pain, conducting experiments on himself in an attempt to work out the distribution of pain fibres in the nervous system and to understand patterns of referred pain.

Lewis fought for full-time clinical research posts to investigate what he called 'clinical science', a broadening of his interests signalled when in 1933 he changed the name of the journal he had founded in 1909 from *Heart* to *Clinical Science*. By the early 1930s, Lewis had become the most influential figure in British clinical research, and his department at University College Hospital was the Mecca for aspiring clinical research workers. He claimed that 'Clinical science has as good a claim to the name and rights of self-subsistence of a science as any other department of biology'.[8]

Britain lagged behind the USA in the funding and organization of medical research. Before the First World War, the medical schools, especially in London, were private and rather disorganized institutions, and there was little encouragement of clinical research. A Royal Commission on University Education in London initiated changes that led to the establishment of modern academic departments in clinical subjects with an emphasis on research. By 1925 five chairs of medicine were established among the twelve medical schools in London.

In the UK, financing of clinical research has come from two main sources – a government-funded agency, the Medical Research Council, and from medical charities, such as the Imperial Cancer Research Fund, the British Heart Foundation, and the Wellcome Trust. From its foundation in 1913, the Medical Research Committee – to become the Medical Research Council (MRC) in 1920 – sought to encourage 'pure' science and also clinical research and experimental medicine.

The MRC also made other major contributions to clinical research, supporting, for example, Thomas Lewis in London.

In the immediate post-war era, the MRC was involved in two vital innovations in clinical research. The first was the introduction of the randomized controlled clinical trial. Advised by Austin Bradford Hill, professor of medical statistics and epidemiology at the London School of Tropical Medicine and Hygiene, in 1946 the council set up a trial of the efficacy of streptomycin in the treatment of pulmonary tuberculosis. The drug was in short supply and it was considered ethically justifiable to carry out a trial in which one group received streptomycin whereas a control group was treated with traditional methods. The MRC trial emphasized the importance of randomization in selecting subjects for study. This, the first randomized controlled trial to be reported in human subjects, served as a model for other such studies.

The second major development was the application of epidemiology to the analysis of clinical problems. The MRC set up a conference to discuss rising mortality from lung cancer. The MRC enlisted the aid of Bradford Hill and in 1948 he recruited the young Richard Doll, later Regius Professor of Medicine at Oxford University, to join him in analysing possible causes of lung cancer. Their painstaking survey of patients from twenty London hospitals showed that smoking is a factor, and an important factor, in the production of cancer of the lung. They went on to establish that the same conclusion applied nationally and, in an important study of members of the medical profession, they demonstrated that mortality from the disease fell if individuals stopped smoking.

These observations were not only important in showing the cause of a commonly occurring cancer in Britain, and subsequently in other countries such as the USA, but also in establishing the position of epidemiology in clinical research. As this last example shows, medical science now knows no bounds; its methods and scope sweep from the laboratory to the social survey, in helping to forge an understanding of the wider parameters of disease.

Roy Porter

CHAPTER 6   *Hospitals and surgery*

Today, surgery and hospitals go hand in glove. Without hospitals, no advanced surgery is possible; without surgery, or at least without a battery of invasive treatments, the hospital would lose its unique place in the medical system. These reciprocal ties reflect modern medical realities, but they provide a wholly misleading picture of the past.

Before 1700, the connections between hospitals and the surgeon's art were slight. The genesis of the hospital had little to do with the meeting of surgical needs; and the rise of surgery owed nothing to any special facilities that hospitals could provide. For centuries, surgery was performed on the kitchen table, on the field of battle, or below deck on the warship. In the eighteenth century and, above all, from around 1850, however, hospitals and surgery grew inseparable: they were destined to become utterly interdependent.

TRADITIONAL SURGERY

Although the surgical art did not undergo revolution until the nineteenth century, surgery is almost as old as humanity. In antiquity and during the Middle Ages, surgeons performed a multitude of minor palliative services, such as lancing boils or bandaging wounds. Before 1850, however, serious surgical operations had to be short and sharp, although they were rarely sweet. Typically, they dealt with the exterior and the extremities while avoiding (except in the direst emergency, as with caesarian section) the abdomen and other body cavities and the central nervous system.

The oldest proofs of surgical procedures are offered by trepaned (or trephined) skulls dating back to at least 10,000 years ago. The skull borings were carefully made with sharpened stone tools. Trepaning – shown here in a reconstruction at the Leiden Museum – was probably a medical procedure designed to permit the escape of evil spirits that were believed to be possessing the head of someone suffering from insanity or epilepsy. It was a well-recognized operation described in Greek and other early surgical texts.

Early surgery in India and China

Early surgery in India seems to have been conservative, although at an ancient date healers were couching for cataract and Ayurvedic healers developed exquisite skills in cosmetic surgery, especially remodelling noses (rhinoplasty). They would cut a leaf-shaped flap of skin from the forehead, making sure that the end nearest the bridge of the nose remained attached. And they pioneered a method of lithotomy (cutting for bladder stones) not introduced into Europe until the sixteenth century AD.

The most important compilation of Indian surgery was known as the *Susrata Samhita* (after Susrata, its author); its composition may be coterminous with the heyday of Greek medicine. Amongst other things, the work lists some 121 different surgical instruments, including scissors, needles, lancets, catheters, tweezers, trochars, knives, and magnets for removing metal objects. Early Chinese surgery for its part developed the technique known as moxibustion, in which a small quantity of combustible plant material was placed on the skin and set alight, causing a painful burn-blister, designed to serve as a counter-irritant.

Archaeology reveals early surgical interventions. Evidence from skulls proves that trepaning was practised at least as early as 10,000 BC. Operators – they may have been shamans – used stone cutting tools to extract portions of the cranium to ease pressure created by depressed skull fracture, or to deliver sufferers from some tormenting 'devil' that had taken possession of the soul. Bonesetting and amputations were performed from early times, although these involved severe risks of haemorrhage, infection, and shock. Egyptian medical papyri dating from the second millennium BC refer to surgical procedures for abscesses and minor tumours as well as disorders of the ear, eye, and teeth.

The Hippocratic writings produced in Greece in the fifth and fourth centuries BC contain much that relates to surgery, including a treatise on wounds (*De Ulceribus*) and another on head injuries (*De Capitis Vulneribus*). In the latter, five different types of injury are recognized and trepaning is described: fractures are to be treated by reduction and immobilization with splints and bandages; the knife is to be used for excising nasal polyps and ulcerated tonsils; and cautery is recommended for haemorrhoids. In general, however, the picture that emerges is conservative: amputation of gangrenous tissue is accepted as a last resort.

The course of plastic surgery in Europe was changed by a nose reconstruction performed in India in March 1793 and still known as the 'Hindu method'. A bullock-driver with the British Army was captured by the forces of Tipu Sultan and had his nose and one hand cut off. After escaping, he turned to a man of the brickmakers' caste, near Poona, to have his face repaired. Two British surgeons witnessed the operation and published a description of it in the *Gentleman's Magazine* for 1794. They reported that the anonymous bricklayer had used a technique superior to anything they had ever seen.

A physician about to cauterize, from an eleventh-century manuscript. Cautery is the treatment of wounds with a burning iron to seal them and to prevent fatal infection. The practice was common in the Middle Ages, was especially advocated by Islamic texts, and remains common in Arab folk medicine to this day. Belief in the necessity of such painful treatments began to be challenged in the sixteenth century. The figure of the patient is not naturalistically drawn. This is not for want of skill; the figure is deliberately schematic, much as would be found in a medical textbook today.

Catheterization is advocated for bladder stone; the removal of stones (lithotomy) is to be left to 'such as are craftsmen therein'. Vascular ligature was apparently unknown to the Greeks.

Hippocratic recommendations for the treatment of wounds proved influential for centuries. The theory was that suppuration was indispensable for healing to take place, because it was believed that pus derived from vitiated blood. This formed the basis for the later influential doctrine of 'laudable pus'.

The Hippocratic Oath (see page 59) stated that physicians should leave surgical interventions to others: this separation formed part of a medical division of labour, but surgery was also clearly viewed as an inferior trade, it being the work of the hand rather than the head. This is reflected in its name: the word 'surgery' derives from the Latin *chirurgia*, which comes from the Greek *cheiros* (hand) and *ergon* (work). Certain Greek physicians paid attention to surgery. Soranus of Ephesus wrote extensively on obstetrics, discussing the use of the birthing-chair and giving instructions for difficult birth positions. Where the fetus was in a transverse position, for instance, he performed the procedure that was later called 'turning the foot' (podalic version), easing a hand into the womb and pulling down a leg, so that the baby would be born feet first. New operations gradually appeared in the literature. In the first century AD, Celsus gave the first full account of lithotomy.

Paul of Aegina in the seventh century, and al-Zahrawi (Albucasis) and Ibn Sina (Avicenna), the illustrious Islamic physicians of the late tenth and early eleventh centuries, discussed cauterizing with a red-hot iron to stop bleeding. The Hippocratic *Corpus* and Celsus had earlier recommended cautery as a means of hindering putrefaction. In his great book, *Altasrif* (Collections), Albucasis discussed a multitude of surgical operations, but placed the greatest faith in cautery.

In the medieval West, the Salernitan school of medicine, which flourished in Salerno in southern Italy from the eleventh century, paid great attention to surgical handicraft, notably the treatment of skull wounds. It introduced the idea of dry wound management, a notion expanded in the distinguished treatises on surgery by the Frenchmen Henri de Mondeville and Guy de Chauliac, whose *Grande Chirurgie* (1363) – for two centuries the most influential textbook – contained discussion of the management of infected wounds. The importance of wound cleansing and closure was stressed, and the old doctrine of 'laudible pus' questioned: dissenting from orthodoxy, Guy de Chauliac suggested that wounds healed faster without pus formation.

The battlefield — the school for surgery

A severe wound to the extremities or the appearance of gangrene was the chief indication for the excision of limbs. Amputation above the knee was rarely performed before the sixteenth century. In time, surgeons grew bolder with amputations, probably because, with the spread of cannon and forearms, war wounds grew more plentiful and dangerous. In severing limbs, experience taught surgeons to remove more bone while preserving the maximum amount of soft tissue, thus permitting the skin to mend over the bone and in due course form a usable stump, to which a wooden leg or a hook might be attached.

Cautery with boiling oil or a hot iron remained a major way of checking haemorrhage until the eighteenth century, although styptics and compression bandaging were tried out as alternatives. Vascular ligature was pioneered by the great sixteenth-century French surgeon Ambroise Paré (see page 206).

From the late Middle Ages, many surgeons learned or developed their art in the army: because warfare presented a vast number of different forms of injury, the battlefield was termed the 'school for surgery'. Not surprisingly, it was army surgeons who wrote the most influential reports of such wound sequelae as hospital gangrene, tetanus, and erysipelas (a streptococcal skin infection) , while making prominent contributions to controversies about infection (contagionism and miasmatism; see page 102).

Growing use of gunpowder changed the character of wounds. Lead bullets and other projectiles tore through flesh, shattered bones, and drove foreign matter deep into wounds. Infections consequently became a major problem, giving rise to the belief, widespread till the eighteenth century, that some kind of 'gunpowder poison' entered the wound. Warfare also led to more amputations, including amputations of the thigh, which were almost always fatal.

A section of Trajan's Column in Rome (AD 113) depicting a field dressing station behind the battle lines, where wounded foot soldiers are receiving treatment. In the Roman Army, buildings were set aside for treating the sick, staffed by *medici* and their assistants. By AD 50, a definite architectural plan had evolved, with individual small rooms round a long corridor, a large top-lit hall, and baths and latrines. Good examples have been excavated at Neuss in Germany and Inchtuthil in Scotland. When military strategy began to change in the third century, large hospitals within permanent fortresses were no longer needed, and the sick and wounded were treated in field hospitals or accompanied the army in carts.

Traditional surgery was performed by regular barber surgeons, for whom hair-cutting and shaving provided a solid day-to-day income. It was also undertaken by itinerants, often called quacks, specializing in one particular (and often intricate or hazardous) operation. Up to the nineteenth century there were itinerant tooth-drawers, precursors of modern dentists; travelling oculists would couch for the cataract; and lithotomists removed bladder stones. Surgical treatment of hernia was likewise long in the hands of such 'empirics' (regular licensed sur-

Intermediary between regular practitioners and outright quacks in earlier centuries were itinerant specialists who pulled teeth, couched for the cataract, cut for the stone, or fitted trusses in the case of hernia. They used some of the methods of the mountebank to attract custom, but often had genuine skills. Until the nineteenth century most towns were too small to support a permanent, resident dentist, so itinerant tooth-drawers flourished instead. *Barbiere del Villaggio* by Heemskerk (1610–80).

geons might be loath to handle hernia, in view of the almost inevitable castration that accompanied it). Itinerant 'hernia masters' were active until the eighteenth century.

From the sixteenth century, however, surgery was showing signs of becoming more methodical. Ambroise Paré, a towering figure, had sections of Vesalius's *De Humani Corporis Fabrica* (1543) translated into French as part of his *Anatomie universelle du Corps humain* (1561), to make the superior anatomical teachings of the Paduan professor available to barber-surgeons who had no Latin. Born in 1510 in northern France, Paré was apprenticed to a barber-surgeon and then saw extensive military service. Many of the treatments described in his *Oeuvres*, published in 1585 when he was seventy-five, were developed as a result of experience with battlefield wounds. The most important of these were the Paré ligature and his development of a substitute for hot-oil cauterizing of open wounds. As related in his *La Méthode de Traicter les Playes Faictes par Hacquebutes* (Method of Treating Wounds) of 1545, Paré concocted an ointment (or 'digestive') from egg yolk, rose oil, and turpentine, which he applied to the wound. The mixture proved successful. Wounds treated with Paré's digestive were less painful, did not swell up, and generally remained uninflamed. Concluding that gunshot wounds did not automatically require cautery – this should be reserved for gangrenous wounds or used as a means of stopping bleeding in infected wounds – Paré abandoned the hot-oil treatment.

Tudor and Stuart England also had competent surgeons. John Woodall's *The Surgeon's Mate* (1617) long served as a manual of naval surgery, and Richard Wiseman became known as the 'father of English surgery'. His *Several Chirurgical Treatises* (1676) dwelt particularly on military and naval surgery, while his *Treatise of Wounds* (1672) advertised itself as being specially intended for ships' doctors 'who seldom burden their cabin with many books'. Nevertheless, wound treatment retained a weird-and-wonderful penumbra. There was much ado, for instance, in the seventeenth century about the 'wound salve' developed by Sir Kenelm Digby and others. Designed to heal rapier wounds, this was an odd mixture of earthworms, iron oxide, pig brain, powdered mummy, and so forth. The salve was applied not to the wound but to the weapon that caused it. The idea clearly traded on magic.

Before the introduction of anaesthesia in the 1840s, all invasive surgery depended on the swift hand, sharp knife, and cool nerve of the operator, so as to minimize pain. Operations that were slow or demanded great precision were beyond the range of early surgeons. A few highly dangerous operations were performed, however, in dire emergency. One of the most controversial was caesarean section, which many authorities, Ambrose Paré included, believed was inevitably fatal. The first properly documented caesarian section was performed in 1610 by Jeremiah Trautman in the German town of Wittenberg. In 1689, in the French town of Saintes, Jean Ruleau performed a successful caesarian on a woman who could not give birth normally because of rickets. There is no record till the 1790s of a successful caesarian being performed in Britain with the mother surviving.

In such circumstances, the bulk of the traditional surgeon's work remained routine, small scale, and fairly safe (if often awesomely painful). It involved everyday therapeutics such as dressing wounds, drawing teeth, dealing with the chancres and sores of venereal disease (common from the sixteenth century), treating skin blemishes, and so forth. The most common surgical procedure – one that served as a symbol of the profession – was bloodletting, often performed at the patient's request (see page 122). The normal method for bleeding (professionally known as 'venesection' or 'phlebotomy') was to tie a bandage around the arm to make the veins in the forearm swell up, and then open the exposed vein with a lancet: this was popularly called 'breathing a vein'. Cupping was another much-used procedure for drawing blood – it was also used to draw boils and similar eruptions; leeches have often been popular for the same purpose. Bleeding agreed with humoral doctrines, especially the theory of plethora – the idea that

ELMODO Ð CAVAR LA CREATVRA VIVA

As the link between Julius Caesar makes clear, caesarian sections have been known since antiquity. But it must be assumed that they were only ever performed in an emergency, when the mother was dying and a desperate attempt was made to save the life of the baby. There is little firm evidence of mothers surviving caesarians until the nineteenth century. This sixteenth-century German illustration is noteworthy for the presence both of a midwife and a male surgeon.

such illnesses as fevers, apoplexy, or headache followed from an excessive build-up of blood. As so often in the history of therapeutics, the 'cure' long outlived its original theoretical rationale, remaining ubiquitous, alongside purging and vomiting, until the mid-nineteenth century.

THE TRADITIONAL HOSPITAL

Although medically advanced, classical Greece had no hospitals. In Hippocratic times, a patient might occasionally be treated in the home of a physician or at shrines of Asclepius, the Greek healing god (see pages 57 and 92). In the Roman Empire, there were also facilities, termed valetudinaria, for the relief of slaves and soldiers and the provision of hospitality for wayfarers. There is no evidence, however, of buildings devoted to treatment of the sick among the population in general until well into the Christian era.

It is no accident that the triumph of the Christian faith brought the rise of nursing and the invention of the hospital as an institution of health care. Christ had performed healing miracles, giving sight to the blind, and driving out devils from the insane. Charity was the supreme Christian virtue. In the name of love, service, and salvation, believers were enjoined to care for those in need – the destitute, handicapped, poor, and hungry, those without shelter, and the sick. Once the conversion of Constantine (died AD 337) made Christianity an official imperial religion, 'hospitals' sprang up as pious foundations, and with them religious orders dedicated to serving fellow humans.

Thus a hospital was founded in 390 by Fabiola, a convert to Christianity who dedicated the rest of her life to charity. A wealthy woman, she mixed among the sick and poor of Rome. Her teacher, Jerome, wrote that she

sold all that she could lay her hands on of her property (it was large and suitable to her rank), and turning it into money she laid out this for the benefit of the poor. She was the first person to found a hospital, into which she might gather sufferers out of the streets, and where she might nurse the unfortunate victims of sickness and want. Need I now recount the various ailments of human beings? Need I speak of noses slit, eyes put out, feet half burnt, hands covered with sores? Or of limbs dropsical and atrophied? Or of diseased flesh alive with worms? Often did she carry on her own shoulders persons infected with jaundice or with filth. Often too did she wash away the matter discharged from wounds which others, even though men, could not bear to look at. She gave food to her patients with her own hand, and moistened the scarce breathing lips of the dying with sips of liquid.[1]

This ideal of nursing and healing as an act of Christian charity remained influential throughout the Middle Ages, giving impetus to the foundation of hospitals.

Some hospitals were outgrowths of religious houses: after all, monasteries themselves needed medical facilities to tend sick brethren. Throughout the medieval centuries, thousands of such institutions were established by pious bequest under the rule of regular religious orders. These 'hospitals' (the term 'hospice' may sound more appropriate to our ears) were often ephemeral, and they were generally modest, with perhaps a dozen beds and a couple of brethren in charge.

Things were different in major cities, where hospitals put down more permanent roots. By the seventh century, there were some hospitals in Constantinople (then the capital of the Roman Empire) that were sufficiently well established to offer separate wards for men and women, and special rooms for surgical patients and for eye cases. The foundation charter (1136) of the Pantokrator hospital in Constantinople (see page 70) assumed that medical teaching would be offered within the hospital. From the tenth century, there were multifunctioned hospitals ('bimaristans') in Cairo, Baghdad, Damascus, and other Islamic cities. Some supported medical teaching. In the early medieval centuries, Byzantium and the Levant were far more medically developed than Latin Europe.

In the Christian West, provision of hospitals expanded from the twelfth century with the growth of population, trade, and towns. Medieval hospitals remained frequently associated with a church or monastery, and life within them

The Hôtel Dieu, a large hospital for the poor in Paris. From the high Middle Ages, hospitals became common in the growing cities of Europe. Almost without exception they were religious foundations, set up for pious purposes and staffed by male and female members of religious orders. Their functions were primarily to care for the sick, the old, the lame, and for others in need of shelter. They would ensure a pious passing for the dying: specifically medical aims and functions were secondary.

was organized around the religious offices. It was more important to ensure that patients died in a state of grace, having received the sacraments, than to attempt heroic medical treatments to prolong temporal life. In medieval England and throughout the rural parts of continental Europe, hospices routinely provided care and hospitality for the indigent, elderly, infirm, and for pilgrims, without predominately being devoted to the sick.

In the twelfth and thirteenth centuries, hundreds of leper asylums were built. By 1225 there were around 19,000 such leprosaria in Europe. A high wall would separate the leprosary from the community, while small huts within provided shelter for the sick. As leprosy declined, the leprosaria were used for persons suspected of carrying infectious diseases, the insane, and even the indigent. Some became hospitals. Thus the Hôpital des Petits Maisons near the monastery of St Germain des Près outside Paris, which began as a leprosarium, was later used for indigent syphilitics and disordered pilgrims. St Giles in the Fields, west of the walls of London, was originally a leprosarium.

When bubonic plague struck Europe in the fourteenth century, the leprosaria were requisitioned as the first plague hospitals. Lazarettos (named after the protective patron, St Lazarus) began to be built in the later years of the century, to safeguard trade and to protect city populations. The first documented pesthouse was built at Dubrovnik (Ragusa) on the Adriatic coast of Croatia in 1377, followed by an infirmary in Marseilles in 1383. Venice built two lazarettos on islands of its lagoon in 1423 and 1468, respectively. Milan completed a pesthouse 20 years later, and the hospital of St Sebastian, built in Nuremberg in 1498, became the model for later German plague hospitals.

A seventeenth-century pesthouse or lazaretto, with its gates and guard, in Rome. The pest cart and its commissioner are in the foreground. Named after the biblical Lazarus, lazarettos were originally designed to house lepers well out of harm's way. With the decline of leprosy in Europe from around the thirteenth century, lazarettos increasingly became requisitioned as pesthouses in times of plague. In either case, their crucial function was to protect the rest of the population.

It was in Italian cities – Venice, Bologna, Florence, Naples, and Rome – that the most distinguished medieval hospitals were established. Unlike small rural foundations, hospitals in the major Italian cities often had a resident medical staff. In Italian urban centres, hospitals played a key part in caring for the poor and sick. Religious confraternities took upon themselves the duty of charity, and some administered hospitals. Severe plague outbreaks and other epidemics spurred the foundation of hospitals, so that by the fifteenth century there were thirty-three hospitals in Florence alone – roughly one for every 1,000 inhabitants. The size of these varied enormously, from under ten beds to 230 at S. Maria Nuova (founded in 1288), the largest and most eminent. These Florentine hospitals were primarily for orphans, pilgrims, widows, and the teeming poor; only seven were principally dedicated to the sick, but these did have medical staffs attached to them. At S. Maria Nuova there were six visiting physicians, a surgeon, and three junior staff members in the fourteenth century.

In England, there were about 470 'hospitals' by the close of the fourteenth century, but they were generally tiny and barely medical. Numbers of inmates varied from around two or three to about thirty, with an average of about ten. Only in London were there hospitals of any significance. The dissolution of the monasteries and chantries during the reformations of Henry VIII and Edward VI (1536–52) brought the closure of practically all such foundations, and the Crown seized their assets. A handful were re-established, however, on a new and secular basis.

Interior of the hospital of S. Maria della Scala, Siena, by Domenico di Barto, 1440–4. The building is still used as a hospital today. Notice the priest. The well-dressed individuals may well be patrons and benefactors who would expect to be included in such a painting, which displays their handsome generosity. The altercation between the cat and dog supposedly emblematizes the less than harmonious relations between physicians and surgeons.

St Bartholomew's (founded 1123) and St Thomas's (founded around 1215), Christ's Hospital, and Bethlem (both thirteenth-century foundations) were sold by the Crown to the corporation of the City of London. St Thomas's and St Bartholomew's expanded as hospitals for the sick poor, and Bethlem catered for the mad (see page 288). Nevertheless, although Stuart London grew into a monster city – it had over half a million people by 1700, making it, with Paris, the largest city in Europe – it had just two medical hospitals of any consequence. And beyond the capital, there were no medical hospitals at all in England in 1700.

In Catholic countries, no equivalent of the reformation of Henry VIII asset-stripped the hospitals, and in Spain, France, and Italy foundations grew in numbers in the sixteenth and seventeenth centuries in response to an increase in population. Religious and lay elements in the hospitals generally worked well

Visitors to a hospital. Bas-relief in enamelled terracotta by Giovanni della Robbia at the Ceppo Hospital, Pistoia, first half of the sixteenth century.

together, although conflicts sometimes arose between physicians, with their medical priorities, and the nursing staff, with their pious ends. Charitable donations to hospitals played a part in local chains of protection, patronage, and family power. In France, the *hôpital général* (similar to the English poorhouse) emerged in the seventeenth century as an institution designed to shelter – or rather confine – beggars, orphans, vagabonds, prostitutes, and thieves, alongside the sick and mad. The Hôtel Dieu in Paris was more specifically designed as a healing institution; this was run by religious orders.

Perhaps the jewel amongst continental hospitals in the eighteenth century was Vienna's Allgemeine Krankenhaus (general hospital), rebuilt by the Emperor Joseph II in 1784. In the time-honoured manner, the Vienna hospital sheltered the poor as well as providing medical facilities for the sick. Planned for 1,600 patients, it was divided into six medical, four surgical, and four clinical sections; eighty-six clinical beds met the teaching needs of its medical staff. As part of Joseph II's grand design for modernizing the Habsburg Empire, provincial hospitals were also built in Olmütz (1787), Linz (1788), and Prague (1789). New infirmaries were also set up in other German-speaking territories, including the Juliusspital at Würzburg (1789), which won praise for its operating theatre.

Berlin's Charité Hospital was built in 1768, and, in the Ukraine, Catherine the Great (1762–96) erected the huge Obukhov Hospital.

Although by European standards early-modern England was exceptionally ill-endowed with hospitals – and also with sister institutions such as orphanages – this lamentable state of affairs changed rapidly in the Age of Enlightenment when philanthropy, secular and religious, raised many new foundations. The new hospitals founded in eighteenth-century England were meant for the poor (although not for parish paupers, who would be dealt with under the Poor Law). Granting free care to the respectable or deserving sick poor would, it was hoped, confirm social ties of paternalism, deference, and gratitude.

London benefited earliest. To the metropolis's two ancient hospitals, a further five were added between 1720 and 1750: the Westminster (1720), Guy's (1724), St George's (1733), the London (1740), and the Middlesex (1745). All were general hospitals. They stirred the founding of institutions in the provinces, where no genuinely medical hospitals had existed at all. The Edinburgh Royal Infirmary was set up in 1729, followed by hospitals in Winchester and Bristol (1737), York (1740), Exeter (1741), Bath (1742), Northampton (1743), and some twenty others. By 1800, all sizeable English towns had a hospital. Traditional cathedral and corporation cities came first, industrial towns, such as Sheffield and Hull, followed.

Augmenting these general foundations, humanitarians also pumped money into specialist institutions for the sick. St Luke's Hospital was opened in London in 1751, making it at that time the only large public lunatic asylum apart from Bethlem. Unlike Bethlem, criticized for its barbarity (see page 296), St Luke's was launched to an optimistic fanfare, its physician, William Battie, asserting that, if handled with humanity, lunacy was no less curable than any other disease. By 1800, other great towns such as Manchester, Liverpool, and York had public lunatic asylums, philanthropically supported. Alongside lunatics, sufferers from venereal disease also became objects for charity – surely a sign of a changing climate of opinion: the harsh religious judgement that such diseases were salutary punishment for vice was evidently on the wane, being supplanted by the Enlightenment view that relief of suffering was the duty of humanity. London's Lock Hospital, exclusively for venereal cases, opened in 1746. It was paralleled by another London charitable foundation, the Magdalene Hospital for Penitent Prostitutes (1759) – less a medical hospital than a refuge where harlots wishing to go straight were taught a trade.

Another new institution was the lying-in hospital. In London, the earliest maternity hospitals were the British (1749), the City (1750), the General (1752), and the Westminster (1765). These met major needs, not least by guaranteeing bed-rest to impoverished women. They also enabled unmarried mothers, mainly servant girls, to deliver their illegitimate babies with no questions asked. Many newborns then ended up in the Foundling Hospital in Bloomsbury, opened in

Extensive hospital building was undertaken in the eighteenth century in Europe. The most notable continental example, shown here, was Vienna's Allgemeines Krankenhaus (general hospital) rebuilt by Emperor Joseph II in 1784 – a perfect expression of the drive towards administrative centralization by the Enlightenment's absolutist rulers. In traditional manner, the Vienna hospital sheltered the poor as well as providing medical facilties for the sick. The central round tower, the Narrenturm, was the lunatic asylum. Six storeys high, it had twenty-eight cells to a floor.

1741. Unwanted children could be deposited there anonymously; they would be educated and taught a trade. The benevolent designs of lying-in hospitals were thwarted, however, by the appalling death rates of mothers and babies alike from what would later be identified as bacterial infections. Nevertheless, they served as sites where medical students could practise obstetric skills.

General hospitals provided treatment, food, shelter, and opportunities for convalescence. By 1800, London's hospitals alone were handling over 20,000 patients a year. But, as with hospitals abroad, they restricted themselves to fairly minor complaints likely to respond to treatment, and they excluded infectious cases. Nothing useful could have been gained by allowing fevers into the hospital: they could not be cured and were sure to spread like wildfire. Separate fever hospitals were, however, set up for those with contagious diseases. London's first fever hospital (euphemistically called the House of Recovery) was opened in 1801. Another new means of healing was the outpatient department, and dispensaries were also founded.

Similar developments took place in North America. The first general hospital was founded in Philadelphia in 1751; some 20 years later the New York Hospital was established. The Massachusetts General Hospital in Boston followed in 1811. All such hospitals catered for the sick poor.

THE START OF CLINICAL ROUNDS

In the eighteenth century, hospitals increasingly opened themselves to medical students, and teachers used instructive cases on their doorstep as training material. In Vienna, the hospital reforms carried through in the 1770s by Anton Stoerck led to clinical instruction on the wards. The success of the Edinburgh Medical School owed much to its links with the city's infirmary. Professor John Rutherford inaugurated clinical lecturing there in the 1740s, and from 1750 a special clinical ward was set up, whose patients served as teaching material for professorial clinical lectures. 'A number of such cases as are likely to prove instructive', noted the medical student, John Aikin, in the 1770s, 'are selected and disposed in separate rooms in the Infirmary, and attended by one of the college professors. The students go round with him every day, and mark down the state of each patient and the medicines prescribed. At certain times lectures are read upon these cases, in which all the progressive changes in the disease are traced and explained and the method of practice is accounted for.' [2] Students were expected to visit patients' bedsides on their own initiative, studying the professors' reports.

Initially, English infirmaries had little to do with teaching. The leading London surgeon-anatomist, William Cheselden, started private surgical lectures in 1711; but in 1718 he moved his lectures to St Thomas's, delivering four courses a year. Clinical instruction was set up, and students were encouraged to follow their teachers round the wards and into the operating theatre. The practice spread. The Philadelphian William Shippen attended London's hospitals in 1759, and recorded in his journal,

> [4 August] saw Mr. Way surgeon to Guy's hospital amputate a leg above the knee very dexterously 8 ligatures … [23 August] attended Dr Akenside in taking in patient and prescribing for them, 58 taken in … [5 September] … saw Mr Baker perform 3 operations, a leg, breast and tumour from a girl's lower jaw inside, very well operated … [7 November] went to Bartholomew's Hospital and saw the neatest operation of bubonocele that I ever saw by Mr. Pott a very clever neat surgeon. [3]

Such accounts show that contemporaries believed that surgical treatment in hospital was improving.

Pupils became a more conspicuous presence in provincial hospitals, and student training was essential to specialist institutions such as maternity hospitals. One such, London's New General Lying-In Hospital, admitted students as pupils to the attending *accoucheurs*, as male midwives were called (see page 222). As a result of all this, by 1800 London was, according to Bristol physician, Thomas Beddoes, 'the best spot in Great Britain, and probably in the whole world where medicine may be taught as well as cultivated to most advantage'. [4]

RELIGIOUS NURSING ORDERS

Hospital nursing had long been provided by religious orders as part of the Christian service ideal – and nursing remained largely the business of religious orders in Catholic Europe until recent times. All monastic orders were charged with caring for God's poor, which included the sick, and each monastery or convent had an *infirmarius* or *infirmaria* who oversaw the infirmary and, with the help of assistants, ministered to the sick. During the Crusades, the Knights of St John of Jerusalem (later called the Knights of Malta, and the progenitor of the St John Ambulance Brigade), the Teutonic Knights, the Knights Templar, and the Knights of St Lazarus were active in nursing as well as hospital building. In seventeenth-century France, a priest, Vincent de Paul, set up the Daughters of Charity primarily as a nursing order.

In the French Revolution, however, as part of the wholesale attack on the Church, religious nursing communities were abolished and charities were nationalized. Revolutionaries confiscated the coffers of religious foundations. In the event, however, political indecision, corruption, and rampant inflation led to a spectacular reduction in the welfare and hospital services being provided for the needy. By choice and necessity, Napoleon largely reverted to the *status quo ante*, with hospitals being financed by pious donations and staffed by religious orders, above all the Daughters of Charity, who flourished in the nineteenth century. Provision of nursing was much more hit-and-miss in Protestant countries. In Georgian England, the stereotypical nurse was a drunken, slovenly battle-axe.

CAMPAIGNS FOR HOSPITAL REFORM

If nursing left much to be desired, the hospital itself, nominally a site of recuperation, readily became a place of disease and death, spreading the maladies it was meant to relieve. The eighteenth century, however, brought campaigns for hospital reform, as part of a broad critique front of outmoded, corrupt, and unhealthy institutions. Moved by humanity, the English philanthropist John Howard (see page 311) turned in his last years from prison reform to the remodelling of hospitals; his extensive travels spread reform on the Continent. He was particularly insistent on the need for cleanliness and fresh air to combat the deadly miasmic effluvia that he and others blamed for sickness and shocking mortality figures in gaols and hospitals.

The medical profession itself was not indifferent to hospital reform. When Louis XVI invited the Académie des Sciences to take up hospital reform, a distinguished surgeon, Jacques Tenon, was sent to visit England. Impressed with the Royal Naval Hospital in Plymouth, and the through-ventilation permitted by its pavilion style, he returned to Paris with noble visions of new buildings. But little came of these rebuilding plans, as the Revolution distrusted hospitals, seeing them as agents of religious indoctrination and oligarchic power. The direct effect of the French Revolution on healing institutions was negative.

SURGERY RISES IN STATUS

Surgery rose in quality and status in Europe during the eighteenth century. For centuries called 'the cutter's art' and disparaged as a manual skill rather than a liberal science, surgery had been subordinate to physic in the medical pecking-order. Surgeons had normally passed not through an academic but a practical education, via apprenticeship not the university. Organized in trade guilds, surgery traditionally carried little status. It could be portrayed as demeaning and defiling; for unlike the clean-handed, bewigged, and perfumed physician, surgeons were habitually dealing with diseased and decaying flesh – tumours, wens (cysts), fractures, gangrene, syphilitic chancres, and such like. Their instruments were terrifying – the knife, cauterizing irons, the amputating saw: they were satirically compared to butchers or torturers.

Butts of satire amongst contemporaries, in the days before anaesthesia, surgeons have traditionally received a bad press from historians, who have tended to represent Old Mr Sawbones as a blundering and bloody operator. The caricature, however, tells but a partial truth, and recent studies of the surgeon's day-to-day trade in the seventeenth or eighteenth centuries have been painting a different picture. The spectacular and frequently lethal operations such as amputations or trepaning on which historians have dwelt were, in truth, the exception rather than the rule. The main business of the average surgeon was minor running-repairs: bloodletting, pulling teeth, managing whitlows, trussing rup-

The year 1540 was an important milestone in British surgery because, in London, the Guild of Surgeons joined the rival Company of Barbers to form a united Company of Barber-Surgeons. In this painting by Hans Holbein the Younger (1541), Henry VIII is shown handing the Act of Union to Thomas Vicary, the first master of the new company. In granting a charter to a medical corporation, Henry VIII was a friend to the medical welfare of his subjects. In many other respects, however, he was not. His reformation permanently closed many monastic foundations and hospitals that gave shelter and aid to the sick.

Early surgical instruments appear to us rather gross and crude, more like tools out of a carpenter's box. These are seventeenth-century knives and lancets for treating abscesses.

tures, treating leg ulcers, patching up fistulas, medicating venereal infections, and so forth. The traditional surgeon had to attend to scores of external conditions requiring routine maintenance through cleansing, pus removal, ointments, and bandaging. The conditions he treated were mostly not life-threatening, nor were his interventions glamorous.

Studies of ordinary surgeons have shown low fatality rates amongst surgeons who sensibly respected their limits. The scope of internal operative surgery they undertook was narrow, because they were well aware of the risks: trauma, blood loss, and sepsis. A dextrous eighteenth-century surgeon would extract bladder stones or extirpate cancerous tumours from the breast. In 1810, the novelist Fanny Burney was cut, without anaesthetic, for cancer of the breast by the great French surgeon Dominique-Jean Larrey, and she survived – although not without experiencing excruciating pain, as this extract from her detailed account of the operation shows:

M. Dubois placed me upon the Mattress, & spread a cambric handerchief upon my face. It was transparent, however, & I saw, through it that the Bed stead was instantly surrounded by the 7 men and my nurse, I refused to be held; but when, bright through the cambric, I saw the glitter of polished steel – I closed my eyes . . .

Yet – when the dreadful steel was plunged into the breast – cutting through veins – arteries – flesh – nerves – I needed no injunctions not to restrain my cries. I began a scream that lasted uninterrmittingly during the whole time of the incision – & I almost marvel that it rings not in my Ears still! so excruciating was the agony. When the wound was made, & the instrument was withdrawn, the pain seemed undiminished, for the air that suddenly rushed into those del-

Surgery long remained a low-prestige occupation, largely on account of its associations with the shedding of blood. It was easy to dub the surgeon 'Mr Sawbones', and to liken him to a butcher. In cartoons, such as this one of an amputation, surgeons were generally depicted as hefty fellows, whereas physicians were seen as more refined. Aquatint by Thomas Rowlandson, 1793.

icate parts felt like a mass of minute but sharp & forked poniards, that were tearing the edges of the wound, – but when again I felt the instrument – describing a curve – cutting against the grain, if I may so say, while the flesh resisted in a manner so forcible as to oppose & tire the hand of the operator, who was forced to change from the right to the left - then, indeed, I thought I must have expired, I attempted no more to open my eyes … The instrument this second time withdrawn, I concluded the operation over – Oh no! presently the terrible cutting was renewed – & worse than ever, to separate the bottom, the foundation of this dreadful gland from the parts to which it adhered … yet again all was not over … [5]

Exploration of the abdominal cavity was strictly for the future. Malfunctions of the heart, liver, brain, and stomach were treated not by the knife but by medicines and management; major internal surgery was not contemplated before the introduction of anaesthetics and antiseptic procedures. Only after 1800 did surgeons begin to perform hysterectomies and other gynaecological surgery, and even then the more conservative members of the profession disapproved of such 'recklessness'.

Improvements were arising, however, in certain surgical fields. Take the treatment of bladder stones. A common traditional procedure, known as the 'apparatus major', had involved dilating and incising the urethra to allow the introduction of instruments to extract the stone. A superior method was introduced around 1700 by the itinerant practitioner, Jacques de Beaulieu, popularly called Frère Jacques (he wore the habit of a Franciscan friar to ensure safety on his travels). This lateral cystotomy involved cutting into the perineum and opening up both bladder and bladder neck. Frère Jacques is said to have performed some 4,500 lithotomies and 2,000 hernia operations.

Two distinguished surgeons, Johannes Rau in Amsterdam and William Cheselden in London, took up Frère Jacques's method with significant success. Cheselden won fame for performing lithotomy with exceptional rapidity – he could complete the excruciatingly painful knifework in 2 minutes flat, whereas other surgeons might take 20. As a result, he commanded huge fees, apparently up to 500 guineas a patient. This example reveals a situation common in early modern medicine: innovations first introduced by itinerants or quacks (who could afford to be daring: they had nothing to lose) in time found their way

Cancer of the breast used to be less common in women than it is nowadays, perhaps because most people did not live long enough for the disease to emerge. However, its fatal consequences were recognized and mastectomy operations recommended, even in the eighteenth century. These illustrations on how to perform the operation, including cautery to seal the wound, are from Johannes Scultetus the elder's *Armentarium Chirurgicum* (1741). Their rather clinical nature hardly masks the painfulness of mastectomy.

into regular practice. The same applies to hernia; traditionally the speciality of travelling itinerants, hernia was increasingly dealt with by regular surgeons, aided by truss-making improvements.

Other operations also underwent refinement. A celebrated French military surgeon, Jean-Louis Petit, developed new practices with amputations at the thigh, inventing an effective tourniquet that controlled bloodflow while the surgeon carried out ligatures as recommended by Ambroise Paré. He also demonstrated the spread of breast cancer to a women's regional lymph glands in the armpit. Military surgery advanced, too, especially the management of gunshot wounds. Endemic warfare and immense colonial and naval expansion created insatiable demands for junior surgeons willing to serve abroad or aboard ship. By the early eighteenth century the British fleet had 247 vessels, each carrying a surgeon and mate. For those with strong stomachs, like the surgeon-hero of Tobias Smollett's novel, *Roderick Random* (1748), naval or military service provided boundless experience and a valuable leg-up into the profession.

Specialist surgeons pioneered new techniques. By 1700 it was recognized that cataract involved a hardening of the lens. A French oculist, Jacques Daviel, discovered a method of extracting the lens of the eye once it had become opaque through cataract, performing the operation several hundred times with good results. Also skilled at the same operation was the British quack oculist, John ('Chevalier') Taylor, who practised with tremendous razzmatazz at many of the princely courts of Europe. According to his enemies, Taylor's overconfidence contributed to the blindness of Bach and Handel.

Other surgeons achieved fame for their dependable skill or innovations. A humane operator, Percivall Pott, a surgeon at St Bartholomew's Hospital in London, published on hernia, head injuries, hydrocele (swelling of the scrotum), anal

Operations for removing bladder stones (lithotomy), from Lorenz Heister's *Institutiones Chirurgicae* (1739). Bladder stones were extremely common in earlier centuries, perhaps because of all the impurities in what was drunk. Notable improvements in lithotomy were introduced around 1700 with the introduction of lateral cystotomy, which involved cutting into the perineum and opening up the bladder and the bladder neck.

fistula, fractures, and dislocations, as well as being the first to observe that chimney sweeps suffer from cancer of the scrotum. Pierre-Joseph Desault, François Bichat's teacher and founder in 1791 of the first surgical periodical, the *Journal de Chirurgie*, improved the treatment of fractures, and developed methods of ligating blood vessels in case of aneurysm. Desault insisted that surgeons should have an understanding of physiology as well as anatomy. Orthopaedics began to emerge, thanks especially to Jean-André Venel of Geneva, who designed mechanical devices to correct lateral curvature and other spinal defects.

Thanks to such improvements in surgery and changes in obstetrical practices, surgery rose in professional standing. This occurred first in France. As elsewhere, French practitioners were initially barber-surgeons – in London, the Barber-Surgeons' Company had been approved by Parliament in 1540 – but they succeeded, thanks to royal favour, in emancipating themselves from the barbers. In 1672, the Paris surgeon Pierre Dionis was honoured by being appointed to lecture in anatomy and surgery at the Jardin du Roi (the Royal Botanical Gardens). Then, in 1687, the misfortune of Louis XIV in developing anal fistula proved a golden opportunity. A successful operation on the Sun King by Charles-François Félix (he had first practised on the poor) contributed to promote surgery's prestige.

From the early eighteenth century, surgery was widely taught in Paris through lectures and demonstrations. The breakthrough came in 1731, when a royal charter established the Académie Royale de Chirurgie; 12 years later, Louis XV dissolved the link between the surgeons and barbers, and, in 1768, the convention of training surgeons by apprenticeship came to an end. Thereafter, surgeons vied with physicians in status, claiming that surgery was no mere manual art. This view of surgery as a science squared with the Enlightenment accent on practical ('empirical') rather than bookish learning. Within such a framework, it became possible to tout surgery as the most experimental and therefore the most progressive branch of medicine.

As a result of these developments, France led the world in surgery for most of the eighteenth century, drawing students from all over Europe. First in Paris and later elsewhere, the hospital became the site of surgical teaching, and the junior ranks of the surgical profession, employed as dressers, found work in hospitals as pupil teachers. The surgeon Pierre-Joseph Desault at the Hôtel Dieu introduced bedside teaching. Moving medical education to the hospital reinforced the links that had been growing between surgery and anatomy since Andreas Vesalius in the sixteenth century, and constituted some steps towards the 'anatomico-localist' or 'patho-anatomical' perspective on disease that became so prominent in the hospitals of post-Revolutionary Paris – a view identifying diseases with specific organs and local pathological changes.

Parallel developments occurred elsewhere. It is significant that the first Alexander Monro, the first incumbent of the chair of anatomy and surgery in the Edinburgh medical school, was by profession a surgeon. Monro helped to found the

The Dr Spocks of the eighteenth century

Obstetrical skills improved in the eighteenth century, as part of a radical transformation of childbirth. Birthing had traditionally been an event exclusive to women: the mother, her female kith and kin, and a midwife, who was often poorly trained if highly experienced. Birth was conducted according to folk and religious customs. But first amongst polite society in England, and, later in North America, the traditional 'granny midwife' became displaced by a male operator, the 'man-midwife' or *accoucheur*.

This new obstetrician claimed superior expertise. As a qualified medical practitioner, armed perhaps with a degree from Edinburgh or some other a prestigious medical school, his anatomical expertise made him confident that he could let Nature do her own work in the case of normal deliveries. Contrary to the claims of some feminist historians, leading man-midwives, such as William Hunter, prided themselves on being *less* interventionist than traditional midwives. Yet *accoucheurs* also possessed, unlike the midwife, surgical instruments – above all, the new obstetric forceps – for use in difficult labours and emergencies. Introduced in the seventeenth century and long kept a secret by their inventors, the Chamberlen family in London, forceps became common property by 1730.

Accoucheurs could claim special expertise because they were frequently attached to the newly founded lying-in hospitals and birth charities sprouting in large towns, or were the proprietors of obstetric schools. In London, the leading instructors were Scots: William Smellie and his pupil, William Hunter. Smellie mastered obstetrics in Paris before teaching it in the 1740s. He devised models for student practice, including a leather-covered manikin. His *Treatise on the Theory and Practice of Midwifery* (1752) proved one of the first great obstetric texts, establishing safe rules for the use of forceps.

For his part, William Hunter underwent 5 years' training at the University of Glasgow, 3 as the pupil of William Cullen, before beginning in 1746 to give private lecture courses in London on dissecting, surgery, and obstetrics (see page 225).

In North America, medical midwifery developed under the inspiration of William Shippen, who had studied with William and John Hunter in London and under William Cullen and the second Alexander Monro in Edinburgh. Shippen taught anatomy and midwifery in Philadelphia from 1763, helping to establish the domination of male *accoucheurs* that became so conspicuous in the USA.

Where *accoucheurs* flourished – it was mainly in Protestant areas – childbirth was transformed from a women-only rite. Fashionable ladies might now have their husbands present at labour. They gave birth in rooms into which daylight and fresh air were admitted. Delivered safely, their newborns would no longer be swaddled: according to new theories, allowing freedom to infant limbs would strengthen bones and promote healthy development. On medical advice, modern ladies also now breastfed their babies: surely mother's milk was best and would encourage good bonding between mother and baby. Enlightened surgeons – the Dr Spocks of their day – played a part in changing the concept of childbirth and baby-care.

William Hunter's *Anatomy of the Human Gravid Uterus* (1774) contained exceptionally lifelike illustrations (below left) of the foetus and womb by Jan van Rymsdyk. The eighteenth century also brought the advent of the man-midwife for normal deliveries. The huge drape over the woman, deployed for modesty's sake, forced the operator to work blind.

Edinburgh Royal Infirmary, and made Edinburgh a major centre for medical training. His *Osteology* (1726), *Essay on Comparative Anatomy* (1744), and *Observations Anatomical and Physiological* (1758) became important anatomical texts.

Monro taught anatomy, but he also gave instruction in surgical operations,
both to medical students and to surgical apprentices. The immense success of
medical education as imparted in Edinburgh began to erode traditional status
divisions, much more tenaciously upheld in England, between physic and surgery.
From 1778, the Royal College of Surgeons of Edinburgh awarded its own diplo-
mas, which were almost as valuable as a degree. Medical students in Edinburgh
found it made sense to equip themselves to practise both skills, particularly if they
expected to become general practitioners, medical jacks-of-all-trades practising
all branches of healing.

The growing prominence of the hospital proved a blessing for surgeons. For
one thing, the new infirmaries attracted accident and emergency cases, which
were treated by surgeons rather than physicians. Moreover, hospitals afforded
supplies of unclaimed dead bodies, predominantly those of the poor, whom surgeons and their students dissected postmortem. Hospitals also provided facilities
for surgeons to lecture to students. Alongside hospitals, the spread of anatomy
schools, first in Paris and then in London, boosted surgery's prestige.

In this nineteenth-century painting by an unknown artist, the despotic surgeon Guillaume Dupuytren is shown demonstrating to Charles X, on a visit to the Hôtel Dieu, the successful results of a cataract operation. Parisian hospitals were famed for their advanced medicine in the eighteenth and nine-teenth centuries, but their impoverished patients were widely treated as experimen-tal materials, upon whom students practised and leading doctors pioneered new techniques.

By 1800 the surgeon had escaped the demeaning association with the traditional barber and bleeder: in London, the Company of Surgeons split from the barbers in 1745. The surgeon's status has continued to improve so that by the twentieth century the surgeon had shot up in status to become, perhaps, the most conspicuous of all the medical practitioners.

THE BIRTH OF THE CLINIC

Particularly with the development, around 1800, of the new medical science typified by physical examination, pathological anatomy, and statistics, the hospital gradually ceased to be primarily a site of charity, care, and convalescence; it turned into the medical powerhouse it has been ever since.

The new anatomical and clinical approach to medicine, pioneered in Paris, was based not on the lecture theatre but on the big, public hospital where direct hands-on experience could be gained in abundance. The 'clinic' (as this hospital medicine was to be called) became central to medicine. It made use of hospital facilities to deploy postmortems to correlate internal manifestations after death with pathology in the living. The huge numbers of patients in the public hospitals meant that diseases were identified as afflictions that beset everyone in the same way, rather than being unique to each case, and statistics were used to establish representative disease profiles. Such an approach was pioneered around 1800 by Philippe Pinel at La Salpêtrière in Paris, by René Läennec at the Hôpital Necker, and by Pierre Louis of the Hôtel Dieu. Their emphasis was not on symptoms but on lesions – that is, the objective facets of disease.

The nineteenth century brought a notable growth in hospitals, in response to population rise: London, for example, expanded from somewhat over half a million people in the early eighteenth century to 5 million by 1900. In 1800, America's population was just over 5 million, with only a tiny proportion of that number living in urban communities. There were, consequently, just a couple of hospitals – the Pennsylvania Hospital and the New York Hospital (founded 1771). By the early twentieth century, the USA had more than 4,000 hospitals, and few towns were without one.

New hospitals were founded to meet rising needs, and medical men started to take the initiative in setting them up – because an association with a hospital became a principal lever of professional advance. From the late eighteenth century practitioners began to found their own institutions, specializing above all in particular conditions. By 1860, London alone supported at least sixty-six special hospitals and dispensaries, designed for outpatients, including the Royal Hospital for Diseases of the Chest (1814), the Brompton Hospital (1841), the Royal Marsden Hospital (1851), the Hospital for Sick Children, Great Ormond Street (1852), and the National Hospital (for nervous diseases), Queen Square (1860).

Specialist hospitals sprang up throughout the developed world. Children's hospitals were set up in Paris in 1802, in Berlin in 1830, St Petersburg in 1934, and

Surgery becomes a science

The private anatomy school established by William Hunter in Windmill Street, Piccadilly, offered instruction in anatomy, surgery, physiology, pathology, midwifery, and diseases of women and children. William Hunter and his younger brother, John, were principally surgeons, but proprietorship of a private anatomy school permitted them to associate surgery with experimentation. John, who became the leading surgeon-physiologist of his age, was a tireless dissector. Whereas William enjoyed being a fashionable *accoucheur* and teacher, John devoted his energies and earnings to research, focusing on comparative anatomy.

Having won his spurs as assistant in the dissecting room to his brother (1748), John Hunter studied surgery at Chelsea Hospital and St Bartholomew's, and in 1754 entered St George's Hospital, becoming house-surgeon in 1756 and then lecturer at his brother's anatomical school. In 1760. he entered the army as staff-surgeon, and served in the expedition to Belle-Ile in the Bay of Biscay and to Portugal. At the peace in 1763 he

John Hunter by Joshua Reynolds, 1786 (detail).

set up his London practice, and devoted much time and money to comparative anatomy.

Hungry for scientific knowledge, John Hunter amassed a huge series of anatomical and biological specimens, about 13,000 of which became the basis of the Hunterian Museum of the Royal College of Surgeons in Lincoln's Inn Fields. He trained many eminent pupils, including Edward Jenner, the promoter of smallpox vaccination, and Philip Syng Physick, the American who imported Hunterian surgery into the New World.

Addressing such key surgical topics as inflammation, shock, disorders of the vascular system, and venereal disease, John Hunter's four main treatises – *The Natural History of the Human Teeth* (1771), *On Venereal Disease* (1786), *Observations on Certain Parts of the Animal Oeconomy* (1786), and *Treatise on the Blood Inflammation and Gunshot Wounds* (1794) – were celebrated by his successors as marking the elevation of surgery from a craft to science.

Vienna in 1837. The Massachusetts Eye and Ear Infirmary was established in 1824, the Boston Lying-In Hospital in 1832, the New York Hospital for Diseases of the Skin in 1836, and scores more. Women's hospitals were also instituted. Specialist hospitals had no broad caring mission; for this reason they became 'medicalized' earlier than the general hospitals, which continued to exercise a charitable role towards the ailing poor. In specialist hospitals, doctors controlled patient admission, appointments, and policy, and pioneered new therapies.

The organized teaching hospital also emerged, often associated with a university. Set up in 1828 as a non-denominational university (Oxford and Cambridge were still exclusively Church of England), University College London established its own hospital in 1834, which became linked to its medical school. King's College was the Anglican response to this development, and King's College Hospital was set up in 1839. With the evolution of the modern hospital, nursing, too, underwent transformation, becoming more professional and acquiring its own career structures.

Nursing becomes professional

The Deaconess Institute, established in 1836 by Theodore Fliedner, the Lutheran pastor of Kaiserswerth near Düsseldorf, marked a significant advance in nursing practice. His institute was designed to instruct women to become nurse-deaconesses so that they could ameliorate the condition of the sick poor. It was a means of channelling respectable ladies into nursing through encouraging ideals of vocation and dedication. By 1864, the school had trained some 1,600 such deaconesses. In 1840, Elizabeth Fry visited Kaiserwerth and on her return to London founded the Institute of Nursing. The women who joined were called Protestant Sisters of Charity — and later, when that term offended Protestant ears, 'nursing sisters'.

In England, it was the Crimean War (1854–56) that roused public awareness to the need for fresh approaches to nursing. The war produced a heroine in Florence Nightingale. Coming from a comfortable background, Miss Nightingale discovered in nursing an outlet for her great need to escape her family and exercise command through service. She studied nursing abroad, staying for 3 months at Kaiserwerth in 1851 and in Paris with the Sisters of Mercy (1853). Her deep convictions about nursing were well known, and when the shocking dispatches sent from the Crimea by *The Times* journalist, W. H. Russell, revealed that Britain's sick and wounded were being looked after by untrained male orderlies, the Secretary of State at War, Sidney Herbert, asked her to put matters right. She arrived with thirty-eight nurses on 4 November at the barrack hospital at Scutari on the Black Sea. Within 6 months and in the teeth of considerable opposition, she had transformed the place and the death rate fell from 40 to 2 per cent.

The extraordinary success of the 'lady with the lamp' produced in 1856 a public subscription of £44,000 to found a nurses' training scheme. Agreements for ward experience and medical teaching were made with St Thomas's Hospital in London, and the first Nightingale nurses started the course in 1860. The Nightingale system emphasized stern discipline, *esprit de corps*, and devotion to nursing as a vocation.

Florence Nightingale conscripted her 'probationers' from young women of respectable character with lower-middle-class backgrounds — such were expected to be easily disciplined. The Nightingale schools became a source for teachers and superintendents (often dragon-like ladies bountiful, with no direct personal experience of nursing, and perhaps more concerned with morality than practicality), who carried the system throughout Britain and into Australia (1867), Canada (1874), and New Zealand.

Her blueprint for nursing was also influential in the USA. Her books, *Notes on Nursing* and *Notes on Hospitals*, helped consolidate her reforms, stressing cleanliness, fresh air, and discipline. Similar reforms were begun in the USA by the redoubtable Dorothea Dix (see page 297), who soon after the outbreak of the Civil War was appointed 'Superintendant of the United States Army Nurses'.

Nightingale schools were the springboard of nursing's modern development. The founding of the Red Cross made a further contribution. In 1859, a Swiss banker, Jean Henri Dunant, witnessed the battle of Solferino between Austria and the Franco-Italian forces of Emperor Napoleon III. His horror at the want of medical support for the wounded led him to institute the International Red Cross in 1864. This association became a powerful influence in developing nurses' training, especially in the less-advanced territories of Europe and in the non-Western world.

In many parts of Europe, religious orders long continued to dominate nursing, and the professional element developed sluggishly. In early twentieth-century Germany there were still 26,000 Roman Catholic sisters and 12,000 Protestant

THE AGE OF ANAESTHESIA AND ANTISEPSIS

The first half of the nineteenth century brought a rise in the standing of the surgical profession, partly thanks to the image fostered by John Hunter of surgery as a progressive science. In France, two decades of war brought military surgeons to the fore, notably Dominique-Jean Larrey, a highly skilful battlefield amputator who developed the first effective ambulance, and Guillaume Dupuytren. In England, Charles Bell and the suave Astley Cooper at Guy's Hospital gained high reputations as skilful surgeons. Cooper's *Anatomy and Surgical Treatment of*

Florence Nightingale in the military hospital at Scutari.
Lithograph by J. A. Benwell, *c.* 1856.

deaconesses out of a total nurse population of about 75,000. After the First World War, however, the Weimar government created a state nursing diploma (1922), and within 10 years lay nurses outnumbered the nursing sisters by nearly two to one. Everywhere, nursing made great strides. Around 1900 Sir William Osler could write that 'the trained nurse has become one of the great blessings of humanity, taking a place beside the physician and the priest, and not inferior to either in her mission'.[6]

Abdominal Hernia published in two parts in 1804 and 1807 became a classic.

More daring operations were attempted, gynaecological surgery developing dramatically. American conditions proved favourable for innovation; there, the medical profession was less regulated, and, in the southern states, surgeons had slaves to practise on. In 1809, the American, Ephraim McDowell, performed the first successful ovariotomy (without anaesthetic) on 47-year-old Jane Todd Crawford, removing 15 pounds (nearly 7 kilograms) of a dirty gelatinous substance from her cyst. The widow not only survived but lived a further 31 years. John

Attlee removed the ovaries of seventy-eight women between 1843 and 1883, with sixty-four recoveries. In 1824, the first British ovariotomy was performed by John Lizars of Edinburgh University. By mid-century the operation was being performed regularly in England by Sir Spencer Wells in London and Charles Clay in Manchester.

Another American surgeon, James Marion Sims, a South Carolinian who settled in Alabama, was responsible for successful treatment (1849) of vesico-vaginal fistula, again on a slave woman. Such operations met mixed reception: the British surgeon Robert Liston denounced them as 'belly rippers', and others argued that such operations were akin to vivisection, being carried out for the sake of scientific curiosity and surgical practice. Surgery was also put to questionable uses. From 1872 Robert Battey popularized an operation he called 'normal ovariotomy', in which normal ovaries were removed to relieve symptoms in women considered hysterical, insane, or peculiar. Unbelievable operations were also performed on 'nymphomaniacs' (see page 104).

Overall, surgery's scope remained limited and its success uncertain, and comprehensive advances were hardly possible before two towering developments: anaesthesia and antisepsis. Anaesthesia – an expression coined in 1846 by an

The American artist Robert C. Hinckley, in an oil painted in 1891–94, here recaptures the first operation performed under ether, on the morning of 16 October 1846. The operation was a milestone in medicine. Thereafter, surgical trauma became bearable and new surgical procedures of all kinds became possible. The 25-minute operation took place at Massachusetts General Hospital, Boston. The surgeon was John Collins Warren, professor of surgery at Harvard Medical School; the anaesthetist William Thomas Morton, a dentist; and the patient making history, a young man with a tumour on his neck, Gilbert Abbot. After the operation, Warren is said to have proclaimed: 'Gentlemen, this is no humbug.'

American, Oliver Wendell Holmes, to indicate the effects of ether – made surgical trauma bearable; the latter breakthrough reduced the otherwise appalling death rate from postoperative sepsis.

Anaesthesia was not entirely new, and medicine had always, of course, used certain analgesics. Early societies were aware of the pain-deadening qualities of opium, hashish or Indian hemp, and alcohol. In the first century AD, the Greek naturalist, Dioscorides (see page 249), suggested the root of the mandrake, steeped in wine, should be given to patients about to undergo surgery. Yet most patients before the reign of Queen Victoria had to face serious surgery with few attempts to deaden the pain (a deeply drugged or drunk patient could be more difficult to handle than an alert one suffering acute pain).

The first gas recognized to have anaesthetic powers was nitrous oxide, the object of self-experimentation in 1795 by the Bristol physician, Thomas Beddoes, and his young assistant, Humphry Davy. After inhalation, Davy reported giddiness, relaxation of the muscles, and a tendency to laugh (hence the popular name, 'laughing gas'). In 1800, Davy published *Researches, Chemical and Philosophical, Chiefly Concerning Nitrous Oxide and its Respiration*. Yet the surgical value of nitrous oxide long went unappreciated.

In January 1842, however, William E. Clarke, a practitioner from Rochester, New York, endeavoured a tooth extraction under ether. The use of ether as a surgical anaesthetic was also developed by a Boston dentist, William T. G. Morton. Another American dentist, Horace Wells, thought of using nitrous oxide for extractions, and he had one of his own teeth painlessly pulled in December 1844, proclaiming a new era of tooth-pulling. Medical scepticism about his claims was to lead Wells to commit suicide shortly after.

Employment of ether as an anaesthetic spread to Europe. On 21 December 1846, Robert Liston, the most acclaimed London surgeon of his day (he was renowned not least for his speed), amputated the diseased thigh of a patient under ether; he called the anaesthetic method a 'Yankee dodge'. Anaesthesia gained approval although ether was soon challenged by the safer chloroform. On 19 January 1847, James Young Simpson of Edinburgh used chloroform for the first time to relieve the pains of childbirth, and it soon began to be used extensively for this purpose, even for Queen Victoria (see page 263).

Acceptance of anaesthesia made more protracted surgery feasible, but it did not by itself revolutionize surgery, however, because of the severe death rate from postoperative infection. The menace of infection was well known. Working in 1848 in the first obstetrical clinic of the Vienna general hospital, Ignaz Semmelweis remonstrated against the dreadful fatality levels from puerperal fever. He observed that the first clinic (run by medical men) had a much higher rate of puerperal fever than the second obstetrical clinic, run by midwives. He became convinced that this was caused by medical staff and students going directly from the post mortem to the delivery rooms, thereby spreading infection. He instituted

The leading American painter of medicine in the late nineteenth century was Thomas Eakins. *The Gross Clinic* (1875), his masterpiece, represents a snapshot of surgical practice in the USA in the 1870s. Samuel Gross, distinguished professor of surgery at Jefferson University Medical College in Philadelphia, demonstrates an operation for osteomylitis, a serious bone infection. The patient is receiving an anaesthetic (ether), but the surgeons wear street clothes, without masks and gloves, and the unsterile surgical equipment lies exposed in an instrument case. Almost a decade after Joseph Lister developed his antiseptic procedures, Gross is still not using carbolic acid to prevent wound infection.

a strict policy of washing hands and instruments in chlorinated lime solution between autopsy work and handling patients, and the mortality rate in the first clinic was diminished to the same level as the second. Opposition to his novel views led him to quit Vienna in 1850. Resentful and frustrated, he died in a lunatic asylum.

Antagonism to Semmelweis was not mere professional closing of ranks but was consistent with the aetiological theories of the time. The leading view was that infections were caused not by contact but by miasmata in the air, emanations given off by non-human sources. Adherents of such views therefore gave priority to ventilation and prevention of overcrowding as preventive measures.

The notion of antiseptics as advocated by Semmelweis was far from unknown, however; the term 'antiseptic' means anything designed to counter putrefaction or corruption. Greek medicine used wine and vinegar in wound dressings. Alcohol gained favour, and around 1820 iodine became popular in France for treating wounds. Other substances used as antiseptics included creosote, ferric chloride, zinc chloride, and nitric acid. There was thus some interest in questions of antisepsis before the labours of Joseph Lister. It was, nevertheless, Lister who introduced effective techniques for antisepsis and who proved a vocal and effective propagandist on their behalf.

By the time Lister retired in 1892, antiseptic surgery had established itself. The carbolic spray, which saturated all concerned and was heartily disliked, came under criticism and Lister himself abandoned it. Other antiseptics came into use. As early as 1874 Louis Pasteur had suggested placing the instruments in boiling water and passing them through a flame; heat sterilization of instruments was accepted by Robert Koch in 1881. The American surgeon William S. Halsted, of Johns Hopkins Hospital, introduced rubber gloves for use in the operating theatre in 1890 – ironically, not for the patient's sake but to protect the operating-room nurse, his fiancée, whose hands were allergic to antiseptics.

By 1900, these and other prophylactic antiseptic and aseptic methods had been put into use by all surgeons. No longer did surgeons operate in blood-caked black frock-coats in dingy rooms with sawdust-covered floors. The introduction of face-masks, rubber gloves, and surgical gowns lessened the risks of infection, and clean and sterile environments were constantly being improved.

As late as 1874, Sir John Erichsen believed that the abdomen, chest, and brain would forever be closed to operations by wise and humane surgeons; and Lister rarely probed into major cavities, mainly setting fractures. But things were changing: as the result of anaesthetics and antiseptic, surgery's horizons widened dra-

Joseph Lister and the first antiseptic operation

Born in Essex of a Quaker family in 1827, Joseph Lister graduated from University College London and became house surgeon at Edinburgh Royal Infirmary, before moving in 1859 to Glasgow as regius professor of surgery. In 1861, he was put in charge of the new surgical block in Glasgow's Royal Infirmary, where he developed his antiseptic technique, somewhat independently of learning, in 1865, about Louis Pasteur's work on fermentation, putrefaction, and bacteria.

Wound infection and putrefaction in wounds had long been accepted as the almost inevitable consequence of exposure to the air. Lister came to the conclusion that carbolic acid would be effective as an antiseptic, a judgment reached after considering its influence in reducing cattle disease and its successful use to combat a typhoid epidemic in Carlisle, Cumberland. Lister undertook his first trial on 12 August 1865 on an 11-year old boy, James Greenlees, whose left leg had been run over by a cart, dressing a compound fracture of the tibia with lint soaked in linseed oil and carbolic (creosote). He kept the dressing in place 4 days, covering it with tinfoil to prevent evaporation. The wound did not become infected; it healed perfectly and the boy walked out of Glasgow's infirmary 6 weeks later. On 19 May 1866, he attempted a graver case, a compound leg fracture. The carbolic treatment was again applied and the wound healed without infection.

In 1867, Lister published three articles in *The Lancet* – 'Illustrations of the antiseptic system of treatment in surgery', documenting his experiences. He stated how his practice depended on two points. First, germs were the causative agents of infections. Second, infection and pus-formation were not normal, still less beneficial, stages in wound healing – despite the old ideas of 'laudable pus'.

Lister was not a profound theoretician, but he was an expert practical surgeon, insisting on basic precautions such as hand-washing, and the technique he invented involved a drill of basic routine steps. Blood was expelled from the wound, which was bathed with carbolic; carbolic-soaked lint was applied to it and a covering of tin foil was taped over the dressing; when a new dressing was required, the tin was lifted and fresh carbolic painted on the lint. Lister's procedures involved both antisepsis (killing infective agents already present in the wound) and what came to be called 'asepsis' (preventing infective bacteria getting into the wound by creating a sterile environment, initially through the use of a carbolic spray).

An early opportunity to put Lister's work to the test came in the Franco-Prussian War (1870–71) when the Prussian military medical staff introduced some of his concepts in treating battle wounds. They gained better outcomes than the French, who neglected Lister completely. In 1875, Lister made a triumphal tour of Germany. But all was not plain sailing, partly because surgeons hated the smell of the carbolic (which could also seriously irritate the skin). In 1882, the American Surgical Association rejected Lister's teachings. Lister also long experienced opposition in Britain, other surgeons claiming similar success rates without using his beloved carbolic sprays.

Joseph Lister (left), one of the true heroes of nineteenth-century medicine. His careful trials with antiseptics were the beginning of the end of postoperative sepsis. The carbolic sprays he advocated (shown in this 1882 engraving) were at first, however, messy and unpleasant.

matically. First in Zurich and then in Vienna, the celebrated Theodor Billroth made important innovations, performing the first total removal of a cancerous larynx, pioneering abdominal surgery, and developing surgery for many forms of cancer, especially of the breast. In the USA, William Halsted devised radical mastectomy, the operation in which the breast, all the lymph glands in the nearest armpit, and the muscles of the chest wall are removed. It long remained the most popular treatment for breast cancer.

Appendectomies became more common in the 1880s: in 1901, Edward VII was operated on when his appendix caused trouble just before his coronation. Removal of gallstones grew common, and cholecystectomy, the removal of the gall bladder itself, was introduced in 1882. Surgery on the small intestine, notably for cancer, was also inaugurated around the same time, and urological surgery developed, especially prostate operations. A prominent figure was Sir William MacEwen, who adopted and extended Lister's antiseptic surgical techniques and pioneered operations on the brain for tumours, abscesses, and trauma.

By 1900 a marked change had occurred in the number and type of operations surgeons were executing. Lister's notebooks record no abdominal surgery up to 1893; but the abdominal surgery practice of William Watson Cheyne at King's College Hospital in London increased steadily in the decade between 1902 and 1912, from fewer than one in twenty cases to around one in six. For so long an emergency treatment or a last resort, operative surgery had become a powerful, even a fashionable, weapon. A surgical revolution had already been wrought by the time of the First World War: conditions such as gastric ulcers became routine targets for the knife.

The new century saw the growth of surgical interventions in tubercular cases. A German, Ernst Ferdinand Sauerbruch, led the field in thoracic surgery, although it was an Italian, Carlo Forlanini, who introduced pneumothorax treatment. Two surgeons were even honoured at this time with a Nobel Prize – Theodor Kocher in 1909 for his work on the thyroid gland, and Alexis Carrel in 1911 for his techniques of suturing blood vessels and work on transplantation and tissue culture.

A professor at Berne from 1871, Kocher developed general surgical treatment of disorders of the thyroid gland, including goitre and thyroid tumours, and elucidated the workings of the thyroid gland. From the 1870s investigations had shown that the thyroid was essential to life; its malfunction was blamed for cretinism, goitre, and various other disorders. As a consequence, enlarged thyroid glands began to be surgically removed – sometimes with disastrous consequences if the thyroid tissue left behind performed inadequately. It was shown that this could be prevented by counterbalancing injections of macerated thyroid tissue. Since delayed growth and slow learning were amongst the features of cretinism, thousands of underachieving children were placed on thyroid extract, and it was recommended for sundry symptoms in adults from constipation and obesity to tiredness and depression.

In a similar way, testicular extract also became popular. On 1 June 1889, Charles-Edouard Brown-Séquard reported to a distinguished scientific society in Paris that he had rejuvenated himself through subcutaneous injections of extracts of guinea-pig and dog testicles. Rejuvenation through gland implants proved, however, a nine-day wonder.

Theodor Kocher's observations on patients suffering the consequences of surgically removing the thyroid gland (total strumectomy) helped elucidate its normal functions, and by the 1890s the isolation of active thyroid hormones made replacement therapy possible. Kocher also pioneered operations of the brain and spinal cord.

For his part, Alexis Carrel, a Frenchman from Lyons, was involved in many aspects of surgery on the blood vessels and heart, and in particular in treating aneurysm. Having migrated to the USA, he showed how parts of the aortal wall could be replaced with a piece from another artery or veins, and found ways of sewing vessels together, thereby initiating vascular surgery. Carrel's work paved the way for many later kinds of surgery dealing with aneurysms, varicose veins, and blood clots.

THE 'GOLDEN AGE' OF SURGERY

The twentieth century was to become the century of surgery. A constellation of advances – far too many to list – followed from the crucial interlinking of pathological anatomy, anaesthesia, and asepsis. From the latter decades of the nineteenth century, surgeons directed their attention to tumours and infections leading to obstruction or stenosis (constriction of vessels), above all in the digestive, respiratory, and urogenital tracts. These could be relieved or cured by fissuring or excision. New operations of this kind included tracheotomy for tuberculosis or throat cancer, and relief of intestinal obstruction caused by cancerous tumours.

Operative surgery entered a 'golden age', when surgeons grew ever more therapeutically active. The habitual performance of operations on the gastrointestinal tract, thyroid, breasts, bones, and blood vessels made surgery safer and more reliable. Abdominal surgery advanced with new methods of extirpation of cancer of the rectum, of hernias, and with treatments for acute appendicitis and disorders of the colon. Herniotomies and appendectomies became routine after 1910. Surgery of the nervous system was almost wholly a twentieth-century advance. The first specialist in neurosurgery was Harvey Cushing, who became professor of surgery at Harvard University in 1912. All the cavities and organs of the body were conquered.

Some surgeons became positively cavalier: the Irish-born William Arbuthnot Lane advocated the removal of yards of the gut for ordinary constipation – or even as a prophylactic measure. Appendectomy not for acute but for so-called 'chronic' appendicitis became fashionable in the 1920s and 1930s, as were the many operations devised to fix abdominal organs, found by X-ray examination to be 'misplaced'. 'Hitching up the kidneys' enjoyed a great vogue. Between 1920 and 1950 hundreds of thousands of tonsillectomies were performed, most quite unnecessary. Hysterectomies enjoyed a similar fad.

Surgical intervention was stimulated by many developments within medicine, but it was also demanded by events in the wider world. The First World War proved crucial. With war wounds occurring on hitherto unimaginable scales, debates raged once more over proper methods of wound management. Experience in the two world wars led to new methods of handling compound fractures; to the development of plastic and reconstructive surgery; and to the establishment of blood and plasma banks (the first were set up in 1935 at the Mayo Clinic in Rochester, New York State). In 1938, during the Spanish Civil War, techniques were developed of administering stored blood by indirect transfusion into the patient from a bottle; these were perfected in the Second World War. Blood transfusions, first pioneered in the seventeenth century, had finally been made safe.

By 1950, better immunological knowledge and the increased availability of drugs effective against bacterial infections had expanded possibilities of operability. Thanks to antibiotics, surgery could be performed on cases hitherto deemed too risky because of danger of infection; for example, interventions in the lung in contact with atmospheric microorganisms. With the pharmacological revolution, such patients could be treated before and after the operation with sulphonamides and later antibiotics.

Surgery entered a new phase, moving from a preoccupation with removal to a subtler concern with restoration. Surgeons developed a growing capacity to control and re-establish the functioning of the heart, lungs, and kidneys, and fluid balance. The first implantation of an artificial apparatus (prothesis) came in 1959 with the heart pacemaker, designed to adjust beat frequency by means of electrical impulses in the case of arrhythmic variations. It was developed by Rune Elmqvist and implanted by Åke Senning in Sweden. Such restorative procedures now range from eye lenses to pneumatic implants to facilitate penile erection.

A fine instance of the switch of surgical approach from excision to implantation is offered by changes in urology. Early on, emphasis lay on the cutting out of malignant tumours. This was challenged by radiotherapy as an alternative procedure: in 1906, an American, Alfred L. Gray, introduced radiotherapy for carcinoma of the bladder, and this was soon used also in the therapy of prostate cancer. Bladder cancer was then one of the first to be successfully treated with hormones (1941), thanks to the work of Charles Brenton Huggins, a Canadian-born American surgeon who undertook investigation of the physiology and biochemistry of the prostate gland. Research on dogs led Huggins to the possibility of using hormones in treating such tumours in human beings and in 1966 he shared the Nobel Prize for his discovery of hormonal treatment for prostate cancer. He also developed the use of hormones in treating breast cancer in women.

Opposite: By the late nineteenth century, surgery had made real advances. In this 1890 painting by Adelbert Seligmann of the great German surgeon Theodor Billroth at work in the Allegemeines Krankenhaus in Vienna, the patient has been anaethethesized and the doctors are wearing white coats over their suits. Yet much still seems highly traditional, not least the total absence of anything resembling the modern operating theatre, and the dependence on daylight. Moreover, nobody is wearing gloves or masks, and it is questionable if the instruments were properly sterilized. German-born, Billroth became director of the Second Surgical Clinic in Vienna, pioneering surgery for gastrointestinal conditions and various cancers. He was a remarkable man, being also a fine writer and musician. Seligmann painted this scene 4 years before Billroth's death.

Hysterectomy operations were developed during the nineteenth century, initially before the introduction of anaethetics, as part of a broad expansion of gynaecological surgery. The operation about to be performed here at London's Middlesex Hospital, reveals the great change that had overtaken the operating theatre by the early decades of the twentieth century. There are surgical gowns, caps and masks, and other precautions to ensure aseptic conditons, as well as a structured surgical 'team'.

Improvements in heart surgery began with the first operation for stenosis of the mitral valve – the abnormal narrowing of the valve between the left auricle and ventricle, which slows down the blood circulation and eventually causes harm. This was performed by Henry Souttar in London in 1925, and was followed in 1947 by operations to relieve pulmonary stenosis (narrowing of the opening between the pulmonary artery and the right ventricle) by Thomas Holmes Sellors and Russell Brock, also in London. Two years later similar operations were undertaken for stenosis of the aorta itself.

In 1942, it was suggested that congenital heart disease (the so-called blue-baby syndrome) could be cured surgically. The operation, first undertaken at Johns Hopkins Hospital in Baltimore in 1944 (see page 8), launched modern cardiac surgery. The pioneer was Helen Brooke Taussig, an American paediatrician who was the first woman to become a full professor at Johns Hopkins University. Taussig worked on congenital heart disease in association with the cardiac surgeon Alfred Blalock. The babies were blue because of congenital anomalies that caused blood to pass directly from the right chamber of the heart to the left without being oxygenated in the lungs; this was then surgically rectified. Their joint efforts helped create a new speciality of paediatric cardiac surgery. Dramatic advances in heart surgery followed.

Operations on the mitral valves increased, but in some cases they initially produced severe brain damage by depriving the brain of oxygen. The idea was then floated of entirely removing the heart from the body, and deploying an alternative system of blood circulation. Such 'open-heart' surgery was made possible by sev-

The first Drinker respirator, or 'iron lung', in 1937. In iron lungs, artificial ventilation is maintained for long periods of time by applying alternating negative and positive pressure to the inside of a rigid metal tank, within which the patient's body, excluding the head, is enclosed. It was developed by an American public health engineer, Philip Drinker, in the 1930s. Iron lungs were life-savers during polio epidemics.

eral key developments. One was the use of hypothermia, reducing through cold the oxygen need of the tissues. Another was the building of the heart–lung machine, maintaining artificial circulation through the great vessels while the heart was bypassed and the operation performed. The machine involved two main components: a 'lung' to oxygenate the blood and a 'heart' pump. Through experience it was discovered that the deeply cooled and bypassed heart could be stopped for up to an hour and started again without suffering damage. Open-heart surgery started in 1952 in the USA with the implantation of artificial heart valves.

A major and highly conspicuous trend has been transplantation. Successful skin grafts were described by the Swiss, Jacques Reverdin, as early as 1869. Such autografts (tissue transplantations within the same patient) were soon used to treat ulcers and burns. Skin grafting led to the rise of reconstructive surgery, first through the work of Harold Gillies on First World War casualties at Aldershot in southern England. During the Second World War, transplantation of non-vital tissue become urgent, to provide 'pacemaker' support for regeneration of connective tissues after severe injuries. The invention of the 'artificial kidney' laid the foundations for the great developments in organ transplantation in the 1950s and 1960s.

The rise of organ transplantation brought inescapable ethical and legal predicaments for medicine. Under what circumstances might living human beings ethically become donors of kidneys and other organs? Should there be a market in organs? Were the dead automatically to be assumed to have consented to the removal of organs? At what point was a person truly 'dead', permitting organ removal?

Partly in view of the demands of transplantation, the general test of death has shifted during the last generation from cessation of breathing to 'brain death', which has the convenience of permitting removal of organs from patients in whom respiration was artificially maintained right up to removal. The issues of

Doctors examining bottles of blood sent from the USA, at the National Institute for Medical Research in London, in the mid-1940s. Blood transfusions were first briefly tried in the seventeenth century. They became properly feasible with the discovery of blood groups early in the twentieth century. Early transfusions were, however, directly from patient to patient. It was only during the 1930s that the principles and practicalities of blood storage were worked out, allowing the development of national blood transfusion services and the vast quantities of blood required for certain modern operations.

Organ transplantation

The invention of the 'artificial kidney' proved a key factor in the development of organ transplantation. A renal dialysis machine was devised during the Second World War by Willem Johan Kolff of the Municipal Hospital at Kampen in the Netherlands. The device, made of aluminium, wood, and Cellophane, was to serve as a model for the kidney machines used throughout the world today. The artificial kidney allowed damaged kidneys time to recover and chronic renal failure to be counterbalanced over a long period. A series of Cellophane membranes remove impurities from the blood that would ordinarily be filtered out by the healthy kidneys. Among Kolff's later achievements were a heart–lung machine and an early artificial heart.

The transplant of organs, however, required a solution of the problem of rejection, a subject highlighted by the investigations of Frank Macfarlane Burnet in Australia and Peter Medawar in England into the tendency of the immune system to reject grafts. For this work, Burnet and Medawar received a Nobel Prize in 1960. Around 1960, the first immunosuppressant drugs were introduced – notably, cortisone, azaserine, and azathioprine. By blocking the production of antibodies without producing susceptibility in the patient to infections, these drugs opened a new era in organ replacement.

Transplants became world headlines on 3 December 1967 when Christiaan Barnard at the Groote Schuur Hospital, Cape Town, sewed a heart from a 24-year-old woman, who had died in a motor accident, into 54-year old Louis Washkansky. Washkansky lived for 18 days. A second patient, Philip Blaiberg, operated on in January 1968, survived for 594 days. Soon, heart transplants were taking place all over the world: within 4 years, 56 teams had carried out a total of 180 transplants.

Many hospitals soon abandoned the operation, however, because few recipients survived for long owing to the immunological problems of graft rejection. These difficulties have now largely been solved, and heart transplants have become routine: by the mid-1980s, hundreds were being conducted each year in the USA alone, with two-thirds of the recipients surviving for 5 years or more.

The first successful kidney transplantation, from one identical twin to another, was done in 1954 by John P. Merrill, Joseph Murray, J. Hartwell Harrison, and Warren Guild in Boston and soon became a routine operation. Liver and lung transplantation, performed since the 1960s, has also become increasingly successful.

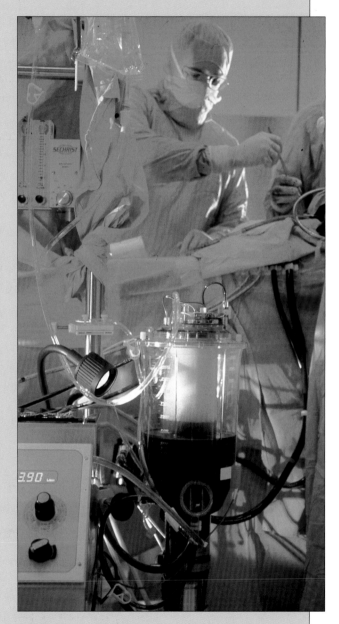

A heart–lung machine. It takes over the functions of the heart while surgeons perform open-heart surgery, such as a coronary bypass or a heart transplant.

Infertility can now be helped by a variety of treatments that bring sperm and eggs together outside the body. With the SUZI (subzonal insemination) technique, fertilization may be achieved by injecting sperm in a micropipette through the outer covering (zona pellucida) of the egg into the space between the zona and the egg cell. This and similar methods of assisted conception, and the related practices of egg and sperm donation and surrogate motherhood, will remain moral problems into the twenty-first century.

patients queuing for organ transplantation and of sorting priorities in the allotment of organs in high demand remain difficult.

Similar moral problems surround the advances in reproductive technology made possible by the advent of the 'test-tube baby'. Here the pioneer was the British gynaecologist/obstetrician Patrick Steptoe. He had long been interested in laparoscopy (a technique of viewing the abdominal cavity through a small incision in the umbilicus) and in problems of fertility. Together with Robert Edwards, a physiologist at Cambridge University, he worked on the problem of *in vitro* fertilization of human embryos. In July 1978, this research resulted in the birth of the first test-tube baby, Louise Brown, who was born by caesarian section in Oldham District Hospital, England, through *in vitro* fertilization and implantation in her mother's uterus.

The ethical issues surrounding test-tube babies remain controversial, but the technique has become more common, as have the related practices of sperm and egg donation and surrogate motherhood. Some of the implications of transformations in reproductive surgery and technology are considered in Chapter 10.

Organ transplants offer an illustration of the move to 'replacement surgery' during the past three decades. At the same time, protheses such as hip joints, middle-ear bones, heart valves, and artificial organs, such as the inner ear, have become routine treatments. A key figure in replacement surgery was the British surgeon John Charnley. After serving as an orthopaedic specialist in the First World War, Charnley devoted himself to the technical problems associated with replacements for badly arthritic hip joints, above all the difficulty of finding a suitable material. Artificial joints made of polytetrafluoroethylene, known by the trade name of Teflon, proved not to wear well in the long term, but from 1962

Charnley, who was then based in Wigan in Lancashire, found that polyethylene was more effective. With scrupulous attention to aseptic techniques, he was able to perfect an operation that gave enhanced mobility to many. Not all implants have been so worthy. Cosmetic surgery has boomed with the fashion for silicon breast implants, a lucrative, if dubious, trade.

Artificial replacements illustrate the increasingly interdisciplinary character of surgery in recent decades, necessitating collaboration with such sciences as physiology, engineering, pharmacology, and immunology – to say nothing of interaction with the electronic, metal, and plastic industries.

Surveying modern surgery, it is possible to picture change in terms of three successive, overlapping, phases of development. The first stage of modern surgery involved an era of extirpation, which pioneered new ways of dealing with tumours and injuries by means of surgical excision. There followed a stage of restoration, in which stress fell on surgical physiology and pharmacology, aimed at repairing impaired or endangered function. The third age has placed greater emphasis on replacement, the introduction into the damaged body of biological or artificial organs and tissues. This last phase requires a more systemic approach

Sir John Charnley carrying out a hip replacement operation in his sterile theatre in Wigan, Lancashire, in the 1970s. The modern hip operation, developed in the 1960s, illustrates the trend away from extirpation, where tumours and injuries are dealt with by excision, towards the 'replacement' of organs and tissues by biological or artificial materials.

to treatment that may be breaking down the time-honoured boundaries between surgery and other medical disciplines.

SURGERY BECOMES HIGH-TECH

The surgical revolution would have been quite impossible without all manner of technological innovations that have come to the aid of surgery, and indeed medicine at large. The breakthrough of greatest symbolic significance was Wilhelm Röntgen's discovery of X-rays, working with vacuum tubes perfected by the English scientist William Crookes (see page 140). X-rays had immediate scientific, technological, commercial, and medical reverberations. Prolonged exposure to X-rays was soon observed to have physiological effects, such as burning the skin, ulcerations, dermatitis, and hair loss. Within a year, Röntgen's discovery had been turned to therapeutic account by a Viennese physician who had used X-rays to burn off a mole from a patient. At the same time, the Danish physician Niels Finsen suggested that ultraviolet light rays were bactericidal and offered promise for treating lupus.

Hard on the heels of these wondrous developments came the discovery in 1896, by the French physicist Antoine-Henri Becquerel, of radiation, associated with heavy elements such as uranium. The husband-and-wife team of Pierre and Marie Curie joined the hunt for other radioactive elements, whose diagnostic and therapeutic implications interacted with surgical interventions in such domains as cancer therapy. By 1900, there were radium institutes, radiology journals and societies, and more than a hundred diseases for which the new miracle cures had

Early X-ray apparatus in use in Germany during the First World War.

been used, although it was for cancer that the new therapies seemed to promise most. Therapeutic enthusiasm outran caution, and the dangers of radiotherapy were only painfully realized. The martyrs to X-rays included many patients and early workers, not least Marie Curie.

In 1903, the Dutch physiologist Willem Einthoven published details of the first electrocardiograph, which picked up electrical activity from the heart, and so led to more effective monitoring of cardiac disorders (see page 141). In the 1930s, the introduction of the electron microscope revealed many aspects of cell structure previously unseen. From around 1955, sonography (ultrasound) was developed in Sweden and the USA; it became surgically applicable in cardiac diagnosis. Nuclear medicine, using radioactive isotopes, became increasingly significant in measuring the functioning of endocrine glands, lungs, and kidneys. The development of catheters of various sorts enabled the investigation of heart and liver functions. Flexible endoscopes, drawing on the use of glass-fibre optics (which enabled light to be sent through a tube by total internal reflection), were developed in the 1970s. These were used not only for diagnostics but soon for therapeutic interventions, not least in connection with lasers.

In 1917, Albert Einstein unveiled the principle of the laser ('light amplification by stimulated emissions of radiation'). Its high-energy waves, capable of being focused to a microscopic point, are sterile and cause minimal bleeding and scarring. Destroying tissue rapidly by heating or by producing photochemical reactions, lasers are 'optical knives' that have proved valuable in eye surgery as well as in internal surgery. With the aid of endoscopes, they can be aimed from within the body.

Visual diagnostics leapt ahead with the introduction in 1972 of the computerized tomograph (CAT) by Godfrey Newbold Hounsfield. An electrical engineer working for the British company EMI, Hounsfield pioneered a system whereby X-ray beams could be resolved with computer assistance to produce a cross-sectional picture of the human body. The result – computer-assisted axial tomography or CAT scanning – was a major breakthrough in the non-invasive diagnosis of disease. Hounsfield shared the Nobel Prize for medicine in 1979 with Allan M. Cormack, the physicist who had established the mathematical principles on which the technique depended. A further development is magnetic resonance (MR), which also shows sections of the body but by using radio waves is also capable of showing metabolic organs (see page 7). Positron emission topography (PET) scanners measure photons coming from radioactive decay of a radioactive tracer administered to the patient. PET scans are especially use-

Marie Curie with her daughter Irène in 1925. Born Marya Sklodowska in Warsaw in 1867, Marie Curie, with her husband Pierre, was the first to discover the radioactive elements radium and polonium. She was always concerned with the medical applications of her work, not least pioneering a mobile X-ray unit for the French army in the First World War and founding a radiological school for nurses. She died aged 67 of leukaemia, undoubtedly as a result of prolonged exposure to high-energy radiation. Irène also became a noted physicist and, like her mother, shared a Nobel Prize for physics with her husband. Marie also won a second Nobel Prize for chemistry.

ful for examining local blood flow and the transfer of chemical information; they are beginning to play a major part in showing the biological basis of psychiatric disorders.

THE TWENTIETH-CENTURY HOSPITAL

The hospital has changed its nature during the last couple of centuries, turning from little more than a poor-house into the nerve centre of modern medicine, and also becoming far more socially conspicuous. In Britain, the number of beds per thousand of the population doubled between 1860 and 1940, and then doubled again by 1980. The astounding modern growth of surgery created a huge rise in absolute and relative hospital expenditure. Vastly important were technological innovations, from the introduction of X-rays through to the electron microscope in the 1930s and the CAT and PET scanners developed in the 1970s.

The creation of tailor-made environments for surgery was equally crucial. From the late nineteenth century, the development of hygienic, well-equipped operating theatres played a major part in turning the hospital from a healing machine for the poor into an institution fit for all classes. The leap in costs began to be seriously felt by the early years of the twentieth century. Between the world wars, surgery became much more intricate, laboratory tests and other investigations were extended, medical technology grew essential, and staff costs rose. Ambulance services made the hospital the nucleus of emergency care.

With costs escalating, hospitals, traditionally funded in Britain and most other countries on a voluntary basis, ran into financial problems. In the USA, hospitals coped with funding difficulties by developing business strategies. In conjunction with insurance schemes, they enticed well-off patients on a paying basis. The absence of the American system of the underpinning of hospital budgets by insurance is one explanation (amongst many) why the post-war British government had little option but to introduce a National Health Service (NHS).

The Second World War had already led to transformations in British hospital organization. The government had made preparations for the massive civilian casualties expected from the Luftwaffe blitz. These emergency plans assigned all hospitals specific tasks, and they were to be remunerated for the beds they set aside. There were two main consequences of such an arrangement: hospitals began to count on government payments, and they became better attuned to cooperation within a state-planned scheme.

In the NHS, hospitals became by far the most significant, and costly, sector. At the time of its establishment (1948), there were more than 900 voluntary hospitals, but many were small – more than 250 had fewer than thirty beds. Most were taken into the NHS, with the ownership of buildings and land passing to the state.

Since then, hospitals have been the basic sites for therapeutic advance. By the post-war period, in the USA and Europe alike, they were seen as quintessentially part of modern medical care: high-tech, invasive, involving skilled coordinated

Wexham Park Hospital in Slough, Buckinghamshire, built in the 1960s to a design by Powell & Moya. The modern hospital is the cutting edge of contemporary medicine. But its costs seem to be spiralling out of control, and it contributes greatly to the 'dehumanizing' atmosphere of medicine today, of which many complain. When it was built, the Wexham Park Hospital was regarded as an excellent example of its type, but it and similar complex modern hospitals embody the paradox at the centre of the medical enterprise.

teamwork amongst many different specialties. Yet from the 1960s critiques of hospitals grew. Particularly in the USA, medicolegal cases and third-party payment fuelled costs; tests and investigations mushroomed; and vast capital sums were spent on medical equipment.

Some critics argued that modern hospital medicine had contributed little except cost: it was public-health measures in the nineteenth century that had actually brought down mortality. In the past, hospitals might even have increased mortality. Whether the medicine of the future can afford the modern hospital remains an unsolved problem. It is conceivable that the huge hospitals of today will soon seem medicine's dinosaurs, and that they will be replaced by simpler and more varied institutions.

CHAPTER 7

Miles Weatherall

Drug treatment and the rise of pharmacology

Pharmacology, the science of drugs, became necessary when the first person to get drunk wondered what was happening to him or her. This occurred long before recorded history. There are records of grape cultivation and wine-making in Mesopotamia and Egypt at least 4,500 years ago but many fermented liquors must have been known long before then, as were other medicinal products. But how did anyone ever identify them?

THE MEDICINES OF EARLY CIVILIZATIONS

One can only guess how the earliest drugs were discovered. Bitter experience taught people which plants were toxic, and, happier events perhaps suggested, more subtly, that some had beneficial properties. Several ancient Egyptian papyruses, dated about 1600–1500 BC, record the medical practices and drugs then in use. Prescriptions were laid out in a form that survived in Western medicine to modern times. But the hieroglyphics are difficult to interpret, and the identity of many remedies is doubtful.

All the major population groups developed their own particular knowledge of local therapeutic and narcotic drugs, and treatments. These reconstructed images of Aztec health and medicine were collected by the scholar Fray Bernardino de Sahagún and appear in the third volume of the *Florentine Codex* of c.1570.

Egyptians attributed medicinal virtues to various familiar fruits and vegetables. They also used tree resins, including frankincense, myrrh, and manna. Extracts of plants still sometimes used as purgatives – senna, colocynth, and castor oil – were recognized. Tannins from plant galls were used for the treatment of burns. Parts of animals were also applied therapeutically, especially fat, and more curious recipes include ox spleen, pig's brain, and tortoise gall (with honey). Antimony, copper, and some other minerals were especially favoured as astringents or antiseptics. But names of remedies must be interpreted carefully; 'ass's heads' and 'pig's teeth' may be no more what they seem than are buttercups 'cups for butter' or foxgloves 'gloves worn by foxes'.

Egyptian practices continued in the civilization of Assyria and Babylonia. Copies of herbals have survived, suggesting familiarity with hellebore, henbane, mandrake, and the opium poppy, all of which contain potent drugs well known today, but the exact purposes for which these remedies were applied are often uncertain or obscure. Other drugs may have been known and mentioned in records that have not survived.

GREEK AND ROMAN REMEDIES

In ancient Greece, a more critical approach developed, based on observation and experience. Much credit is given to Hippocrates of Cos and his followers (see page 58). As in China, simplicity was sought by inventing a small number of basic principles, this time the four temperaments – the blood, the phlegm, the yellow bile, and the black bile, giving the sanguine, the phlegmatic, the jaundiced, and the melancholic temperaments – and in attributing disease to an excess or deficiency of the wet and dry, hot and cold humours responsible for these temperaments. Treatment gave more weight to diet and lifestyle than to drugs as a means of restoring a healthy balance. Surviving ancient Greek texts include references to books on drugs, and to suppliers of medicinal plants, but no great ancient Greek schedule of drugs is known to exist.

In the more regulated civilization of Rome, Galen of Pergamum has become the most famous, and for many centuries was probably the most influential, medical

Medicines of ancient China and India

In ancient China, treatment before about 1100 BC seems to have been dominated by philosophical ideas of disease. In the golden period that followed, treatment was more empirical and based on direct observation: medicines were given because they were seen to have worked before, not because they were supposed to summon a god to help. Then orthodoxy became unpopular, with a growing influence of Buddhism and Indian ideas, and increasing reliance on charms and magic.

Attempts to understand a complex world by very simple principles led to the notions of *yin* and *yang* – complementary influences that were balanced in health and disturbed in disease. Therapy was directed to restoring harmony between the principles, and drugs, it was thought, might be supposed to act in this way. The great Chinese herbal, the *Pen T'sao*, was long reputed to be very ancient, perhaps from about 2700 BC, but probably dates from about 200 bc. It is known only by quotations, and is said to have included 240 vegetable and 125 other remedies.

Symbol of *yang* and *yin* (above) with tiger (below). *Yin–yang* relations are fundamental in traditional Chinese medicine.

In India, an empirical and rational system, Ayurvedic medicine, displaced earlier magico-religious practices between 600 and 100 BC. No medical books from the Veda period have survived, but as far as is known the medical materials then used resembled those of Egypt and Mesopotamia, augmented by many indigenous Indian plants. In later Brahmanical texts (AD 100–700), a basic theory of seven elements appears – chyle, blood, flesh, fat, bone, marrow, and semen – and perhaps gave a basis for explaining the actions of some medicines.

A few ancient Eastern remedies have received a new lease of life from twentieth-century research. The Indian plant *Rauwolfia serpentina*, or snake-root, was introduced to European medicine during the 1950s as a sedative and to treat high blood pressure. Its active constituent, an alkaloid called reserpine, was isolated in 1952 in the Ciba laboratories in Basle. It is still used but it can cause severe depression and other side-effects and has not become popular. Most traditional remedies have not yielded potent ingredients.

The 'botanical garden' of Tuthmosis III (fifteenth century BC) in the Temple of Amun at Karnak. The relief depicts plants and animals encountered by the Egyptian pharoah in Asia. The ancient Egyptians attributed medicinal properties to many familiar fruits and vegetables.

writer (see page 62). Other authors sheltered under the cover of his authority, just as they had after Hippocrates, and the probably diverse medical practices of centuries became consolidated in a Galenical system, which related more to the individual patient than to the formal classification of disease. The most important record of drugs then in use came from Dioscorides, physician to the Emperor Nero (reigned AD 54–68), or at least a doctor in Nero's army.

The accumulated experience of Greece and Rome became mingled in the medieval Arabic world with that of Muslims. Among the works of this period are a systematic treatise on poisons written in the eighth century by the Arabic alchemist Jabir ibn Hayyan. The noted scientist and philosopher Ibn Sina (Avicenna) also included a book on medicaments in his *Canon on Medicine* published in the eleventh century, a text that continued to serve for 500 years. Much medical knowledge was reintroduced to Europe after Muslim conquests in North Africa and Spain, especially through the medical schools established at Salerno in Italy and at Montpellier in France in the eleventh and twelfth centuries.

PARACELSUS AND THE FIGHT AGAINST AUTHORITY

Through many centuries, thought and actions in Europe were dominated by the opinions of authority. Then came the great outburst of independence and originality in the 'rebirth of learning' or the Renaissance. In medicine, rejection of orthodoxy began gradually, and was made conspicuous by the flamboyant character Philippus Aureolus Theophrastus Bombastus von Hohenheim, who was born near Zurich and adopted the name Paracelsus in recognition of the Roman medical writer Celsus.

Dioscorides

The five-volume herbal produced by Pedanius Dioscorides of Cilicia (southern Anatolia) in the first century AD became a basic source of knowledge about plants and medicines for at least fifteen centuries. Although written in Greek, and translated into a variety of languages over the years, it is best known by its Latin title *De Materia Medica.* About 500 plants are included in the treatise, many of which can be identified from their descriptions.

The earliest versions of the herbal were probably not illustrated, and only fragments of them have survived. Some 400 years after Dioscorides compiled the work, however, a specially illustrated copy (now called the *Codex Vindobonensis*), with nearly 400 full-page coloured botanical paintings, was prepared by a Byzantine artist in Constantinople. For many of the illustrations, the artist copied drawings made in the first century BC by a Greek physician called Krateuas. This manuscript, which is now in the Austrian National Library in Vienna, was a present from the reigning Roman Emperor in the West, Flavius Anicius Olybrius, to his daughter Juliana Anica in AD 512. More than a thousand years later, Dioscorides' work was 'Englished' by a John Goodyer in 1655, but not published. This manuscript remained in the Library of Magdalen College, Oxford, until 1934, when it was at last printed with an appendix by Robert W. T. Gunther.

Goodyer translated all five books, which cover 'aromatics, oils ointments and trees', 'living creatures, milk and dairy produce, cereals and sharp herbs', 'roots, juices and herbs', 'herbs and roots', and 'vines and wines, metallic ores'. The classification seems strange to us, but the plants described and illustrated cover an extensive range of those familiar today. The 'aromatics' include saffron (in Dioscorides' time, as today, expensive and particularly liable to adulteration), cinnamon, and mustard;[3] the 'trees' of particular interest are the fig and the date.

The medicinal applications, written long before any modern concepts of disease had been formulated, are essentially symptomatic treatments. Most plants are claimed to cure almost every ill. The bramble ('batos', *Rubus fruticosus*), according to Dioscorides,

> binds and drys; it dyes ye hair. But the decoction of the tops of it being drank stops ye belly, & restrains ye flux of women, & is convenient for ye biting of ye Prester. And the leaves being chewed do strengthen ye gums, and heal ye Apthae. And ye leaves being applied, do restrain ye Herpetas, & heal ye running ulcers which are in ye head, & ye falling down of the eyes . . .[1]

Forty-four drugs mentioned by Dioscorides survived into the twentieth century in offical European pharmacopoeias, according to the historian Charles Singer, passing 'to us through the Middle Ages, some continuously and some through the Arabian physicians in translations prepared between the thirteeth and fourteenth centuries'. Of these, Singer commented in 1927, 'only about a quarter have any definite pharmacological action. The remainder are diluents, flavouring agents, emollients and the like'.[2]

To our eyes, this illustration of Galen (centre) in conversation with Dioscorides in the *Codex Vindobonesis* may show the early medieval lack of a sense of history, because Dioscorides was alive around AD 60 whereas Galen was not born until AD 129. But the force of the illustration is chiefly symbolic, with the greatest diagnostician of antiquity shown to be on good terms with the greatest master of herbal lore and pharmacy.

A page from a pseudo-Galen 'Book of Antidotes', from northern Iraq, AD 1199, showing labourers at work on the cultivation of herbs. Partly because of advances in chemistry and alchemy, herbal medicine flourished amongst the Arabic inheritors of Greek philosophy and science.

Opposite: In this thirteenth-century manuscript, a child is being given a fomentation (poultice) for internal pain and a woman a herbal potion for nausea.

Martin Luther had shown his defiance of authority by burning a papal bull and a copy of canon law, and Paracelsus followed his example by burning the books of Galen and Avicenna. Appointed town physician of Basel in 1527, he also taught medical students there for a year. Later, after he had lost a lawsuit against a canon of the cathedral, he became a wandering practitioner. He treated patients, but also made chemical experiments and reported novel observations, many of which have been repeatedly confirmed.

Paracelsus noted that air was necessary for wood to burn and he claimed that without air all living things would die. He recommended various minerals as medicines, and may have introduced mercury for syphilis, as well as advising the use of antimony, arsenic, copper, iron, and lead for various purposes. His secret remedy, laudanum, probably depended mainly on opium for its benefits (see page 258). Although Paracelsus was a good observer, he also was a great theorist. He sought a small number of simplifying principles, but these belonged to several sets. He invented a mystical philosophy of gnomes, sylphs, nymphs, and sala-

Cibum puleium ctum cum aqua aü aceto in. ad nausum stomachi.
potu dib nausiam stomachi sedat.

Cibum puleum mittis in aqua feructe ma[ ]un. advetu pruriginem.
centu diu donec bib: possit optimü e.v. adventq dolore.
Cibtu pulegu comasticato ei in umbilicu religat oti nuo q dolore tollit.

PARACELSUS.

Paracelsus, the radical sixteenth-century medical thinker and practitioner, stressed the spiritual side of illness but also advocated the use of mineral, metallic, and chemical remedies. When he introduced chemical remedies, his experiments were alchemical. He divided all substances into types of sulphur, mercury, and salt. Sulphur stood for the combustible, mercury for the volatile, and salt for the unchangeable constituents in natural objects. By trial and error, he discovered methods of detoxifying chemicals so that they could be used medically.

manders, which corresponded to the elementals of earth, air, water, and fire, but also related in some way to the chemical elementals of combustible sulphur, volatile mercury, and residual salt.

Paracelsus's doctrines shocked many respectable physicians of the time, who clung, sometimes with great bigotry, to Galenical doctrine in the face of Paracelsian heresy. It is so much easier to assert authority than to investigate facts, and the time was one of original ideas but not yet of their experimental evaluation. Nor was understanding of ill health sufficiently advanced to distinguish what now we call one 'disease' from another.

Injuries – broken bones, and wounds with accompanying sepsis, fevers, and tumours – were obvious enough. Certain patterns of fever could be recognized, such as tertian and quartan agues in which the fever (probably malarial) recurred on the third or fourth day. But accurate diagnosis of internal disorders was non-existent, and had little basis for developing until the elements of physiology and pathology were established in the seventeenth and eighteenth centuries by, among others, William Harvey (see page 159).

The choice of drugs for treating sick patients thus depended on a mixture of authority, tradition, and philosophy (or metaphysic, or superstition). The idea of bodily humours, which caused diseases if they were out of balance, provided reasons for getting fluids out of the body, by sweating, bleeding and purging, and led to unfounded ideas – not extinct even today – that purgation provides relief from a great many ills, even political:

What rhubarb, senna, or what purgative drug,
Would scour these English hence?

Macbeth, 5.3

A REMEDY FOR EVERY DISEASE

Those who believed that the world was made for humanity's benefit were inclined to think that there must be a remedy for every human disease, and that it must be labelled so that it could be recognized. Thus the doctrine of signs or signatures evolved gradually over the centuries. Yellow plants, notably saffron crocus (*Crocus sativus*) were chosen for jaundice. Red substances, such as rust or red wine, were good for bloodlessness. More subtly, the white spots on the leaves of lungwort (*Pulmonaria officinalis*) showed that the plant was good for lung disease.

Sometimes, it was argued that remedies had been put in convenient places for people to use. So, in England, the bark of the white willow (*Salix alba*) was tried for agues, because the tree grows in moist or wet soil, where agues chiefly

In this miniature at the beginning of Nicolaus Myrepsus's alphabetical formulary in Greek of 1399, a patient consults a physician who is examining his urine. In Greek and medieval medicine, the balance of the humours was the source of health or sickness. Humoral balance was best judged by the careful inspection of urine. The pharmacist with his remedies at hand is on the right.

abounded, as the Revd Edmund Stone, of Chipping Norton in Oxfordshire, observed in his report to the Royal Society of London in 1763:

> the general maxim, that many natural maladies carry their cures along with them, or that their remedies lie not far from their causes, was so very apposite to this particular case, that I could not help applying it; and that this might be the intention of Providence here, I must own had some little weight with me.[3]

There are, in fact, active compounds in willow bark (one is salicin, the precursor of salicyclic acid and the basis of aspirin) (see page 261), which are useful in dispelling some fevers, but reliance on a helpful providence has not often been so rewarding.

Herbals, or accounts of plants and their culinary and medicinal properties, were popular sources of remedies throughout medieval Europe. As medicine became more scientific, however, they began to be supplemented and superseded by pharmacopoeias, which described how drugs in regular use should be prepared and defined what materials were acceptable. Municipal authorities in Europe started issuing such standards in the sixteenth century. In London, the Royal College of Physicians produced a pharmacopoeia in 1618; fresh editions appeared with increasing frequency until the last in 1841. After that, as a result of the Medicines Act of 1858, a *British Pharmacopoeia*, produced under the auspices of the General Medical Council, became the national standard of reference. Other nations similarly set up their own standards – Brandenburg in 1698, Russia in 1778, Portugal in 1794, and so on. The first edition of *The Pharmacopoeia of the United States of America* appeared in 1820, although its standards were not legally enforceable until an act was passed in 1906.

NEW MEDICINES FROM OVERSEAS

Information about drugs was much needed, because explorers, missionaries, and colonizers were returning to Europe with unknown plants, many with supposed medicinal properties. The most notable, Peruvian or Jesuit's bark (*Cinchona offic-inalis*), was introduced into Europe between 1630 and 1640 and was promoted by Jesuit priests, who gave the powdered bark to those suffering from fever. Later, it was shown that it was specific for malaria, and that quinine, an alkaloid, was one of its constituents (see page 257).

A legend grew up that the bark was introduced to Europe in 1641 by the Spanish viceroy of Peru, after his wife, the Countess Anna del Cinchon, was cured by it, and the remedy was called cinchona. But the story is full of inconsistencies, as are several other claims for credit, which probably belongs to the traders of the time or to Jesuit missionaries in South America. Peruvian bark is a powerful remedy for malaria and, when diagnosis was imprecise, was widely in demand for fevers of all kinds, and as a tonic. It was introduced into the *London Pharma-copoeia* in 1677. Supplies were limited, however, and the search for new sources and alternative remedies became important. No effective substitutes were found until the nineteenth century after great advances had been made in the science of chemistry.

Other introductions to Europe from the Americas included the practice of smoking the dried leaves of the tobacco plant, *Nicotiana*, brought to England by Sir Walter Raleigh in the sixteenth century, primarily as a medicine. Thus began the long history of a valuable and much-abused drug, nicotine, one of the plant's constituent alkaloids. Adventurers also brought home ipecacuanha (*Cephaelis*

A warehouse in Amsterdam with cases of cinchona (Peruvian or Jesuit's bark) – the source of quinine, an anti-malarial drug. From the sixteenth century vast quantities of drugs were imported into Europe – especially opium from the east and cinchona from South America. Great ports such as London and Amsterdam became and remained markets for dealing with these products and for their pharmaceutical prepara-tion. By 1750, druggists in London were despatching hundreds of different medi-cines worldwide.

ipecacuanha) from Brazil, where the shrub was known as a powerful medicine. The dried root is useful against certain kinds of acute diarrhoea (such as amoebic dysentery), is an effective emetic in some cases of poisoning, and, in small doses, is used as a cough expectorant. Belief in the drug's effectiveness is emphasized by its current inclusion in many national pharmacopoeias.

In the past, ipecacuanha was famous because it was commonly prescribed in a powder with opium to provoke sweating, according to a recipe invented by a piratical physician from Warwickshire called Thomas Dover. He was second captain on the privateer *Duke* on Woodes Roger's expedition to South America in 1708–11. His powder is commemorated in this anonymous rhyme from St Bartholomew's Hospital, London, published in 1923:

> Oh, Dover was a pirate and he sailed the Spanish Main.
> A hacking cough convulsed him; he had agonising pain.
> So he mixed hisself a powder, which he liked it more and more.
> Ipecac. and opium and K2SO4.4

THE FIRST CLINICAL TRIALS

While exploration flourished abroad, scientists in Europe were starting their search for objective evidence of medicines by doing experiments. Direct evaluation of medical treatment in a scientifically respectable way began to be advocated prominently – that is, by comparing the effects of a treatment with the consequences if the treatment was not applied (either successively in the same patient, or by comparison between comparable patients). Famous trials were conducted by the English naval surgeon James Lind, who showed that lemon juice prevents scurvy, while careful analysis and enumeration of clinical records by the French physician Pierre Louis (see page 174) undermined the classical belief in the efficacy of bleeding. Lind and Louis were not the first to attempt the difficult practice of evaluating remedies. Although they made great advances, good practices of evaluation or re-evaluation did not become established. But the dawn of clear judgement was beginning to replace the dark night of treatment by the unquestioned authority of a priest or a physician.

THE CHEMICAL BASIS OF MEDICINES

During the eighteenth century, the science of chemistry, fundamental to understanding all living matter, began to take shape. Antoine Lavoisier, one of several men called the father of modern chemistry, thought – in part at least – of the living body as a well-knit piece of chemical machinery. Some of his experiments showed that animal heat was produced by chemical action on the food consumed – that is, there was no basic difference between bodily warmth and the production of heat by burning coal or wood. This was a most important advance, but Lavoisier's ideas could not be developed in detail until much more was known

Scurvy – an early clinical trial

James Lind, the so-called 'father of naval hygiene' and conductor of the first serious clinical trial, qualified in medicine in Edinburgh before being appointed physician at the Royal Naval Hospital at Haslar, Gosport. While serving as a naval surgeon in the West Indies and elsewhere, he saw that scurvy was disabling many seamen. He investigated carefully what was known about the disease, and then did carefully controlled experiments at sea and on land.

Lind's first therapeutic trial took place in 1747. He divided a dozen scurvy sufferers into six groups of two, treating each pair with a different remedy for 14 days. The two sailors given two oranges and a lemon each day recovered best. His *Treatise of the Scurvy* published in 1753 is lengthy and leisurely by our standards, but it is a model of what such a record should be, and his conduct and interpretation of his clinical trials leaves nothing to be desired.

Scurvy preventives were known to Captain James Cook, who kept his men healthy on his long circumnavigations by feeding them fresh fruit and vegetables. Joseph Banks, the young naturalist on board Cook's *Endeavour* on the first voyage (1768–71), had first-hand experience of the value of lemon juice when in the South Sea in April 1769:

> The ship was supplied by the Admiralty with sower crout [sauerkraut] which I eat of constantly till our salted cabbage was opened which I preferd as a pleasant substitute wort was servd out almost constantly. Of this I drank of a pint or more every evening but all this did not so intirely check the distemper or to prevent my feeling some small effects of it. About a fortnight ago my gums swelled & some small pimples rose on the inside of my mouth which threatened to become ulcers. I then flew to the lemon juice which had been put up for me according to D[r] Hulmes method described in his book & in his letter . . . Every kind of liquor which I used was made sour with the lemon juice N[o] 3 so that I took near 6 ounces a day of it. The effect of this was surprising. In less than a week my gums became as firm as ever & at this time I am troubled with nothing but a few pimples on my face, which have not deterred me from leaving off the juice intirely.[5]

Three 'mixes' of orange and lemon juice were supplied to the *Endeavour* by Nathaniel Hulme 'by order of Dr [John] Fothergill'. The cask of the first contained 6 gallons of lemon juice evaporated down to less than 2 gallons; the second, 7 gallons of orange juice and 1 gallon of brandy; and the third, 5 quarts of lemon juice and 1 of brandy. 'When you come to use of the juice which is in the casks, Hulme wrote to Banks on 1 August 1768,

> do not open the bunghole but draw it off at the end of the cask, by means of a wooden-cork, and make a vent hole at the top of the cask, with a peg in it, and always observe this method when you draw off your juice which you keep in casks . . . It would not be amiss then, if you were to take out with you several *wooden corks*, least any should be lost or broken; and perhaps 2 or 3 strong iron-bound casks, holding ten gallons a piece, might be very useful for taking in a quantity of orange, lemon, or lime juice, when you touch at any place abroad where these fruits grow.[6]

Many years later, in 1795, the Admiralty finally took heed of the findings of Lind and others, and lemon or lime juice was routinely included in the navy's diet. For a time scurvy ceased to obstruct the navy's business, and during the Napoleonic Wars, for example, the British navy had far less scurvy than the French. The lime juice regime became so well known that British sailors were called limeys. In the late nineteenth century, for good economic reasons, the Admiralty changed its source of supply of limes. The new limes were less effective, and it was wrongly supposed that the fruit juice theory was unsound.

Biochemical research from 1910 onwards showed beyond doubt that fruit juices did contain varying amounts of a substance that prevented scurvy. The substance was called vitamin C. It was isolated in 1928 and named ascorbic acid in 1932 by a Hungarian chemist called Albert von Szent-Györgyi, who later (1937) received the Nobel Prize for his discovery.

A man with scurvy, early twentieth century.

about the organization of living bodies, until the science of physiology was properly established.

Chemical methods were more immediately useful in purifying and identifying the ingredients of substances used as medicines. Clinical science was far too rudimentary to judge reliably whether a drug actually did a patient any good (or harm), but the new art of physiological experiments made it possible to show and even measure effects of potent medicines on animals in a laboratory. These investigations were immensely beneficial, because they threw new light on the way the body worked and they identified the active principles – constituents – of some important medicines. An active principle was no longer a philosopher's intellectual construct; it was there to be looked at, a crystalline substance of known chemical composition carefully preserved in a glass tube.

The great French physiologist François Magendie collaborated with an outstanding pharmacist Pierre-Joseph Pelletier in the first half of the nineteenth century in researches to isolate pure drugs. A small Indian tree called *Strychnos nux-vomica* yielded strychnine; and ipecacuanha from Brazil gave emetine. Pelletier, with his colleague Joseph Caventou, also improved the purification of morphine from opium, and isolated quinine from Peruvian bark and caffeine from coffee beans. All these substances reacted like alkalies with acids to form salts, and so were called alkaloids. Chemical analysis showed that they consisted of carbon, hydrogen, oxygen, and nitrogen and the proportions of these elements differed significantly in different alkaloids. But the structure of complex carbon compounds – the way the numerous atoms were joined to each other – was not understood until well on in the nineteenth century.

HOW DRUGS WORKED

François Magendie was primarily concerned with the normal workings of the body and drugs were his tools to separate one function from another. His one-time assistant at the Collège de France, Claude Bernard (see page 181) who took over Magendie's job in 1852, did more towards explaining exactly how drugs acted. Bernard showed that certain drugs acted at strictly localized and well-defined sites, a profoundly important fact that began to displace vaguer notions that drugs had some sort of general influence throughout the body. He discovered that the poison used by South American Indians called curare (a tree resin) works where a nerve joins the muscle on which it acts, and nowhere else. It prevents the nerve impulse from making the muscle contract, and so causes paralysis as long as the curare persists. Injected into an animal – on the tip of an arrow, for instance – the poison is carried by the bloodstream to all the muscles of the body and causes paralysis and death when the muscles of respiration are made inactive.

The discovery paved the way to the chemical understanding that Antoine Lavoisier had foreshadowed a century earlier. Clearly, there was some special

Opium and laudanum

Opium is the dried juice of the unripe seed capsules of the poppy *Papaver somniferum* (the plant's specific name means sleep-inducing). Capsules of this poppy have been found in burial chambers in Granada believed to be 5,000 years old, and the plant was important in the medicine of ancient civilizations in Babylonia, Egypt, Rome, and Greece. It is generally believed to be the principal ingredient of a secret remedy promoted by Paracelsus in the sixteenth century and called laudanum – basically, opium dissolved in alcohol. The seventeenth-century English physician Thomas Sydenham commended its use and it became an important remedy for the relief of pain, sleeplessness, and diarrhoea.

Fanny Trollope, and many other writers of the eighteenth and nineteenth centuries, took laudanum as a matter of course:

> At fifty-five, Mrs Trollope re-established her routine of writing her books by night, helped by laudanum and green tea. The famously drug-addicted writers of the period such as de Quincey and Coleridge were not exceptional except in degree. Harriet Martineau, writing in her autobiography about the 1830s and 40s, claimed that a 'clergyman who knew the literary world well' told her that 'there was no author or authoress who was free

from the habit of taking some pernicious stimulant; either strong green tea, or strong coffee at night, or wine or spirits or laudenum. The amount of opium taken, to relieve the wear and tear of authorship was, he said, greater than most people had any conception of, and all literary workers took something.' (Except of course the high-principled Miss Martineau.) [7]

Opium taken by mouth or by smoking gives very pleasurable effects and is, of course, highly addictive. Extensive legal controls have been applied to the drug, and been extensively defied by traders, governments, and consumers.

Opium contains several alkaloids, of which morphine is the most important; it was isolated in 1806 by a 22-year-old German apothecary's assistant in Paderborn, Frederick Sertürner, who did not at first appreciate the potency of the material he isolated and nearly killed himself with an overdose. Codeine was isolated in 1832 by Pierre-Jean Robiquet and papaverine in 1850 by G.F. Merck. Simple chemical treatment of morphine converts it to diamorphine or heroin, advertised as 'a magnificent sedative' for laryngitis by the Bayer Company in 1898, but now recognized as more potent than morphine with a worse reputation for causing addiction.

Opium was widely smoked in China and other oriental nations for therapeutic and recreational reasons. Much was imported from British India. When the Chinese government attempted to stop the trade in the 1840s, Britain went to war in defence of 'free' trade. The scenes in an opium factory in India (opposite) appeared in *The Graphic* in 1882.

THE EXAMINING HALL

THE MIXING ROOM

THE BALLING ROOM

THE DRYING ROOM

THE STACKING ROOM

OPIUM FLEET DESCENDING THE GANGES ON THE WAY TO CALCUTTA

THE INDO-CHINESE OPIUM TRADE: NOTES AT AN OPIUM FACTORY AT PATNA structure or substance that was inactivated by the curare; and similar specific points of action were recognized for other drugs. These specific structures or substances, of then unknown composition, came to be called 'receptors', and the study of drug receptors became a mainspring of fundamental pharmacology. So the reactions of drugs with bodily constituents began to be seen to be chemical events, best understood in terms of chemical knowledge.

These, however, were the ideas of the laboratory scientist, and only the wisest doctors of the time saw how important the science of chemistry was becoming to the practice of medicine. One who did was Sir William Osler, a Canadian who graduated at McGill Medical School in Montreal, became professor of medicine at Johns Hopkins University in Baltimore (see page 182), and built up the first organized clinical unit in any Anglo-Saxon country. In 1905, he became regius professor of medicine at the University of Oxford. In his address to McGill University in 1894, he commented: 'the physician without physiology and chemistry flounders along in an aimless fashion, never able to gain any accurate conception of disease, practising a sort of popgun pharmacy, hitting now the malady and again the patient, he himself not knowing which'.[8]

PHARMACOLOGY COMES OF AGE

The initiatives of Pierre Pelletier and Joseph Caventou, and of François Magendie and Claude Bernard, spread from France to Germany, and more slowly to Britain and later the USA, and by the 1850s the experimental science called pharmacology had become widely established. It is a curiosity of history that the first chair of pharmacology was established, not in France, Germany, or Britain, but in the university at Dorpat, now called Tartu, in Estonia. Dorpat was at that time a particularly active university. It had strong links with Germany, and recruited from Leipzig an able young doctor, Rudolph Buchheim, who had already translated the classic English textbook on pharmacology – Jonathan Pereira's *The Elements of Materia Medica and Therapeutics* (1839–40). Buchheim developed the subject and was duly created a professor. His pupil, Oswald Schmiedeberg, succeeded him, and, in 1872, moved to a new department at Strasbourg. There he attracted many young doctors and scientists, who later left to develop the subject in other parts of the world.

Scottish medical schools had a strong tradition of teaching 'materia medica', largely as a branch of botany, and the departments of materia medica were well placed to take up the new science of pharmacology under the old name. These academic departments were mainly concerned with medicinal plants, and began isolating their active constituents and discovering exactly how they worked, in terms of the growing knowledge of normal physiology. Robert Christison, a medical professor in Edinburgh from 1822 to 1877, wrote a textbook on poisons and described experiments on his own heart and blood vessels with a poisonous bean from Calabar in West Africa, noting the muscular weakness or paralysis that the

Help for headaches and fever

The aspirin family of medicines, introduced by the German chemical industry mostly between 1884 and 1894, provided new ways of treating pain and fever. All were synthesized in the laboratory as by-products of coal-tar distillation. They included phenazone (Antipyrine), acetanilide (Antifebrine), and phenacetin. Some did not survive long. Studies on toxicity in animals were, by modern standards, almost non-existent, and several compounds were withdrawn because they caused ill-effects in too many patients. However, several had longer lives. For example, paracetamol, derived from acetanilide, was first used medically in 1893 and became a popular over-the-counter-painkiller (bufferin, acetaminophen, etc.) after the Second World War. Amidopyrine started to fall into disrepute in the 1930s but was eventually replaced by the related compound phenylbutazone. This was introduced in 1949 but became increasingly unpopular, especially in the 1980s.

While these antifever drugs (antipyretics) were being discovered and put to use, the most familiar of all, aspirin (acetylsalicylic acid), was lying unappreciated on a chemist's shelf. In 1838, salicyclic acid was manufactured from salicin, an ingredient of willow bark (see page 252) and used to relieve fever and rheumatic pain. Fifteen years later, a relative of salicin, acetylsalicyclic acid, was synthesized by the German chemist Charles Gerhardt. Only in the 1890s, however, was this compound checked for antirheumatic effects. The Bayer laboratories in Elberfield first tested animals, then arranged for clinical trials. Their work, published in 1899, showed that the compound was indeed effective in controlling pain and inflammation both in rheumatism and other conditions, and in reducing fever as well. Bayer patented the production process, and named the new drug Aspirin.

The lapse of nearly half a century before aspirin was recognized as a useful medicine may seem surprising, but not unusual. It is difficult, tedious, and not without risk to discover whether a substance has unpredicted medical properties, and the odds against any particular compound being useful are enormous. Aspirin became probably the most widely used of all synthetic medicaments in the Western world, and nowadays competes for favour with paracetamol, the chief survivor of the coal-tar antipyretic analgesics.

Substances judged highly dangerous today, including heroin, were freely on sale around 1900 when this advertisement appeared.

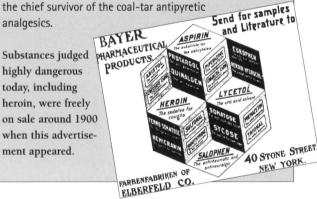

bean gradually induced. His successor, Thomas Fraser, isolated the bean's active constituent – an alkaloid, which he named eserine. Both researchers threw much light on the working of the autonomic nervous system. In the USA, still then a young country, developments came on similar lines, if a little later, with a profitable flow of people and ideas between the developing American universities and the established laboratories of Europe.

SPINOFFS FROM CHEMISTRY

Chemistry also developed rapidly in the nineteenth century, and young chemists in training had great opportunities. At the Royal College of Chemistry in London, an ambitious young student, William Henry Perkin, noted that quinine was described as $C_{20}H_{24}N_2O_2$. He thought of a simple reaction by which it could be synthesized by oxidizing allyltoluidine, a compound available to him. It looked all right on paper, but he was quite wrong. The attempt produced a coloured precipitate, certainly not quinine but exciting enough to suggest further experiments,

The properties of anaesthetics were in part found out by accident, as is indicated in this rendering of the discovery of chloroform by the Scottish obstetrician James Young Simpson on 4 November 1847. The artist is unknown.

which produced other coloured substances. Aged only 18, Perkin realized that one of them might do as a dye, and with great persistence he arranged for the material, called mauveine, to be made on a larger sale, and, finally, marketed.

Mauveine became famous as the world's first synthetic dye, and Perkin's work thus started the great dyestuff industry that developed, mainly in Germany, in the later nineteenth century. Many special chemical skills were developed in this industry, and by the end of the nineteenth century these were being applied to the manufacture of new drugs as well as dyes. Perkin's ambition to develop medicinal substances was, in a long roundabout way, fulfilled, and, after his death, on a vastly wider scale than he is likely to have foreseen.

The early history of these new substances, and especially how some came to be recognized as potential medicines, is obscure. German industrial firms worked in great secrecy, and did not reveal how they tested their new products to see if they were medicinal, or harmless, or poisonous. Some new drugs came initially from academic chemists, others from by-products of heavy chemical manufacture – pain-relievers (analgesics) and antifever drugs (antipyretics) from coal-tar distillation – and, later, from producers of fine chemicals, especially dyestuffs. Practising doctors, either on their own initiative or requested by industry, tried hitherto unknown substances on themselves, on animals, and on patients, sometimes with little more than guesswork about what the substances might do, either of benefit or of harm.

Among the most rash experiments were those with nitrous oxide, ether, and chloroform, all of which were found to cause reversible loss of consciousness. Nitrous oxide ('laughing gas'), first made by Humphry Davy about 1800, was taken up by showmen at fairgrounds to provide entertainment. Its use as an anaesthetic was inspired by observing that a man who fell and injured himself while under its influence suffered no pain at the time. Ether was more difficult to inhale, but experiments suggested that it could be more effective, and after some hesitations both substances were adopted as anaesthetics. So one horror – surgery without anaesthesia – was abolished, and new surgical procedures of all kinds became possible (see page 229). Chloroform followed soon afterwards; easiest to give but more hazardous, it was for long a controversial drug.

The introduction of anaesthesia was not looked on favourably by everyone. Some thought it was unnatural and wrong to alleviate the suffering inflicted on mankind by God as a retribution for his sins. However, by the time Queen Victoria received chloroform – administered by John Snow – for the birth of Prince Leopold on 7 April 1853, the protests were medical, on the grounds of safety, rather than theological. The editor of *The Lancet* thundered, 'In no case could it be justifiable to administer chloroform in perfectly ordinary labour',[9] and went on to the special iniquity of taking risks with the Royal Sovereign. But the Queen was delighted ('The effect was soothing, quieting and delightful beyond measure', she wrote in her journal[10]) and on the next (and last) occasion, the birth of Princess Beatrice in 1857, the critics were silent.

'GERMS' AND THE START OF CHEMOTHERAPY

For most doctors at the end of the nineteenth century, the 'germ theory of disease' was more important than anaesthesia or any other benefits of pharmacology. The revolutionary work of Louis Pasteur and Robert Koch and their followers is described in Chapter 5 (page 184); its significance cannot be overrated. The new knowledge of 'germs' started new studies of immunity and of ways in which infections could be prevented or overcome. So vaccines and antitoxins were devised. They were, by modern standards, crude and impure materials, containing complex substances far beyond the chemical knowledge of the time, and not encouraging thought on chemical lines about how they acted.

However, such thought was possible, and led the great German medical scientist Paul Ehrlich to the idea that much simpler substances might act powerfully against microbes without harming the patient. In the early part of his career, Ehrlich worked with Koch and Emil Adolf von Behring in studies of tuberculosis and diphtheria, and had an important role in the production of diphtheria antitoxin (see pages 137 and 191). He contracted tuberculosis himself, but recovered, and became Director of the German State Institute for Serum Research in Berlin, and later of specially endowed research laboratories. In 1908, he and the Russian Elie Metchnikoff shared a Nobel Prize for their work in immunology. By then, Ehrlich's thoughts on defence against bacteria had turned to chemical aspects, and he was investigating what he called 'chemotherapy' – the cure of bacterial infections with substances of known chemical identity.

In his student days Ehrlich had studied the staining of microbes and animal cells by dyestuffs, necessary for their observation under the microscope. It sounds

Paul Ehrlich, the leading pharmacologist and immunologist of his day, photographed around 1900, probably shortly after he became director of a new state research institute in Frankfurt am Main.

an obscure subject, of purely technical interest and unrelated to the discovery of new drugs, but it was in fact fundamental. Why do dyestuffs combine with particular cells, or particular parts of cells, and not with others? Does not this question arise about any substance, coloured or not, that act as drugs? Dyestuffs are convenient because they can be seen to be fixed by particular cells. But the chemical problem is the same whether the reagent is a visible dye or an invisible drug. It is the problem originally raised by Claude Bernard's studies. Ehrlich was particularly enthusiastic about the word 'receptor' for the submicroscopic structures that 'received' a dye or a drug. Developments from his lines of thought have been fundamental to pharmacology ever since.

Ehrlich looked for substances – dyes at first, other germicides later – that were fixed by microbes but not by the human or animal host of the microbe. Disinfectants and the like were effective killers but destructive also of host tissues, and he thought of modifying them chemically so that they were fixed by receptors in the microbe but not by those in the host.

The 606th compound Ehrlich studied became the famous drug called Salvarsan or arsphenamine. It was active against syphilis in rabbits, monkeys, and human beings, and was the first synthetic drug with practically useful 'chemotherapeutic' activity. It created great excitement when Ehrlich formally announced its discovery in 1910 because syphilis was at that time a socially unmentionable condition, a disease acquired immorally and ending in paralysis and insanity, and no previous remedy was curative. Ehrlich's hope that Salvarsan would kill the spirochaete bacterium that causes syphilis promptly and completely was too optimistic, but the power of the drug was undoubted and attracted the name 'magic bullet'. Salvarsan was difficult to use because it was unstable and needed to be dissolved immediately before use, and because it was active only when injected directly into the bloodstream. At that time injecting anything into a vein was unheard of except as a serious surgical procedure.

Improvements on Salvarsan were therefore looked for, and several related compounds in due course replaced it. Salvarsan and its successors attacked few other microbes, and no more magic bullets were discovered until the sulphonamides and penicillin (see pages 270–1). Ehrlich's work was followed by a period of pessimism; his success against syphilis was dismissed because the spirochaete that causes it is a very unusual organism, and many people said that antibacterial chemotherapy was an impossible dream.

THE FUNCTIONS OF DUCTLESS GLANDS

Meanwhile, physiology was making progress. From the 1830s onwards, scientists were concerned about various 'ductless' glands in different parts of the body – the thyroid and parathyroid glands in the neck, the adrenal or suprarenal glands near the kidneys, and the pituitary at the base of the brain. Some islets of tissue in the pancreas did not connect with the pancreatic ducts, and these also counted as a ductless gland. Gradually, the functions of the ductless glands were identified – by clinical observation of conditions in which the glands were enlarged or damaged or destroyed, and by seeing the results of their removal in experimental animals.

Was it possible that the glands contained materials that were essential to life? In 1891, the English physician George Murray, then in Newcastle upon Tyne, prepared extracts of the thyroid gland of sheep and fed them to a patient with myxoedema (underactivity of the thyroid). She got better, and was kept in good health for 28 years by treatment with thyroid preparations. Like the discovery of diphtheria antitoxin at about the same time, this discovery was a major advance; one of the occasions on which a completely effective treatment superseded a state in which no cure was known. Then, in 1927, material identical with the thyroid hormone was synthesized and used to treat a patient. The treatment succeeded, and no difference whatever was found between the natural and the synthetic hormone. Magical though the effect of thyroid hormone appeared to be, there was no need to attribute its benefit to any mysterious vital principle.

Other hormones presented greater difficulties. The connection between the pancreas and sugar diabetes was discovered in 1876, about the time when the thyroid was recognized as important. But feeding pancreas by mouth did not help diabetics. An injectable active pancreatic principle was sought for a long time, with several near misses. During 1921, however, Frederick G. Banting and Charles H. Best in Toronto University isolated material from the pancreases of dogs and used it to keep diabetic dogs alive. On 11 January 1922, they gave the first injections of this substance, which they named insulin, to a 14-year-old boy dying of diabetes; almost immediately his blood-sugar level

Frederick G. Banting and Charles H. Best on the roof of the medical building at the University of Toronto with one of the first diabetic dogs to have been kept alive with insulin, and the laboratory where they developed their technique for making the hormone. The laboratory is preserved in the Museum of Technology and Sciences in Toronto.

Large-scale production of extracts of the tubercle bacillus in Emil von Behring's laboratory in Marburg (watercolour by Fritz Gehrke, 1906). Tuberculosis worsened in the nineteenth century but the cause remained unknown until the German bacteriologist Robert Koch tackled the problem. On 24 March 1882, he reported that he had identified a certain bacillus that was invariably present in tuberular lesions in animals and humans; that he had cultivated the bacterium; and that he had produced the disease in healthy animals by inoculation.

fell. In 1923, with the help of a biochemist, James B. Collip, the pancreatic extracts were purified sufficiently to reduce the side-effects from the treatment. That same year, a Nobel Prize was awarded to Banting and to John J. R. Macleod, in whose physiological laboratory the research was done; Best, Banting's assistant, was overlooked. Banting was so furious at the omission of Best that he shared his half-prize with him; Macleod shared his with Collip.

Tremendous excitement was created by this discovery and there was an enormous demand for insulin, but its manufacture in sufficient quantities was far beyond the capacity of any university laboratory. Only the collaboration of the Connaught antitoxin laboratories in Toronto and the pharmaceutical business of Eli Lilly in Indianapolis made large-scale production (using pig pancreas) possible. Thereafter, diabetes in young people became no longer a death sentence but a condition entirely compatible with leading a normal life.

Hormones have been isolated from other glands, each with their own special and curious problems and consequences. The testes and ovaries were found to secrete hormones as well as producing sperm and ova, and their hormones, mostly isolated in the early 1930s, were of great value in the management of sex-

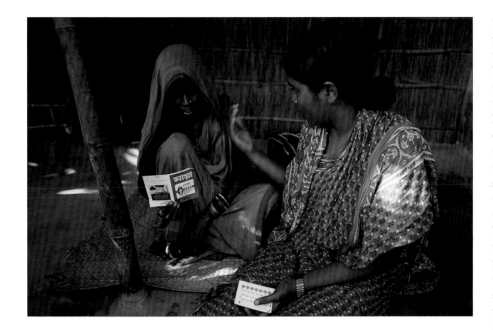

Distributing the contraceptive pill in Bangladesh. More importantly than any sexual license, the pill gives women the freedom to space their families or to choose not to have children at all. The idea of a perfect female contraceptive was pioneered by early-twentieth-century feminists such as Margaret Sanger in the USA. Later hormonal research was to make it feasible. By 1951, Gregory Pincus in the USA had shown that progesterone inhibited ovulation, and began a search for synthetic hormones. Further research on a pill by Pincus, John Rock, and Carl Djerassi led to successful clinical trials in Puerto Rico in 1956. By 1960, 'the pill' was on sale in the USA, and soon afterwards worldwide.

ual and reproductive disorders. That they could also be used to control fertility was long suspected, but needed many experiments and trials to be realized practically. Twenty years later, a biologist at the Worcester Foundation for Experimental Biology in Massachusetts called Gregory Pincus, with Carl Djerassi and others, developed an oral contraceptive for women. It was not until the 1960s, however, that the 'pill' became widely available. It is interesting to speculate, but difficult to get evidence, whether discovery of oral contraceptives was an important factor in the great increase in sexual licence at the time. It is perhaps more important to appreciate their potential for allowing women to space their families and reducing world population.

CHEMICAL OR ELECTRICAL MESSENGERS?

Hormones are not the only way in which substances secreted by certain cells influence the activity of other cells. After experiments by Luigi Galvani and others in the eighteenth century (see page 167), the main controlling part of the body, the nervous system, was recognized as working by some kind of electricity. But evidence accumulated that nerves acted on other cells, and even on each other, by chemical means, by substances bridging the tiny gaps between adjacent cells.

'Of known natural processes that might pass on excitation, only two are, in my opinion, worth talking about', wrote Emil du Bois-Reymond in 1877: 'either there exists at the boundary of the contractile substance a stimulatory secretion in the form of a thin layer of ammonia, lactic acid, or some other powerful stimulatory substance; or the phenomenon is electrical in nature.'[10] Some striking resemblances between hormones and nerve transmitters (the latter were sometimes called local hormones) had been noted. The hormone adrenaline, secreted by the medullary part of the adrenal glands, acted very like the sympathetic nervous system. Could it be, physiologists wondered, that the nerves themselves released adrenaline at their endings, and that the adrenal medulla served to reinforce the effects of all the sympathetic nerves? The same question was asked about the parasympathetic nervous system, because an unstable substance called acetylcholine acted just like parasympathetic nerves. Was it the transmitter at those nerve endings? As summarized in Chapter 5, experiments by neurophysiologists such as Otto Loewi in Graz, Henry Dale and his colleagues (who included several refugees from Nazi persecution in Germany) in London, Walter B. Cannon in Cambridge, Massachusetts, and Ulf von Euler in Stockholm turned these ideas into hard fact and provided the basis on which an astonishing number of new drugs were discovered.

Chemical transmitters make muscles contract and start glands secreting, and set into train more elaborate processes. All kinds of chemical transmission (and so chemical control of particular cellular activities) can be imitated by substances that resemble the natural transmitters closely. This principle was first made to work in the USA in about 1930 in Pennsylvania, when two new drugs, carbachol and methacholine, were synthesized at the Merck laboratories and used medicinally. They imitated acetylcholine, but the effects lasted longer, so they were used for their action on the bladder to overcome postoperative retention of urine. The application was comparatively trivial, but the principle was sound and is the basis of most of the blood-pressure drugs in use today.

VITAMINS

A new kind of medicine arrived with the discovery of vitamins. Although nutritional deficiency diseases were known since the work of James Lind and others, the different chemical identities of the substances causing the diseases were not discovered until the twentieth century. The term 'vitamin' was coined in 1912 by Casimir Funk, a chemist working at the Lister Institute in London. It was partly his research that helped clarify the distinctive functions of vitamins.

When Funk started his work, it was known from clinical studies that certain human diseases were caused by a deficiency of specific vitamins: for example, beriberi for lack of thiamine (vitamin B_1) (see pages 45 and 192); scurvy, long known to be prevented by a sufficiency of citrous fruits, for a lack of ascorbic acid (vitamin C) (see page 256); and so on. It was realized that where there was a lack of a particular vitamin in the diet, treatment with that vitamin was life-saving. Once this became known, there were no further doubts about how to treat specific deficiency diseases.

Regrettably, however, superstition grew fast about vitamins, and they promptly acquired a reputation as magical cure-alls. Manufacturers were quick to exploit the myth, baffled physicians were relieved to adopt it, and comfort-seeking patients were (and are) all too willing to believe it. Evidence for minor benefits from various vitamins is hard to obtain and generally of the anecdotal and unconvincing kind. But poisoning by excess, particularly of the fat-soluble vitamins, is well known: nervous disturbances and birth defects are produced by an excess of vitamin A, and excess of body calcium and kidney stones after too much vitamin D. But vitamins remain a popular and heavily promoted form of therapy, rarely (in prosperous countries) with any rational basis. They are probably more rewarding to the shareholders of manufacturing companies than to most of the people who consume them.

Whether vitamins are drugs is a matter of the use of language, and need not be pursued. The term vitamin, contracted mistakenly by Casimir Funk from 'vital amine', is misleading, because most accessory food factors are not amines, and whether they are vital, meaning essential for survival, differs from species to species. But the name has come to stay.

The way vitamins act in living cells throws much light on the ways cells work, and knowledge of this activity has been used to design drugs for specific purposes, especially antibacterial agents. The detailed biochemistry of vitamins was worked out largely in microbes – much more convenient and socially acceptable research subjects than mammals. From the knowledge so gained it was a simple step (although few saw the great possibilities) to go on to designing antibacterial drugs that interfere with the way microbes use their essential foods. Remarkable results followed.

MODERN PHARMACEUTICALS EMERGE

Before the development of such antibiotics, however, there was a discovery made on more classical lines. It took place in the laboratories of the Bayer Company in Elberfeld, Germany, in the early 1930s. A German biochemist, Gerhard Domagk, appointed to direct Bayer's research in 1927, continued Paul Ehrlich's approach of investigating dyestuffs, and presently showed that a red dye, later named Prontosil, was extraordinarily effective in curing streptococcal infections in mice. Clinical trials followed, and by 1935 the drug was used in patients with great success. One of the first to receive the new medicine was Domagk's daughter, who made a dramatic recovery from a streptococcal infection caused by a needle prick.

Prontosil proved especially effective in treating women with childbirth fever or puerperal sepsis, which is mostly streptococcal in origin and, until that time, took a sorry toll of deaths of young mothers. The discovery deserved a Nobel Prize; indeed, Domagk was nominated for one in 1939, but was forbidden by the Nazi government to accept it. When Germany was no longer at war, the Nobel rules forbad him to have the prize money after such a delay.

Meanwhile research at the Pasteur Institute in Paris showed that only a part of the molecule of Prontosil was necessary to defeat streptococci, and the active component, named sulphanilamide, soon superseded Prontosil – no doubt to the chagrin of all concerned in the Bayer Company, which held the patents for Prontosil. Sulphanilamide was a well-known substance; it was first synthesized in 1908 during studies on dyes and for nearly 30 years lay among the stores of many organic chemists, because no one knew or suspected that it could save lives.

When Gerhard Domagk and his Bayer colleagues found that sulphanilamide checked streptococcal bacteria in mice, they, and many others, naturally wondered how the drug worked. Their question was answered remarkably soon. Clinical trials with human patients showed that the drug did not work in abscesses filled with pus. Test-tube experiments showed that pus and also other materials, including yeast extracts, protected the germs against sulphanilamide. The protective principle in both pus and yeast was identified: it was a simple compound called *p*-aminobenzoic acid (PABA), very closely related to sulphanilamide itself. PABA was soon found to be an essential nutrient for some microbes, and these turned out to be just those species that were sensitive to sulphanilamide. Clearly, the two compounds competed. The sulphanilamide got in like PABA, but then jammed the works. The process, named 'competitive antagonism', was studied closely, and, in spite of the labyrinthine complexity of the details, provided a huge advance in understanding how drugs acted, how drugs might act, and how new and useful drugs could be invented.

The clinical trials of sulphanilamide were not elaborate by more recent standards, but the drug had dramatic effects and left little doubt about its merits. However, it also had ill-effects, altering blood pigments so that patients looked blue, and occasionally damaging the blood-forming tissues so that white blood cells disappeared. Hence the search began for better compounds, mostly from the family called sulphonamides, to which sulphanilamide belonged. Within a few years more than 5,000 sulphonamides had been examined and perhaps 50 found clinically useful against bacteria of various kinds and some other organisms. The earliest sulphonamides – sulphanilamide itself and the sulphapyridine from May and Baker (once famous as M & B 693) – were discarded when numerous safer agents were discovered.

The distinction between antibiotics and chemotherapeutic drugs is a historical accident. Several antibiotics have been prepared synthetically, and no distinction whatever has been found between these and those prepared from 'natural' fungal material. However, penicillins (there were several varieties in the materials originally extracted) are difficult to prepare synthetically, and are more economically made from cultured moulds. Nonetheless, the original penicillins have been modified chemically and with advantage for various specific purposes, and clinical practice today depends heavily on such semisynthetic materials.

Unhappily for humans, strains of bacteria resistant to drugs have emerged. Microbes pass through many generations in a matter of days or weeks, and so they evolve very rapidly. As soon as antibacterial agents were widely used, microbes that resisted them had a great advantage for survival, while their less-resistant cousins and competitors were quickly eliminated. Bacteria resistant to antibiotics

Antibiosis and penicillin

Soon after the sulphonamides restored the tarnished hopes for 'chemotherapy' in the 1930s, a quite different kind of antimicrobial agent arrived. It started from a phenomenon known since the late nineteenth century and called antibiosis – the killing of one kind of organism by the products of another. Bacteriologists knew how certain microbes on a culture plate could stop other kinds from growing, and some innovators tried to isolate the 'antibiotic' materials responsible. As early as the 1870s it was realized that *Penicillium* moulds checked the growth of bacteria. The famous surgeon and bacteriologist Joseph Lister (see page 231) treated a patient soon afterwards, but no record is known of the consequences except that the patient survived for many years.

Other antibiotic substances were soon found in bacteria as well; one was prepared from the organism then called *Bacillus pyocyaneus* (now known as *Pseudomonas pyocyanea*), and marketed in Germany early in the twentieth century. However, these early antibiotic materials were too unstable to be relied on, and were abandoned.

In 1922, Alexander Fleming at St Mary's Hospital in London observed that human nasal secretions were antimicrobial and called the active substance, an enzyme, lysozyme. It could not, however, be prepared in concentrated form. A few years later, in 1928, Fleming made a more famous observation, when one of his culture plates of staphylococci was contaminated by airborne spores of an unusual *Penicillium*. He noticed that the bacteria were killed near the mould. Spoilage of a culture like this is usually seen as a regrettable nuisance, but Fleming fortunately thought the event worth investigating. He did not have the chemical skills or resources to isolate pure penicillin (the name he gave to the bactericidal) but he used crude preparations of it for some clinical studies – which, in the event, proved unrewarding – and as a tool for identifying bacteria.

Penicillin is a difficult substance to isolate in pure form because it is unstable. It was not until the early 1940s that concentrated penicillin was obtained by the biochemist Ernst Chain, working with

the Australian pathologist Howard Florey and their colleagues in the Dunn School of Pathology, Oxford. Clinical trials of Chain and Florey's material were, however, hampered by great difficulties in producing enough material. Although penicillin was obviously an effective antibiotic, the trials were too small to persuade many people that it had remarkable curative properties. No pharmaceutical company in war-torn Great Britain was prepared to commit substantial resources to manufacturing an awkward product on such slender evidence. Florey therefore sought help from the Rockefeller Foundation in New York, which was already supporting his work, and a leading American pharmacologist, A. N. Richards, who had formerly worked with Florey in England, helped him in finding drug companies in the USA that would risk the necessary investment. Merck, Squibb, and Pfizer hence became deeply involved. Success followed, and enough penicillin was available by 1944 to treat battle casualties in North Africa and Europe and severe infections among civilians. In 1945, Fleming, Florey, and Chain were awarded a Nobel Prize for their work on penicillin.

Penicillin attacks the same microbes as the sulphonamides, and many others. Unlike the sulphonamides, however, it is virtually non-toxic. (Sensitization to penicillin is uncommon, although very serious, and was not discovered for some time.) The dramatic success of the new agent aroused widespread enthusiasm, and other antibiotics were sought in many parts of the world and in many laboratories. The first success was streptomycin. This was isolated from a microbe living free in the soil by Selman Waksman, an Ukrainian-born American. In 1944, he demonstrated its effectiveness against the hitherto incurable tuberculosis. High hopes were soon damped, however, when streptomycin was found to be liable to cause deafness and permanent giddiness. More seriously, tubercle bacilli adapted quite quickly to the antibiotic and became resistant to it.

Alexander Fleming in his laboratory in 1943, and (above) his famous culture plate.

such as penicillin thus steadily became more common, and so the dream faded that a few antibiotics would put an end to humanity's infectious diseases.

Some respite has been achieved by using combinations of antibacterial agents, because resistant strains have less chance of emerging if microbes are attacked by two or more drugs at the same time. Important new antibiotics are especially those that control resistant strains of familiar germs. But the conflict between humans and microbes is not resolved, nor is likely to, and continued research is essential if new and dangerous strains are to be kept under control.

ANTIVIRAL AGENTS

Finding agents against viruses has proved difficult. Most success has been obtained with vaccines, and especially the first vaccine (pioneered by Edward Jenner at the end of the eighteenth century), which made possible the elimination of a once universally feared deadly or disfiguring disease, smallpox. Vaccines against other viruses, notably that of yellow fever, have also been successful. Viruses are, however, intracellular parasites, difficult of access, and the intimate association between the metabolism of the virus and the host has for long challenged any chemical solution. Only in the past 20 years has striking progress been made, illustrated by the remarkable properties of acyclovir.

Acyclovir (Zovirax), discovered in the Wellcome laboratories in the USA and in England in the 1970s is potent against herpes zoster (shingles), cold sores, and other herpes infections. Acyclovir is converted in cells infected with the herpes virus to a metabolic blocking agent, and so is of minimal danger to healthy tissues; the problem of toxicity to the host is largely overcome. Other viruses have been less amenable, or less intensively pursued; influenza viruses continue to be a recurrent hazard, especially the human immunodeficiency virus (HIV), which paves the way for AIDS. Zidovudine (Retrovir), a somewhat distant chemical relative of acyclovir, is the first drug to be recognized by regulatory bodies for the treatment of HIV infection.

THE CHEMOTHERAPY OF CANCER

A different kind of chemotherapy began with the discovery that substances called nitrogen mustards selectively kill a particular kind of cancerous cell. The story is a fine example of a trail that reached a valuable conclusion quite different from the intended objective. It began in the Second World War, when research was resumed, for obvious reasons, on chemical warfare agents. Whatever the ethics of their use, no nation could afford to be ignorant of their properties or be unprepared to treat whatever casualties might occur. In the USA, substances closely related to mustard gas were studied in depth by the pharmacologists Louis Goodman and Alfred Gilman at Yale University and found, among other properties, to destroy white blood cells (lymphocytes). When one was administered to a mouse with a lymphoma (a large solid tumour of the lymph cells) the tumour shrank dramatically, in a way never seen before. The experiment was reproducible, and so patients with lymphocyte tumours were treated with nitrogen mustards, naturally with extreme caution, but soon with considerable success.

The path was opened to the discovery of other agents for cancer chemotherapy. One promising approach was to synthesize compounds that resembled folic acid, which is used in the formation of new blood cells, including the excessive proliferation in leukaemia. Folic acid analogues were made, especially at the Lederle Laboratories. One of them (aminopterin) was shown in the 1940s to cause striking remissions in childhood leukaemia. Another approach depended on studying the pathway by which nucleic acids are synthesized. Here, too, the tactic was used of making analogues that could jam some particular part of the works without non-specific disastrous consequences. George Hitchings and Gertrude Elion at the Wellcome laboratories then in New York produced a sequence of new drugs in this way in the 1940s and 1950s. They included 6-mercaptopurine, which was also found to cause remissions in some leukaemia patients.

More fortuitous discoveries included the anthracycline antibiotic called daunorubicin, derived from a *Streptomyces* fungus and active against a variety of solid tumours as well as acute leukaemias, and the alkaloids called vincristine and vinblastine, obtained from periwinkles (*Vinca*). All of these substances are highly toxic and their use calls for specialist expertise at every stage. Many leukaemias responded well, and these conditions, once invariably fatal, now often have a prospect of recovery. But cancer cells, like microbes, become resistant to chemotherapy. Repeated courses of treatment are all too often less and less effective, and drugs, whether natural or synthetic, have, so far, proved more often palliative than curative.

GROWTH OF THE PHARMACEUTICAL INDUSTRY

After the war of 1939–45, the pharmaceutical industry expanded greatly. By the 1980s around ten companies were usually among the top fifty major corporations in the USA, and there was similar growth in Britain and elsewhere in Europe. Research laboratories grew even faster than the companies; typically, the old-established American firm of Smith, Kline & French had a research staff of eight in 1936, which grew to hundreds in the 1950s and now is enlarged by amalgamations with other enterprises into Smith Kline Beecham.

In such laboratories millions of compounds were synthesized and tested for pharmacological and antimicrobial properties. The search was conducted in various ways, some rational, and sometimes more speculative or quite random. Many useful drugs resulted from each kind of approach; luck as well as judgement is crucial to success in research. Often, several drugs were discovered with closely similar properties, and complaints were made about the waste in such 'me-too' discoveries. However, among major series of drugs, such as sulphonamides and corticosteroids, the original agents have been completely superseded by successors widely regarded as having a better overall performance. A 'me-too' drug is not necessarily worse, and may be distinctly better than its competitor.

DOES IT REALLY WORK?

It has always been much easier to believe optimistically in a remedy than to prove its worth in even a faintly scientific way. Extensive clinical research has been applied to discovering how best to use the powerful new remedies produced by the pharmaceutical laboratories, to discovering which of similar drugs is preferable, and indeed to discovering whether their use is, in the long run and in spite of superficial appearances, beneficial at all. Bedside observation of individual patients under treatment has been supplemented by collection of facts about as many as possible of the patients treated in one way or another. Sometimes it then turns out that, however excitingly some sufferers appear to recover, most of the patients being treated actually do worse than those who are left alone or receive other treatments.

Not only do new remedies need evaluating: many traditional remedies must also be questioned, as the eighteenth-century naval physician, James Lind, observed in the preface to his *Treatise on Scurvy* (1753). His wisdom remains all too true but is often forgotten:

> It appeared to me a subject worthy of the strictest inquiry: and I was led upon this occasion to consult several authors who had treated of the disease; where I perceived mistakes which have been attended in practice, with dangerous and fatal consequences. There appeared to me an evident necessity of rectifying those errors, on account of the pernicious effects they have already visibly produced. But as it is no easy matter to root out old prejudices, or to overturn opinions which have acquired an establishment by time, custom, and great authorities; it became therefore requisite for this purpose, to exhibit a full and impartial view of what has hitherto been published on the scurvy; and that in a chronological order, by which the sources of those mistakes may be detected. Indeed, before this subject could be set in a clear and proper light, it was necessary to remove a great deal of rubbish. [11]

James Lind, who pioneered early clinical trials that demonstrated the efficacy of citrus fruits in combating scurvy, discredited many traditional remedies.

History of the use of medicines reveals, over and over again, how much trust is placed in medical beliefs that particular remedies are effective and that it is negligent or worse to withhold them. And yet, years or centuries later the remedies have fallen into disuse, if not positive disrepute, because their lack of good or their positive harm has at last been revealed by careful accumulation of evidence and refusal to be swayed by casual anecdotes.

The principles and value of good clinical trials were shown most lucidly when the efficacy of streptomycin in the treatment of tuberculosis was evaluated just after the Second World War by the British Medical Research Council, advised by Sir Austin Bradford Hill of the London School of Hygiene and Tropical Medicine.

Very little of the new drug was available when the trial started in 1946 – just enough for a small proportion of the patients who might have benefited. It was therefore considered ethically justifiable to carry out a trial in which one group received streptomycin whereas a control group was treated with traditional methods. The randomized controlled clinical trial, the first of its type, provided clear evidence about which treatments were more effective than others and set a model for many subsequent studies of new drugs. It has become unacceptable to claim benefit for a new drug without clinical trials. Unfortunately, not all trials are conducted well enough to be reliable.

UNWANTED EFFECTS

The toxicity of many new agents has been discovered only after they were in regular use. The harm caused by thalidomide in the 1950s was particularly distressing and aroused powerful demands for safe drugs. Testing drugs for toxicity, however, is an insoluble problem; the number of ways in which a drug may be toxic is unlimited, and attempts to detect them all in advance have consistently been defeated, whenever new hazards have been discovered.

In recent years, the introduction of life-saving drugs has often been delayed while tests of regrettably uncertain value are done. In the 1970s, the phrase 'drug lag' became familiar, especially in the USA, to describe the delays imposed by authorities. It has been claimed that several thousand American citizens would die of heart failure between the time a drug that would prevent their death become available in European countries and the time it was licensed in the USA. Special procedures, sometimes called the 'fast track', were designed to overcome the lag. Gradually, it has been accepted that the most valuable safeguard rests on adequate recording of all uses of new drugs and reporting of all adverse effects.

SOCIETY AND DRUGS

Since the Second World War, in at least industrialized societies, people have become more preoccupied with health, illness, and medicine than ever before. Certainly, the media endlessly draw attention to medicines and drugs and arouse enthusiasm or anxiety often on very slender grounds. How far popular attitudes are fuelled by broadcasting, or by the advertising of drug manufacturers, is no part of this chapter, nor are the social processes that led to the rise and decline of the 'permissive society' and the use of 'recreational' drugs with all the hazards of toxicity, impurity, and abuse.

One of James Sowerby's illustrations for William Withering's *Account of the Foxglove and Some of its Medical Uses etc.; With Practical Remarks on Dropsy and Other Diseases* (1785). Withering, an Edinburgh-trained physician who worked at Birmingham General Hospital, demonstrated that digitalis (a constituent of foxglove leaves) had a powerful stimulant action on the heart, increased urine flow, and was effective in reducing oedema.

The thalidomide disaster

Thalidomide was introduced as a safe sleeping tablet, at a time of popular concern about suicides caused by barbiturates taken in overdose. It was indeed difficult to take enough of thalidomide to cause death, and it was widely used in Europe. Scientific assessors in the US Food and Drug Administration, however, had doubts about other aspects of its safety, and the drug was never licensed in the USA.

In 1961, after the drug had been on the market for 2 years, obstetricians in several parts of Europe observed that babies were being born unusually often with a rare deformity – the failure of the limbs to develop. It took 2 years of extensive research for the cause to be identified as thalidomide, taken at a particular, brief period in early pregnancy to ease the discomforts of morning sickness. Nearly 500 babies were born with deformities in Britain alone; worldwide, there were many thousands.

Naturally, after the thalidomide disaster there were widespread demands for 'proper' testing of drugs. Drug-regulatory authorities already existed in the USA, and committees with similar purpose were set up in other countries. In Britain, the Dunlop Committee functioned well with the voluntary cooperation of the drug industry, but was superseded by bodies set up under the Medicines Act of 1968.

Toxicity testing is not simple. One cannot predict what a drug will do in so complex an organism as a mammal by test-tube experiments and biochemical guesswork. Moreover, in testing a drug in this way, one is concerned with what it will *not* do. The test systems of the 1960s, required by the regulatory authorities, depended on feeding large doses of potential new drugs to dozens of animals of various species and looking for ill-effects. Experience showed that these experiments did not necessarily reveal serious ill-effects in humans, and even with the most meticulously tested drugs, such as Practolol, fresh tragedies occurred.

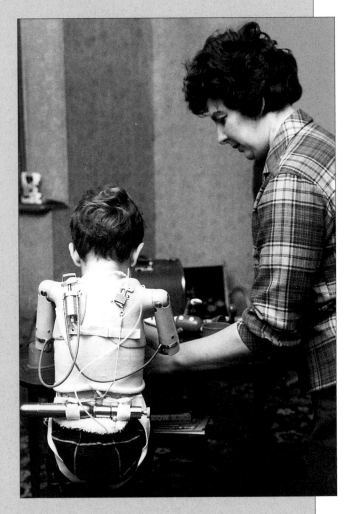

The human disaster of thalidomide children created an emotional public outcry. A cylinder of compressed gas powered the artificial arms of this boy.

One may note how enthusiasm for 'science' has given place to scepticism, and particularly in medicine how the pursuit of technical improvements has got in the way of compassion and caring. There is an interesting parallel in the history of China. In about 700 BC, medical practice had become increasingly based on direct observation and was to that extent comparable to 'scientific medicine'. Then it gave way to new, or resuscitated, systems in which superstition, magic, and charms played a large part. Whether the change had any significant consequences for the health of the Chinese of the time is not certain, and only time and reliable statistics will tell whether the current confusion and distaste for 'scientific medicine' is having measurable results.

As far as drugs are concerned, the important 'alternative' or 'complementary' therapies are homeopathy and herbalism. The tenets of homeopathy (see page 114) involve rejecting the whole basis of orthodox physics and chemistry, and the homeopathist's use of medicines does not depend on their actions as studied by pharmacologists but on an unconventional system of beliefs. Herbal remedies existed long before any evaluation of medicines was thought about. From herbs have come many important drugs, including belladonna, curare, codeine, digitalis, ipecacuanha, and nicotine. All these are potent, and the plants that produce them are recognized as poisonous. Many other herbal remedies remain of unproven worth, at least by scientific standards.

Without a demonstrable action, no active ingredient can be identified. Many herbal preparations available 'off the shelf' do not contain any potent substances and, like homeopathic medicines, give comfort if they please the patient. However, quite a number of garden plants are poisonous, and any self-treatment with such plants is dangerous. With the penchant for a 'green' way of life, accidental self-poisoning with 'natural' herbs is being recorded more frequently. Even seemingly mild herbal teas may cause harm if taken regularly for long periods of time. Also, herbal remedies are occasionally adulterated with 'chemical' drugs to achieve greater potency, regardless of safety, and the lack of control of the sale of herbal remedies is a cause for growing concern. Homeopathy and herbalism, like faith in vitamins, have been favoured chiefly for conditions in which symptoms rather than objective changes are prominent. Measurement of benefit is difficult, and evaluation by properly controlled trials is rare.

Potent drugs are as dangerous as a surgeon's sharp knife, and must be handled with equal care if they are to do good. The proper use of orthodox medicines has brought about great triumphs in prolonging life and relieving suffering, and it is silly to despise or underrate this achievement. The greater the power of the remedy, the greater the hazards of misuse.

Chapter 8

Mental illness

Roy Porter

Madness is an enigma. Being 'mad' is part of common speech. Especially in American English, 'mad' means 'angry' ('he'll get real mad!') and we speak of being 'mad about' someone, or crazy in love. In such usage, madness is a mood or feeling. Most people, medical and lay alike, also accept that madness (or mental illness, psychiatric disorder, and so forth) can be an authentic medical condition. I emphasize 'most', because leaders of the antipsychiatry movement launched in the 1960s – notably Ronald Laing in Britain and Thomas Szasz in the USA – denied the reality of mental illness in the strict sense of the term, denied that madness was a disease like measles or malaria. According to Szasz, writing in 1974, madness was a witch-hunting label pinned on 'deviants' or scapegoats for the purpose of psychiatric empire-building and to exercise social control.

The relations between being mad as extreme emotion or eccentric behaviour, and (on the other hand) madness as a medical diagnosis are complex and controversial. Even those satisfied that madness is a disease, contest what it is, what causes it, and what may be done about it. To understand how madness has grown so maddeningly confusing, its history must be explored.

THE GREEK TRADITION

Pre-Classical cultures certainly identified madness, but it is with the Greeks that madness first became an object of rational inquiry and literary depiction. In Greek myths, the heroes grow demented, driven wild with frenzy or beside themselves with rage or grief.

DIONYSUS: The reason why I have chosen Thebes as the first place
To raise my Bacchic shout, and clothe all who respond
In fawnskin habits, and put my thyrsus in their hands –
The weapon wreathed with ivy-shoots – my reason is this;
My mother's sisters said – what they should have been the last
To say – that I, Dionysus, was not Zeus's son;
That Semele, being with child – they said – by some mortal,
Obeyed her father's prompting, and ascribed to Zeus
The loss of her virginity; and they loudly claimed
That this lie was the sin for which Zeus took her life.
Therefore I have driven those same sisters mad, turned them
All frantic out of doors; their home now is the mountain;
Their wits are gone. I have made them bear the emblem of
My mysteries; the whole female population of Thebes,
To the last woman, I have sent raving from their homes.
Now, side by side with Cadmus' daughters, one and all
Sit rootless on the rocks under the silver pines.

Euripedes, *The Bacchae*

A Maenad, one of the god Dionysus's followers. She bears a knife with which she has cut off the head of a wild animal that she will eat raw. A Roman bas-relief.

The *Iliad* reveals the remnants of archaic attitudes towards madness; it does not display insanity as later understood by medicine and philosophy, for Homer's heroes do not possess psyches or forms of consciousness comparable to that of Sophocles's Oedipus, still less to that of Hamlet or Sigmund Freud. Homer's epics give their characters no sensitive, reflective, introspective selves. Greek heroes are puppetlike, at the mercy of forces from Beyond: gods, demons, the fates, and furies. They do not have what modern authors call 'intrapsychic' existences.

The introspective mentality emerged at the height of Athenian civilization in the fifth and fourth centuries BC; and an American psychiatrist and historian, Bennett Simon, argued in his book *Mind and Madness in Ancient Greece* that the idea of the psyche then developing was to set the mould for Western reasoning about minds and madness ever since. Sigmund Freud said as much by labelling infantile psychosexual conflicts the 'Oedipus Complex', thereby paying homage to Sophocles's tragedy, *Oedipus Rex*.

The Romantic artist Théodore Géricault (1791–1824) was closely associated with the Paris psychiatrist Etienne-Jean Georget, a pioneer in the humane treatment of the insane. He made a series of studies of mad people, following the diagnostic categories in use at the time yet also bringing out their individual characteristics. The studies were made during the last years of the artist's life in 1822–3, while he was dying of what seems to have been cancer of the spine, aged only thirty-three. His studies of women lunatics in particular, of which this murderesss of children is considered a masterpiece, are terrifying images.

Socrates, Plato, Aristotle, and other Greek thinkers of their day systematically reasoned about nature, society, and consciousness. They probed the unknown, seeking to grasp the order of things and to depict the rational self as exemplary, creating ideals of ethical man or political man. Through self-knowledge (as in the adage 'know thyself'), reason could fathom human nature and thereby master enslaving appetites. Thus philosophy ennobled reason.

In their pursuit of reason, Greek philosophers did not deny the reality of what was not rational. On the contrary, the store they set by reason attests the dangerous power they ascribed to passions and the mysterious forces of fate, just as they were also fascinated by the transcendental 'fire' that consumed geniuses and artists. Nevertheless, Plato and his followers defined the irrational as the enemy of human dignity and freedom; and the polarity between the rational and the irrational, as with supremacy of mind over matter, became cardinal to Classical moral and medical values, remaining influential down to the present day.

If the rise of philosophy enabled the Greeks to reason on madness, how did they explain that calamity of the soul? How did they expect to prevent or cure it? There were two leading traditions through which they made sense of madness. One lay in culture, expressed in rhetoric, art, and theatre. Greek tragedians dramatized the primeval conflicts of life – the fate of the individual crushed by ineluctable destiny, the torment of divided loyalties, the rival demands of love and hatred, pity and revenge, duty and desire, mortals and deities, family and polis. And they showed these conflicts becoming (contrast Homer's puppet-like heroes) conscious objects of reflection and inner conflict, censure and guilt. Madness had become the condition and fate of minds divided against themselves. The heroes of Sophocles and Euripides were conscious of having brought madness on themselves; psychic civil war thereby became intrinsic to the human condition.

But drama also suggested resolutions, or, in Bennett Simon's phrase, theatre became therapy. As with Oedipus, desperate suffering could engender a higher wisdom, blindness could beget insight, bloodshed could purify, and public drama could stage collective catharsis. Enacting madness, forcing the unthinkable to be spoken, bringing into the open the monsters of the mental deep, reclaimed the emotional battleground for reason, all passion spent.

Thus madness could be the tormented soul, which art could capture. Yet the Greeks also developed a quite different way of grasping madness: a medical tradition. As explained in Chapter 2, the style of medical thinking expressed in the Hippocratic writings in the fifth century BC and dominant thereafter insisted that disease was natural and hence amenable to empirical and rational inquiry. Of particular relevance, a Hippocratic treatise, *On the Sacred Disease,* insisted that the falling sickness or epilepsy – heretofore regarded as a supernatural disorder – was a regular ailment like any other, a routine malady produced by normal bodily processes. So if the so-called 'sacred disease' was natural, by implication all other abnormalities of behaviour, all madness, equally fell within medicine's bounds. Explanations of insanity should thus be couched in terms of physical causes and effects, emphasizing the heart or brain, blood, spirits, and humours; and treatments would rely on regimen and medicines. To the scientific temper, insanity was not a dilemma or a drama but a disease.

As discussed more fully in Chapters 2 and 3, mainstream Greek medicine proposed internal, constitutional causes for illness. Health hinged on the four 'humours' or body fluids. These were also the key to mental disturbance. An excess of yellow bile (*choler*) would overheat the system, causing mania or raving madness: by contrast, surplus black bile (*melancholia*) would induce dejection. Aretaeus, a contemporary of Galen active in the second half of the second century AD in Alexandria, gave particularly detailed accounts of melancholy and mania in his *On the Causes and Signs of Diseases.*[1] 'Sufferers are dull or stern: dejected or unreasonably torpid, without any manifest cause: such is the commencement of melancholy', he observed:

and they also become peevish, dispirited, sleepless, and start up from a disturbed sleep. Unreasonable fears also seize them; if the disease tends to increase, when their dreams are true, terrifying and clear; for whatever, when awake, they have an aversion to as being an evil, rushes upon their visions in sleep . . . But if the illness become more urgent, hatred, avoidance of the haunts of men, vain lamentations are seen: they complain of life and desire to die; in many the understanding so leads to insensibility and fatuousness that they become ignorant of all things and forgetful of themselves and live the life of inferior animals.

As Aretaeus's discussion of fear, loathing, and suicidal urges makes clear, in Classical medicine melancholy was far from the delicious langour it became for eighteenth-century churchyard poets. It was a dangerous condition that bred devastating delusions. 'The patient may imagine he has taken another form than his own', commented Aretaeus:

> one believes himself a sparrow; a cock or an earthen vase; another a God, orator or actor, carrying gravely a stalk of straw and imagining himself holding a sceptre of the World; some utter cries of an infant and demand to be carried in arms, or they believe themselves a grain of mustard, and tremble continuously for fear of being eaten by a hen; some refuse to urinate for fear of causing a new deluge.

Comparable stereotypes – the man fearful of urinating, and the patient convinced he was made of glass, at any second liable to shatter – remained widespread until the eighteenth century.

Paralleling melancholia, Aretaeus depicted mania, marked by uncontrollable ferocity and visible in 'furor, excitement and euphoria'. In grave forms of mania (the Latin term was *furor*), the sick person 'sometimes kills and slaughters the servants'; in less-severe cases, he would became grandiose: 'without being cultivated he says he is a philosopher'. Rationalist by temper, Aretaeus also drew attention to manifestations of religious mania involving possession by a god (divine furor), especially among those trapped in frenzied goddess cults. In 'enthusiastic and ecstatic states', devotees of Cybele (Juno) would engage in orgiastic rituals, and occasionally 'castrate themselves and then offer their penis to the goddess'. All this, Aretaeus considered, betrayed 'an insanity . . . in an ill, drunken and confused soul'. As is evident, Aretaeus linked disturbance with the changed physical states caused by intoxication, through 'ingestion of wine, mandrake or black henbane'. Mania was typically the product of excessive heat, originating from the heart (the seat of vital heat) and sympathetically connected with the brain.

In short, through a philosophy that made man the measure of all things, Classical thinkers humanized madness. They then specified divers schemes for explaining derangement. On the one hand, insanity might be mind at the end of its tether, tortured by the pitiless Fates, at war with itself. Or mental disorder might be somatic, a fever-like delirium, caused by bad blood or bile. The dichotomy between psychological and somatic theories of madness was left for the inheritors of the Greek legacy – and finally us – to resolve.

MEDIEVAL AND RENAISSANCE MADNESS

Ideas about madness in the Middle Ages and the Renaissance drew heavily on motifs inherited from antiquity. Melancholia and mania (often in English just called 'madness') provided a convenient scheme of opposites. Denys Fontanon, a professor at Montpellier, one of Europe's leading medical schools, argued in his *De Morborum Interiorum Curatione Libri Tres* (Three Books on the Cure of Internal

Diseases, 1549) that mania, 'arises from stinging and warm humours, such as yellow bile, attacking the brain and stimulating it along with its membranes. It sometimes even originates in incorrupt blood which may even be temperate but which harms the brain by its quantity alone'.

His younger Montpellier contemporary, Felix Plater, similarly depicted mania as a condition of excess. Maniacs, he wrote in *Praxeos Medicae Opus* (1650), would 'do everything unreasonably'. 'Sometimes they . . . express their mental impulse in a wild expression and in word and deed . . . Some of them intensely seek sexual satisfaction. I saw this happen to a certain noble matron, who was in every other way most honorable, but who invited by the basest words and gestures men and dogs to have intercourse with her.'

The contrasting models of mental alienation developed by the Greeks – madness as moral perversion, madness as disease – were assimilated within Christendom. But the Church added another conviction: religious madness as the expression of divine providence, regarded as a symptom of the warfare waged between God and Satan for the soul. Religious madness was generally viewed as a diabolical contagion, spread by witches, demoniacs, and heretics. In his celebrated *Anatomy of Melancholy* (1621), Robert Burton, an Oxford clergyman, identified Satan as the true author of depression, despair, and self-destruction. Spiritual maladies, Burton believed, had to be treated by spiritual means, especially prayer and fasting.

Although often viewed as a divine affliction – witness Herod's fate – religious madness was occasionally honoured as a wondrous revelation of holiness. A faith founded on the madness of the Cross, which celebrated the innocence of babes

Renaissance artists commonly depicted madness in the form of Folly, marked by the pinwheel that he carries on a stick, traditionally a child's toy and a jester's device. The mad were usually represented half naked and dressed in hides and with straw in their hair, all emphasizing their sub-human status. It was common belief that lunacy was not a hidden condition but made itself manifest to all. Woodcut from Hans Holbein the Younger's *Icones Historiarum Veteris Testamenti* (1547).

and sucklings, valued the spiritual reveries of hermits and mortification of the flesh, and prized faith over intellect. Such a creed could hardly avoid seeing gleams of godliness in the simplicity of the idiot or in the wild transports of mystics. Strands of medieval, Reformation, and Counter-Reformation theology therefore believed that Folly might be a medium for divine utterance and bade it be heard.

MADNESS IN THE AGE OF REASON

From the seventeenth century, powerful cultural forces changed attitudes towards madness. The Scientific Revolution attacked humoral medicine as part of its all-out assault on the theories of Aristotle and his followers (see Chapter 5). The fashionable view of the body as a machine promoted long-term research into its solid parts, notably the cardiovascular and the nervous systems. Anatomists laid bare the hydraulic system of pipes and the circuitry of wires coordinating the limbs, spinal cord, and cortex, and began exploring the role of the nervous system in governing sensations and motion. Within this mechanical model of the body, confused thoughts, feelings, and behaviour became attributed to some defect of the sense organs (eyes, ears, etc.) and their nervous networks. Eighteenth-century doctors popularized the term 'nerves' and coined the word 'neurosis'. For long, 'neurosis' denoted a physical lesion of the nervous system; only during the nineteenth century did 'neurosis' come to mean a mild, non-specific anxiety state, as distinct from 'psychosis'.

'I *think*, therefore I am', claimed the philosopher René Descartes in 1637; and the Enlightenment in turn endorsed the Greek faith in reason that had been poured into new bottles by the seventeenth-century Rationalists. Reformers in the age of reason set about criticizing beliefs and institutions considered unreasonable or irrational. The progress of science and technology, the development of the professions and bureaucracy, the expansion of the market economy with its laws of supply and demand, and the spread of literacy and education all contributed to the privileging of 'rationality', as understood by the right-thinking elite in the eighteenth century. Capitalist economies and centralizing states needed order, regularity, predictability, and self-discipline; abnormality provoked anxiety.

From the mid-seventeenth century, similar processes of redefinition were afoot within the Church, Catholic and Protestant alike. Traditional teachings about religious madness came under scrutiny. Popes, prelates, and preachers grew as sickened as other elites by the carnage caused by endless dogmatic faction-fighting, by witch-hunts and heresy trials. The grand apocalyptic struggles during the Reformation and Counter-Reformation between God and the Devil for the possession of souls had evidently produced only chaos; the idea of life as a spiritual Great War became repellant and was rejected. And so the reality – or at least the validity – of religious madness came into question. Especially after 1650, claims by self-styled prophets to speak with divine tongues were treated with the utmost

In praise of folly

In the secular sphere, court jesters were also sometimes allowed a licensed folly, turning normality topsy-turvy and uttering in jest truths prohibited to politic courtiers: Desiderius Erasmus's *Encomium Moriae* (The Praise of Folly, 1511) and other Renaissance feasts of paradox pointed to a crazy wisdom superior to that of worldly wisdom.

Complementing this idea – 'it's a mad world, my masters' – moralists such as Michel Eyquem de Montaigne in sixteenth-century France chose to call the whole world crazy, or at least to hint that all humans, since the Fall, lived in jeopardy of Reason's shipwreck or the poison of the passions.

As is shown in Shakespeare's plays featuring mad and mock-mad people – notably *King Lear*, *Hamlet*, and *Twelfth Night* – madness played many parts in early modern times: moral and medical, negative and positive, religious and secular.

> HAMLET: How long hast thou been a grave-maker?
> 1ST CLOWN: Of all the days i'th'year, I came to't day that our last King Hamlet overcame Fortinbras.
> HAMLET: How long is that since?
> 1ST CLOWN: Cannot you tell that? Every fool can tell that: it was that very day that young Hamlet was born – he that is mad, and sent into England.
> HAMLET: Ay, marry, why was he sent into England?
> 1ST CLOWN: Why, because 'a was mad: 'a shall recover his wits there; or, if 'a do not, 'tis no great matter there.
> HAMLET: Why?
> 1ST CLOWN: 'Twill not be seen in him there: there the men are as mad as he.
> HAMLET: How came he mad?
> 1ST CLOWN: Very strangely they say.
> HAMLET: How strangely?
> 1ST CLOWN: Faith, e'en with losing his wits.
> HAMLET: Upon what ground?
> 1ST CLOWN: Why, here in Denmark. I have been sexton here, man and boy, thirty years.
>
> William Shakespeare, *Hamlet* (1604)

Numerous scholars, notably the late Michel Foucault, have suggested that the status of madness plummeted in subsequent centuries, a development to be understood as paralleling the rising policy of confining the insane in institutions.

Madness and dancing were linked: both involved loss of bodily control.

suspicion by the authorities. Such 'Fifth Monarchists', 'Ranters', and 'Convulsionaries', it was now said, were probably nothing but blind zealots, suffering from delusion or disease, perhaps epilepsy. At the close of the 'century of revolution', John Locke found it time to reassert *The Reasonableness of Christianity* (1695). Even religion, it seemed, now had to be rational.

A similar shift applied to witches. Across Europe from the fifteenth century, authorities had treated witches as confederates with the Devil. But the witch-hunt got out of hand, creating rather than quelling anarchy. By 1650, ruling elites wanted to wash their hands of it. They argued that witchcraft was

A Representation of the Manner in which the infatuated Mob cruelly Murded Ruth Osborne on Marlston Green in the Parish of Tring in Hertfordshire.

The Mob tying Osborne and his Wife's Great Toes and Thumbs together, their Legs and Arms being first cross'd.

Colley in y Marlston Mere turning & Pulling y poor Woman about and Humbles and Red Beard holding y Ropes that they drawd her in by.

In the great witch-craze of the sixteenth and seventeenth centuries, witches were believed to be authentically possessed by Satan and to have diabolical powers; hence it was essential that they should be put on trial and, if found guilty, punished, often with death. By the eighteenth century, the intellectual tide was turning. So-called 'witches' were increasingly regarded as misled old women, and their persecutors, as in this case from Tring in Hertfordshire, came to be depicted as ignorant, supersti-tious, and 'infatuated' peas-ants. In the Enlightenment, progressive opinion dubbed many old-fashioned religious beliefs as crazy.

not a real Satanic plot but a gigantic delusion. So-called witches were not truly diabolically possessed but deluded, and their victims were merely prey to per-sonal and collective hysteria. What was once attributed to Satan was increas-ingly seen as sickness; so-called witchcraft and demonism were (according to the fashionable physicians and philosophers who joined London's newly founded Royal Society) merely psychopathological, symptoms of mental ill-ness. In eighteenth-century England, magistrates widely believed that the fer-vent excesses of Methodist converts, swooning in sermons, were fit cases for the mad-doctor. An Anglican clergyman and a healer of the sick at heart,

William Pargeter, had stronger reasons than most for denouncing Methodism as a form of mass hysteria.

> *Fanaticism* is very common cause of Madness. Most of the Maniacal cases that ever came under my observation, proceeded from religious *enthusiasm*; and I have heard it remarked by an eminent physician, that almost all the insane patients, which occurred to him at one of the largest hospitals in the *metropolis,* had been deprived of their reason, by such strange infatuation. The *doctrines* of the *Methodists* have a greater tendency than those of any other sect, to produce the most deplorable effects on the human understanding. The brain is perplexed in the mazes of mystery, and the imagination overpowered by the tremendous description of future torments.[2]

The redefinition of religious madness as essentially psychopathological widened the gulf between 'society' – those promoting polite reason – and the strange. This was a deep-seated process. In numerous ways, affluent, polite, and literate society was distancing itself from those who did not comply with its norms – criminals, vagrants, the religious 'lunatic fringe' – and was calling them irrational, crazy, or mad. Finding such outsiders disturbing it was easy to call them disturbed. Madness thus became a term of opprobrium.

But it would be glib to suggest that the notion of the irrational was simply turned into a stick with which to beat the masses. For within elite culture, fashionable eccentricity was to enjoy a long vogue. It was the done thing, throughout the eighteenth and nineteenth centuries, for certain young ladies to have fits of hysterics and for artists and poets to be morbidly oversensitive, suffering nervous breakdowns, or, like the composer Robert Schumann, going insane. Romanticism glamourized the mad genius, and nineteenth-century Bohemianism cultivated a dandified degenerateness.

CONFINEMENT OF THE INSANE

What was the fate of the mad? In medieval and pre-modern times, most of those regarded as lunatics or idiots, mentally strange, or spiritually afflicted were taken care of – all too often a euphemism for 'neglected' – in local and familiar surroundings. In England, the immediate family was expected to shoulder responsibility for crazy relatives. The insane were generally kept at home, locked in a cellar or barn if dangerous, perhaps tended by a servant. Failing the family, the parish generally assumed control, sometimes boarding out the lunatic to a local carer. The presence in Charlotte Brontë's *Jane Eyre* (1847) of the first Mrs Rochester, raving mad and hidden away in the attic, suggests that such informal procedures continued into the nineteenth century.

Nevertheless, institutions gradually emerged for the confinement of the insane. The earliest specialized lunatic asylums had been established under religious auspices in fifteenth-century Spain – in Valencia, Zaragoza, Seville, Valladolid,

Toledo, and Barcelona (Islamic models may have been influential). In London, the priory of St Mary of Bethlehem, established in 1247, was specializing in housing lunatics by the fifteenth century: it later became famous, or notorious, as Bethlem ('Bedlam'). The Netherlandish town of Geel, which had the healing shrine of St Dymphna, grew celebrated as a refuge for the mentally disturbed.

Throughout urban Europe and along the Eastern seaboard of North America, the eighteenth and nineteenth centuries brought a proliferation of schools, prisons, houses of industry and correction, workhouses, and, not least, madhouses to deal with troublesome people. The centralized state sometimes took the initiative. In 1961, the French intellectual Michel Foucault argued in *La Folie et la Déraison* that the rise of absolutism, symbolized by Louis XIV (1638–1715), inaugurated a Europe-wide 'great confinement'. Elements in society identifiable with 'unreason' found themselves at risk of being locked away. Paupers, the aged and ill, ne'er-do-wells, petty criminals, prostitutes, and vagabonds formed the bulk of this horde of 'unreason'. But their representative leaders were lunatics and imbeciles. Already by the 1660s some 6,000 undesirables – mad people included – were locked away in the Hôpital Général in Paris alone. Similar hospitals were soon set up in major French provincial cities.

Foucault argued that this 'great confinement' amounted to far more than physical sequestration. It represented a degradation of the status of madness. Hitherto, by dint of peculiarity, the mad person had possessed fascinating power: holy fools, geniuses, and jesters had uttered deep if obscure truths. Madness had spoken and society had listened. Once institutionalized, however, madness was robbed of all such allure, eerie dignity, and truth. It was reduced from a positive state ('madness') to a negative condition ('unreason'). Locked up in madhouses, lunatics resembled wild beasts caged in a zoo. It was easy to view them not as sick people but as animals.

There is a certain truth in Foucault's characterization of the age of reason 'shutting up' the mad, in every sense of the term; but it is overstated. The reign of the Louis XIV saw a surge of institutionalization in Paris. Throughout the *ancien regime*, French absolutism continued to exercise a centralizing control over the insane; later, under the later Napoleonic Code, provincial prefects assumed these duties. Families could have mad relatives legally confined on obtaining a *lettre de cachet* from royal officials; such warrants deprived the lunatic of legal rights.

But elsewhere the picture is highly varied; policies differed, and often there were no policies at all. In Russia, almost no public receptacles for the insane existed before the second half of the nineteenth century. Before then, the mad, if

From Greek times, poets, painters, and other geniuses were often regarded as being touched by some kind of 'divine' madness. Van Gogh was one of many artists who ended up in lunatic asylums in the Romantic era; another was the English painter Richard Dadd. A similar fate befell the poet John Clare. Van Gogh was emotionally intense throughout his life; coupled with financial failure, the result was growing mental disturbance that led to his being voluntarily committed in 1889 to the Asylum of St-Paul de-Mausole at St Rémy. A year later, after a bout of feverish painting, he cut off his ear; he was moved to another asylum at Auvers near Pontoise, where he shot himself, fearing that his madness was incurable.

Bethlem Hospital in the mid-sixteenth century. Bethlem developed out of a religious house founded in the thirteenth century by Bishopsgate, beyond the walls of London. From the fifteenth century, Bethlem became a refuge for lunatics. Surviving the dissolution of the monasteries in Henry VIII's reign, the asylum was rebuilt after the Fire of London a little to the west at Moorfields, before moving early in the nineteenth century to Lambeth, and during the twentieth century to Beckenham in Kent.

confined at all, were kept in monasteries. Across great swathes of rural Europe – Poland, Scandinavia, or the Balkans, for instance – few people were institutionalized before 1850. At the close of the nineteenth century, two lunatic asylums sufficed for the whole of Portugal.

In spite of being densely populated and highly urbanized, even England does not easily square with Foucault's model of a 'great confinement' launched by act of state. Confinement through legislation came late. It was not until 1808 that an Act of Parliament was passed, permitting public money to be raised for county lunatic asylums, and only in 1845 – almost two centuries after Foucault's 'great confinement' supposedly began – were such asylums made compulsory. Figures are necessarily unreliable, but it appears that no more than around 5,000 people (out of a national population of some 10 million) were being held in specialized lunatic asylums in England around 1800, with perhaps as many again in workhouses and jails. In other words, there is little evidence that the English ruling elite felt insanity or 'unreason' posed a shocking threat to public order.

Indeed, in England, the rise of the lunatic asylum is better seen not as an act of state but as a service industry within a flourishing commercial society. In 1800, lunatics were mainly secured in for-profit private asylums operating within the free market economy, forming part of what contemporaries bluntly called the 'trade in lunacy'. As late as 1850, more than half the confined lunatics in England were still housed in private institutions, some good, some bad, some indifferent.

Private madhouses had taken root by the mid-seventeenth century, although evidence is scanty (owners and families alike had a vested interest in secrecy). When George Trosse, a young merchant from Exeter, went mad around 1650 (drink was probably to blame) his friends carried him off, strapped to his horse, to a fellow in Glastonbury in Somerset, who kept a house for boarding mad people. Not long after this, London newspapers begin to carry advertisements for private madhouses.

Several superior madhouses offered *de luxe* conditions for patients paying hefty fees. At Ticehurst House in Sussex, founded in 1792, the rich could live in separate houses in the grounds, install their own cooks, and ride to hounds. But most early madhouses provided at best Spartan and at worst brutal conditions for their inmates, especially the poor. Bethlem was widely criticized. But it might be unjust and anachronistic to depict institutionalization as essentially punitive. Its main role was segregation. The asylum's rationale, first and foremost, lay in the belief that sequestration was in the interests of dangerous lunatics, giving them security and maximizing prospects of cure. From the mid-eighteenth century, a new faith was emerging in psychotherapeutics. Lunatics, the argument ran, ought to be confined, because intensive treatment would restore them. As advocates of the mechanical philosophy and of a medical model of disease, eighteenth-century doctors investigated the bodily seats of insanity.

In the Middle Ages, saints' shrines became associated with healing. That of St Dymphna at Geel in Belgium was believed to cure insanity. The sanctuaries of St Mathurin at Larchant and St Acairius at Haspres in northern France were also dedicated to the insane.

'PSYCHIATRIC' TECHNIQUES

Controlling and restoring the system through drugs and mechanical restraint loomed large in treatments of mental disorder from the eighteenth century; a rather rough-and-ready psychopharmacology remained popular on both sides of the Atlantic through the Victorian era. But the segregative environment of the asylum held out the potential of more 'psychiatric' techniques of mastering madness, ones that would directly command the mind, passions, and will. Such approaches especially appealed to critics who attacked mechanical restraint (manacles and chains) as cruel and counterproductive, provoking in the patient the

Medicine for the mad

Ever since the heyday of humoralism, the guts had their champions as the prime site of lunacy, perhaps because of the powerful associations between digestive disorders and hypochondria, gluttony and nightmares, and drink, drugs, and hallucinations. Another favoured site was the heart or the blood; popular culture, afterall, spoke of broken hearts and boiling blood. People grew fascinated by 'nervous' symptoms (swooning, weakness, paralyses, and such like) in the eighteenth century and suggested that the nervous system held the secret. Collapsing into madness, King George III insisted that he was not mentally ill but only 'nervous'.

Many specialist 'mad doctors' – asylum keepers, soon to be known as 'alienists' and later still as 'psychiatrists' – adopted the organic model of madness and pursued medical courses of treatment. They bled patients to deplete the system. They used drugs – opiates to sedate maniacs, brandy to stimulate melancholics; and they purged the constitution through vomits and laxatives. Mechanical devices such as manacles and strait-waistcoats were designed to calm the mind through restraining the body.

The technological inventiveness of the industrial revolution left its own mark on treatments of the insane. Cold-water douches were devised, to shock the system back into sanity, and rotatory chairs, whirling at up to a hundred revolutions per minute, were contrived to dislodge *idées fixes*. Mechanical restraint, medicines, and isolation in the sheltered environment of the asylum gave mad doctors new control over the insane.

In the late eighteenth century, William Perfect deployed a battery of physical techniques at his private asylum at West Malling in Kent. He had recourse to opium, solitary confinement in darkened rooms, cold baths, a 'lowering' diet, blood-letting, purgatives, and bitters. These would first pacify and then strengthen the body. Depleting the frenzied constitution was a means to calming the mind, and thus rendering it receptive to reason.

A gentleman, aged fifty-eight, was, in the beginning of January 1770, put under my care for insanity. The cause of his disorder was attributed to a sudden transition in his circumstances, which, from being easy and comfortable, were become doubtful and precarious; his complaints were great pain in the head, almost a continual noise in his ears, and, at intervals, a melancholy depression, or a frantic exhaltation of spirits ... he passed whole nights without sleep, sometimes raved and was convulsed, and his attention was invariably fixed to one object namely, that he was *ruined, lost,* and *undone!* ... Strong purges, antimonial vomits, ammoniac draughts, sagapenum, steel, and both kinds of hellebore had alternately been exhibited; issues, venæsection, a seton, and vesicatories had been tried ... ; bathing, and, in short, almost everything, seemed to have been done without the least visible alteration for the better ... When I undertook the care of this person, he appeared very impatient of contradiction ... my curative plan ... began by making a seton between his shoulders, and confining the patient to a still, quiet, and almost totally darkened room; I never suffered him to be spoken with, either by interrogation or reply, nor permitted any one to visit him but such whose immediate business it was to supply him with his aliment, which was light, cooling, and easy of digestion.[3]

George III in his final illness. The king showed signs of madness in autumn 1788, becoming irritable, sleepless, aggressive, delirious, and increasingly obscene in speech, and was treated by a specialist 'mad doctor', the Revd Dr Francis Willis. He recovered, but he had several subsequent bouts before finally becoming senile in 1811. Modern opinion believes he suffered from the metabolic disorder porphyria. Engraving by Charles Turner.

frantic violence they were meant to allay. In the name of Enlightenment, new regimes were touted from the 1750s, accentuating 'moral' (or, in modern terminology, 'psychological') methods – kindness, reason, and humanity. Alienation of mind, claimed proponents of moral treatments, was not a physical disease like smallpox, but a psychological disorder, the product of wretched education, bad habits, and personal affliction – a traumatic bereavement, bankruptcy, or religious horrors like fear of hell. It needed a distinctive psychotherapeutics.

As already hinted, these new psychological approaches had deeper foundations on which to build. From Sophocles to Shakespeare, playwrights has dramatized the passions, showing the inner torments of desire and duty, guilt and grief, that tore personalities apart. In the seventeenth century, Descartes' *cogito ergo sum* ('I think, therefore I am') highlighted the role of consciousness in forging identity. His great English successor and critic, John Locke, depicted madness as the product of faulty logical processes or uncontrolled imagination (a view later underlined by Samuel Johnson). 'The defect in *Naturals*', Locke wrote in 1690,

> seems to proceed from want of quickness, activity, and motion, in the intellectual Faculties, whereby they are deprived of Reason: whereas *mad Men*, on the other side, seem to suffer by the other Extream. For they do not appear to me to have lost the Faculty of Reasoning: but having joined together some *Ideas* very wrongly, they mistake them for Truths; and they err, as Men do, that argue right from wrong Principles. For by the violence of their Imaginations, having taken their Fancies for Realities, they make right deduction from them.[4]

And the *enfant terrible* of the Enlightenment, Jean-Jacques Rousseau, anticipated Sigmund Freud's *Civilization and its Discontents* (1930) by suggesting that the pressures of modern civilization alienated man from his soul, creating a divided self.

Thus emerged the building-blocks of a psychological way of reading derangement. Insanity could best be corrected, thought advocates of this model, by intense interpersonal dynamics between patient and doctor who would overcome derangement; and the right place for these close encounters was the lunatic asylum, an environment totally under the doctor's regulation. So-called 'moral managers' made great play of reclaiming the deranged through charisma, relying on force of character and inventive psychological tactics, outwitting the wilful perversities of the disordered. First, patients had to be subdued; then they had to be motivated through manipulation of their passions – their hopes and fears, their need for esteem.

The point was to revive the dormant humanity of the mad by working on residual normal emotions still capable of being awakened and trained. Such ideas were taken several stages further around 1790 by the emancipatory visions of Vincenzio Chiarugi in Italy, Philippe Pinel in Paris, the Tukes at the York Retreat, and, perhaps more ambiguously, by Johann Reil and other Romantic psychiatrists in

The York Retreat – concentrating on the mind

The York Retreat was opened in 1796 by a group of Quakers, led by a York tea-merchant, William Tuke, to provide a refuge for mentally disordered Friends. By 1813, when Tuke's grandson, Samuel, wrote the Retreat's manifesto, *Description of the Retreat, an Institution near York for Insane Persons of the Society of Friends Containing an Account of its Origin and Progress, the Modes of Treatment, and a Statement of Cases*, he felt obliged to confess that the medicines they had used had proved worthless. The key to the Retreat's success had lain in 'moral therapy', concentrating on the mind, as this case history from the Tukes's hospital shows:

> Some years ago a man, about thirty-four years of age, of almost Herculean size and figure, was brought to the house. He had been afflicted several times before; and so constantly, during the present attack, had he been kept chained, that his clothes were contrived to be taken off and put on by means of strings, without removing his manacles. They were however taken off, when he entered the Retreat, and he was ushered into the apartment, where the superintendents were supping. He was calm; his attention appeared to be arrested by his new situation. He was desired to join in the repast, during which he behaved with tolerable propriety. After it was concluded, the superintendant conducted him to his apartment, and told him the circumstances on which his treatment would depend; that it was his anxious wish to make every inhabitant in the house, as comfortable as possible; and that he sincerely hoped the patient's conduct would render it unnecessary for him to have recourse to coercion. The maniac was sensible of the kindness of his treatment. He promised to restrain himself, and he so completely succeeded, that, during his stay, no coercive means were ever employed towards him.[5]

The Tuke family aimed to make the Retreat a wholly domestic environment, so as to avoid the brutalizing effects of institutional settings. Finding that medicines did little good, they believed that insanity could be cured by reason, mildness, and the support offered by a true sense of community: the mad ought to be treated rather in the manner of young children. At the start, almost all patients were Quakers, like the Tukes themselves, but later the Retreat took patients of all religious persuasions.

Germany. With their 'moral therapy', which valued kindness, calm, and rationality, such reformers aimed to treat their charges as human beings capable of regeneration. Pinel's 'French revolution' in psychiatry would free the mad from their chains, literal and figurative, and restore their rights as rational citizens.

Drawing on Locke's theory of the human understanding, such reformers stressed that the madman – unlike the idiot – was not utterly bereft of reasoning power. Madness was essentially delusion, argued the Tukes at the York Retreat, springing from error in the intellectual processes (the 'software', in a more modern jargon). Mad people were trapped in fantasy worlds, outgrowths of unbridled imagination. They needed to be treated like obstreperous children, who required rigorous mental discipline and retraining in thinking and feeling. The madhouse should thus become a reform school.

Such psychotherapeutics around 1800 were launched on a wave of noble optimism. The madhouse was not just to secure but to cure. Moral therapy led to schemes for redeeming lunatics that were implemented on a massive scale during the nineteenth century: after all, if enlightened asylums restored the insane, wasn't it society's duty to place them in such institutions? Throughout Europe and North America, the state accepted enlarged responsibilities for legislating and caring for the mad, and a new psychiatric profession emerged to manage them. The lunatic asylum became the mad person's home. Despite reformers' best intentions, all too often it proved a prison.

NINETEENTH-CENTURY MUSEUMS OF MADNESS

The nineteenth century prided itself on being in the van of psychiatric progress. In the not-so-distant past, recalled Charles Dickens in 1852:

> coercion for the outward man, and rabid physicking the inward man were . . . the specifics for lunacy. Chains, straw, filthy solitude, darkness, and starvation; jalap, syrup of buckthorn, tartarised antimony and ipecacuanha administered every spring and fall in fabulous doses to every patient, whether well or ill; spinning in whirligigs, corporal punishment, gagging, 'continued intoxication'; nothing was too wildly extravagant, nothing too monstrously cruel to be prescribed by mad-doctors.[6]

Lunatics' Ball at the Somerset County Asylum. If in Renaissance pictures dancing was associated with a lack of physical control, in the Victorian era the lunatics' ball was use to convey the supposed happiness and harmony of the progressive institution, where physical shackles and punishments had ceased and the emphasis was on 'non-restraint'. The annual ball provided an opportunity for patients, staff, and wellwishers to be seen to be part of one big family. Often, however, it was little more than a publicity occasion, masking the tedium and penny-pinching economy that marked the routine of the rest of the year in the new (and increasingly huge) public asylums.

All had changed! Cruelty had been quelled, Dickens declared, kindness was the watchword. Traditional institutions like Bethlem, reminders of the bad old ways and days, were investigated and transformed. Private asylums came under strict regulation. The eighteenth-century madhouse had been a secret space, hidden from public scrutiny. Nineteenth-century reformers subjected it to the full glare of publicity. Exposés such as John Mitford's *The Crimes and Horrors in the Interior of Warburton's Private Madhouses at Hoxton and Bethnal Green* (1825) roused desires for the remedy of abuses.

Institutionalization of the mad was transformed from an *ad hoc* expedient into a system with goals and ideals. In France, for example, the reforms of Philippe Pinel and the legal stipulations of the Napoleonic Code were systematized in the epochal statute of 1838. This required each *departement* either to establish its own public asylums or to ensure provision of adequate facilities for the mad. To prevent illicit confinement, it established rules for the certification of lunatics by medical officers (although for pauper lunatics the prefect's signature remained sufficient warrant). Prefects were given powers of inspection. Similar legislation was passed in Belgium in 1850.

A comparable reform programme was enacted in England, in the teeth of opposition from vested medical interests who feared the profitability of private asylums would be threatened. Scandals revealing felonious confinement of the sane had already led to one important legislative safeguard. The Madhouses Act of 1774 had set up rudimentary licensing and certification. Under its provisions, all private madhouses had to be licensed by magistrates. Annual renewal of licenses would depend on satisfactory maintenance of admissions registers. Magistrates were empowered to carry out visitations (in London, the inspecting body was the Royal College of Physicians). Most importantly, medical certification was instituted for all but paupers. (Scotland had a different system for both the ayslums and the public administration of them.)

Further reforms in England followed after scandalous revelations led to parliamentary committees in 1807 and 1815 investigating madhouses. Evidence of gross mismanagement at Bethlem (where the recently deceased surgeon, Bryan Crowther, had himself been so deranged as to require a straitjacket) led to dismissals. The 1774 Act was strengthened by a succession of laws passed from the 1820s, which above all established the Commissioners in Lunacy, first for London (1828) and then for the whole realm (1844). The Lunacy Commissioners constituted a permanent body of inspectors (doctors, lawyers, and officials) charged to report on asylums. They had powers to prosecute and to withdraw licenses. They also possessed a remit to standardize and improve conditions of care and treatment. The Commissioners ensured eradication of the worst abuses by insisting on proper patient records and the recording of all cases of physical coercion.

Safeguards against improper confinement were further tightened. Under a consolidating Act of 1890, two medical certificates were required for all patients,

The new 'science' of asylum management

Important innovations were pioneered in the nineteenth-century asylum. In England, the new philosophy of non-restraint was introduced from the 1830s – above all, thanks to the initiatives of Robert Gardiner Hill at the Lincoln Asylum and John Conolly at the huge Middlesex asylum at Hanwell on London's western outskirts. Extending the programme of moral therapy, Gardiner Hill and Conolly abolished all forms of mechanical coercion, not just manacles but even straitjackets. Perfect security could be achieved, they claimed, through surveillance by vigilant attendants and a regime of disciplined work and exercise designed to stimulate the mind, tire the body, and foster self-control. Gardiner Hill claimed that non-restraint was a huge success. At the Lincoln Asylum in 1834, 647 incidents had occurred that required manual restraint; by 1838, there were none at all – and this had been achieved without any deaths or suicides.

In spite of Philippe Pinel's striking off the chains from the insane at the Bicêtre in Paris, total non-restraint was seen by continental reformers as a peculiarly English fixed idea, an instance of doctrinaire liberal individualism run riot, and it was little imitated. But reformers in France, Germany, and Italy made inventive use of the asylum environment.

Work therapy, in horticulture and agriculture, was widely favoured. Sited in the countryside, the nineteenth-century asylum typically became a self-sufficient colony, running its own farms, laundries and workshops, partly for economy's sake, partly to achieve cure through labour. In France, spa treatments were favoured. Everywhere, care and cure of the mad became associated with the new 'science' of asylum management; asylum keepers united to create the nucleus of the psychiatric profession, and specialist journals were established. The new profession became preoccupied with the pragmatic issues of managing the well-run asylum.

Questions of architecture were of cardinal importance. Asylum design had to ensure maximum security, ample ventilation, efficient drainage, optimal visibility (Jeremy Bentham's goal of panopticism – that is, total surveillance), and, not least, differential classification and housing of distinct grades of lunatics. Males had to be separated from females, incurables from curables, the violent from the docile, the clean from the dirty, and pathways of progress established to enable improving lunatics to move, stage by stage, nearer the exit (and chronic cases to occupy the back wards). Such aims had to be achieved without prejudice to order, economy, efficiency, and discipline.

Like his contemporaries the Tukes in England, the French physician Philippe Pinel repudiated severe mechanical restraints and outdated medical treatments, and stressed the efficacy of 'moral' means in caring for the insane. He gained a reputation in the nineteenth century as the founder of modern psychiatry. But dramatic gestures, such as the one here showing Pinel at the Bicêtre, were the stuff more of myth than reality. Painting by Charles Muller, c. 1840–50.

including paupers. In the long run, this legalistic concern to prevent asylums being abused as carceral institutions may have proved counterproductive. For, by insisting that only formally certified lunatics be quartered in asylums, it delayed the transformation of the asylum into a more flexible 'open' institution, easy of access and exit. Instead the mental hospital was confirmed as the institution of last resort; certification thus became associated with prolonged detention. The result was a failure to provide institutional care appropriate for temporary insanity, partial insanity, or mild mental disturbance.

In Europe and the USA alike, the nineteenth century witnessed a phenomenal rise in the number of mental hospitals and the patient population. In England, patient numbers rose from a few thousands in 1800 to some 100,000 in 1900 (the national population increased at less than half that rate). In the USA, similarly, there were fewer than 5,000 asylum patients in 1850 but more than 150,000 in 1904. By 1950, some 150,000 mental patients were institutionalized in Britain, half a million in the USA. Patient numbers also rocketed in the new nation states. In Italy, for example, some 18,000 were behind walls in 1881; within 35 years the number had more than doubled. Such increases are not hard to explain. Bureaucratic and utilitarian mentalities vested great faith in institutional solutions, in bricks and mortar. Reformatories, prisons, hospitals, asylums – all these, it was claimed, would solve the intensifying social problems induced by rise in population, urbanization, and industrialization.

Asylums, however, never lacked critics. From early days, Bedlam became a by-word for man's inhumanity to man. Patient protests grew, complaining of brutality and neglect, as in the dramatic *Address to Humanity, Containing a Letter to Dr. Thomas Munro: A Receipt to Make a Lunatic, and Seize his Estate; and A Sketch of a True Smiling Hyena*, issued in 1796 by a former patient, William Belcher. And a radical fringe within the medical profession always doubted the efficacy of herding the insane together. But champions long outnumbered critics, and the asylum movement was buoyed up on waves of optimism.

This was to change; in the last third of the nineteenth century, a new pessimism spread. Statistics demonstrated that expectations that asylums would prove engines of cure had been unfounded. Cure rates seemed to be dipping, and public asylums were silting up with long-stay patients. Psychiatrists had become victims of their own opinions. They had warned that society was riddled with masses of hitherto unknown psychiatric disorders – whom they, and they alone, could treat. Developing such categories as 'monomania', 'kleptomania', 'dipsomania', and 'moral

William Norris, an American marine kept at Bethlem Hospital for at least 10 years in a brutal restraining contraption. Reformers discovered him in 1814 and publicized his case as evidence of the cruelty of unreformed Bethlem. The public outcry helped lead to the House of Commons Inquiry of 1814 into the conditions in madhouses. The Bethlem staff claimed that severe restraint was necessary for Norris because he was the most violent maniac they had ever encountered. Etching by G. Arnald after his drawing, 1814.

insanity', they had maintained that much aberrant conduct traditionally labelled vice, sin, and crime were, in truth, mental disorders, that should be treated psychiatrically in the asylum. Magistrates were encouraged to divert difficult recurrent offenders from the workhouse or jail. But asylum superintendents were to discover to their cost that regeneration posed more problems than anticipated. Furthermore, the senile and the demented, along with epileptics, paralytics, sufferers from tertiary syphilis, ataxias, and neurological disorders were all increasingly warehoused in the asylum. For such conditions, the prognosis was gloomy. The asylum became a last resort for hopeless cases.

The mounting number of chronic patients gave cause for alarm. Perhaps madness was more menacing than imagined. No sooner were asylums built than they overflowed with those judged to be disturbed: alcoholics, habitual masturbators, sex maniacs, neuropaths, those suffering from general paresis of the insane, and other neurological deficits. Furthermore, bitter experience proved that the insane did not recover as predicted; the asylum was changing character, from being the retreat for regeneration to a dustbin for derelicts. Critics alleged that the asylum might be not the solution but the problem, creating the illnesses of institutionalization. Was faith in the asylum itself a form of delusion?

Defenders retorted that the true problem lay not in the asylum but in the patients. If psychiatry's best efforts didn't work cures, did this not show that many forms of mental disorder were authentically incurable? Such views encouraged the development, towards 1900, of new biomedical theories that pictured insanity as a hereditary taint, a blot on the brain. To generations of psychiatrists whose daily occupation lay in watching the living death of asylum zombies, or who pursued research into the neuropathologies of various mental disorders, sober realism pointed to 'degenerationist' theories: disorders were ingrained, they got worse over the generations. Such conclusions matched the mood of a sociopolitical elite anxious about the menace of the mass society and mass democracy (see page 326).

Dorothea Lynde Dix. Born in 1807 in Maine (USA) and working and a schoolteacher, Dorothea Dix took up the cause of improving the conditions for patients in almshouses, prisons, and lunatic asylums. Her passionate commitment and vast energies led to reforms being passed through Congress and state legislatures. Later in life, she extended her reformist campaigns to Britain and Europe.

DEGENERATION AND SCHIZOPHRENIA

Heroic efforts were made to analyse and classify mental disorders. Such nosological endeavours were stimulated by the emergence of the asylum, the rise of psychiatric specialists, and the progress of neurology. The profession needed to justify itself to society by cracking the secrets of psychosocial disorders; hence it undertook the task of psychopathologizing deviancy. Psychiatry successively staked greater territorial claims to 'discovering' mental disease where it had not been suspected before. Inordinate drinking became medicalized as alcoholism, sexual abuses such as sodomy were psychiatrized into 'homosexual neurosis', and many other erotic 'perversions' were captured by psychopathology in and after the pathbreaking *Psychopathia Sexualis* (1886) by the German psychiatrist Richard von Krafft-Ebing: bestiality, coprolagnia, exhibitionism, fetishism, flagellation,

The talking cure — Freud and psychoanalysis

In the twentieth century, new hope for the mentally ill has sprung from many quarters. Sigmund Freud was one. Psychoanalysis offered a startling new way with the disturbed: the conviction that, if the patient simply 'told all', using the method of free association, the unconscious repressions that Freud considered the basis of neuroses would find release.

Freudian psychoanalysis — its elements were in place by the time he published his seminal work *Die Traumdeutung* (The Interpretation of Dreams) in 1900 — claimed that the disturbances of neurotics typically stemmed from unresolved sexual conflicts experienced in early childhood and subsequently repressed and endlessly elaborated. Freud was not the first to highlight the importance of sex. It had long been maintained that erotic denial provoked mental unbalance; spinsters succumbed to hysteria, and medical folklore traditionally recommended marriage as its remedy. Freud's teacher, Jean-Martin Charcot (see page 129), a great student of hysterical neurosis, had observed, *à propos* of hysterics, '*c'est toujours la chose génitale*'. But it was Freud who set sexual desires and denial stage-centre in the understanding of psychiatric problems.

Freud was a realist. He insisted that only mildly disturbed people could be treated by his methods (neurotics, not psychotics or schizophrenics), for psychoanalysis made heavy demands on patients' cooperation. Aware of the inescapable pressures of civilization, and developing, during the First World War, the idea of the 'death wish', Freud certainly expected no miracle cures. And he was right: none came.

By trial and error, Freud developed the practice of getting patients to recline on a couch and 'free associate'; that is, say whatever came into their heads. The notion was that total and free disclosure would bring to the surface the repressed memories that were the causes of traumatic neuroses. Freud was to discover that various complications hindered this therapeutic approach, not least 'transference' —

the tendences of clients to project their feelings on to the analysis (Freud never seems to have acknowledged 'counter-transference', that process in reverse).

Sceptical contemporaries of Freud, including the Viennese satirist Karl Kraus, argued that psychoanalysis revealed less about the unconscious minds of patients than of the fantasy world of Freud himself. Such a view is contained in the modern criticism that psychoanalysis failed to transform itself into a properly scientific body of knowledge and methods.

Although the psychoanalytical movement developed, branched, and flourished, the close of the twentieth century finds orthodox psychoanalysis in disarray, riven with scandals and losing ground. Not least, psychoanalysis proper always remained somewhat of a pastime for the rich and leisured. Nevertheless, Freud's insights into unconscious processes, infant development, and family dynamics have proved immensely fruitful in generating psychotherapeutic initiatives and communities, particularly in child and family therapy.

Although trained as a doctor and fancying himself as a scientist, the mature Freud argued, against orthodox medical psychiatrists, for a psychogenic theory of neurosis: disturbance arose in the psyche, out of personal experience. Freud's concept of the struggles between unconscious and conscious principles that led to neurosis entailed a reworking of the old Platonic doctrine of the tripartite soul divided against itself, but one that took a particularly frightening form. Whereas Plato had optimistically concluded that harmony would reign when reason ruled the passions, Freud saw the relations between *id, ego*, and *superego* as generating ceaseless psychic civil war.

Freud suspected that reason itself was a charade, a mask, a defence, or a mystifying power of resistance. Reason might be the apex of civilization, but it was also rationalization,

sadomasochism, transvestism, and so forth. Abnormal children, women, 'inverts' (homosexuals) and other 'perverts' were deemed mentally ill and often confined.

Degenerationist psychiatry also saw mental disease in the decadent effusions of literary geniuses and artists such as Impressionists and Cubists, whose sensory systems, some psychiatrists suggested, must be pathologically disordered. And fears grew, above all, about the dangerous degeneracy of the rabble, who were, many psychiatrists warned, endangering civilization with mental imbecility prethe agent of false consciousness, a form of self-deception providing protection from inadmissible desires and unendurable memories. Why else did mankind still live by such illusions as religion?

Worse still, personal drives were forever at loggerheads with social demands. To explain the discontents of civilization, Freud suggested late in life, in works such as *Totem und Tabu* (1913), that it was founded upon parricide and animated by a death instinct. By the close of his career, his doubts even about the therapeutic potential of his own techniques were stated more publicly. A final word on that subject came in a paper titled 'Die Endliche und die Unendliche Analyse' ('Analysis terminable and interminable') published in 1937. As well as possessing great insight into

The early psychoanalytical movement operated like a family group, with strong personal bonds tying its members together. Freud (front left in this photograph taken at Clark University, Worcester, USA, in 1909) assumed the role of 'father'; his close associates included Ernest Jones (back centre), Sándor Ferenczi (back right), and Carl Jung (front right). Abraham Brill (back left), William James, and Stanley Hall (front centre) were sympathetic Americans.

individual patients, Freud supremely captured the quandary of twentieth-century culture. God was dead, as the philosopher Friedrich Nietzsche had pronounced, but reason was also dethroned.

cisely at a time when Social Darwinism was dictating that only fit societies would survive. Enlightenment optimism had peaked in the French Revolutionary aspiration that the mad could be freed from shackles and restored to reason. A century later, however, psychiatry had grown more pessimistic. A token of this lies in the formulation by the German psychiatrist Emil Kraepelin of *dementia praecox* (literally, precocious dementia), shortly to be termed schizophrenia by the Swiss doctor, Eugen Bleuler. As depicted by Kraepelin in *Einfürung die Psychiatrische Klinik*

(Lectures in Clinical Psychiatry) in 1901, the archetypal schizophrenic was not stupid; on the contrary, he might be alarmingly intelligent and astute. Yet he seemed to have renounced his humanity, abandoned all desire to participate in human society, withdrawing into an autistic world of his own. Describing schizophrenics, Kraepelin used such phrases as 'atrophy of the emotions' and 'vitiation of the will' to convey his conviction that such patients were moral perverts, sociopaths almost a species apart.

The more lurid fantasies of degenerationist psychiatry – its egregious racism, hereditarianism, and sexual prurience – were denounced by Sigmund Freud and other champions of the new dynamic psychiatries arising around the beginning of the twentieth century. And the therapeutic innovation at the heart of psychoanalysis proposed yet another optimistic new deal: the talking cure.

MODERN PSYCHOLOGICAL MEDICINE

The twentieth century has brought efforts to fathom psychiatric diseases, establish their taxonomy and investigate their causes. Specially significant has been the grand differentiation between psychoses (severe disturbances, involving loss of contact with reality) and neuroses (relatively mild conditions). That has been popularly seen as the grounding for distinctions between conditions with real organic aetiologies and ones that are psychological. Among the psychoses, a further cardinal contrast has been established between manic-depressive (or bipolar) conditions and schizophrenia.

Nevertheless, delineation and classification of mental illnesses remains fiercely contested. A glance at sucessive editions of the *Diagnostic and Statistical Manual* (*DSM*), the profession's diagnostic handbook produced by the American Psychiatric Association, shows just how fluid the characterization of mental illness continues to be. Requiring energetic revision every few years, and itself the subject of controversy, *DSM* reveals a proliferation of different, and often incompatible or overlapping terminologies, some disappearing and reappearing from edition to edition. A notorious postal-vote poll, held by the American Psychiatric Association in 1975, led to homosexuality being belatedly removed from its list of mental afflictions. It is not only cynics who claim that politico-cultural, racial, and gender prejudices continue to shape diagnoses of what are purportedly objective disease conditions.

Partly because of hostility to violent treatments such as insulin therapy and ECT, the new psychotropic drugs becoming available after 1950 were enthusiastically greeted. Psychopharmacology had long been burdened with worthless weapons such as bromides and croton oil (a powerful purge that put the patient out of action). From the 1950s, neuroleptics such as chlorpromazine (Largactil), used on schizophrenics, and lithium, for manic-depressive conditions, had remarkable success in stabilizing behaviour. They made it possible for patients to leave the sheltered but numbing environment of the psychiatric hospital.

Quick-fix procedures

The failure of the nineteenth-century asylum to fulfil its promise led to a renewal of more direct medical interventions, not least a succession of high-tech, quick-fix, procedures, each enjoying its brief hour of glory.

First, fever therapy: induction of a dose of malaria was touted for treating general paralysis of the insane (GPI), the outcome of tertiary syphilis — a procedure that won a Viennese psychiatrist, Julius Wagner-Jauregg, the Nobel Prize in 1927. Then insulin therapy was developed. Manfred Sakel, also Austrian, claimed that the coma induced by hefty insulin injections could supply schizophrenics with a break in consciousness that would provide release from mental oppression. Coma therapy was widely used between the mid-1930s and the early 1950s.

Another panacea emerged at the same time: electroconvulsive therapy (ECT), or, as it is known in the USA, electroshock therapy. First used by an Italian, Ugo Cerletti, in 1938 it is still occasionally used today. Here Cerletti describes the strain of the first experiments with it:

> Two large electrodes were applied to the frontoparietal regions, and I decided to start cautiously with a low-intensity current of 80 volts for 0.2 seconds. As soon as the current was introduced, the patient reacted with a jolt and his body muscles stiffened; then he fell back on the bed without loss of consciousness. He started to sing abruptly at the top of his voice, then he quieted down.
>
> Naturally, we, who were conducting the experiment were under great emotional strain and felt that we had already taken quite a risk. Nevertheless, it was quite evident to all of us that we should allow the patient to have some rest and repeat the experiment the next day. All at once, the patient, who evidently had been following our conversation, said clearly, and solemnly, without his usual gibberish: 'Not another one! It's deadly!'.
>
> I confess that such explicit admonition under such circumstances, and so emphatic and commanding, coming from a person whose enigmatic jargon had until then been very difficult to understand, shook my determination to carry on with the experiment. But it was just this fear of yielding to a superstitious notion that caused me to make up my mind. The electrodes were applied again, and a 110-volt discharge was applied for 0.2 seconds.[7]

Also in the 1930s, lobotomy was developed by the Portuguese physician, António Egas Moniz, and popularized by the American neurologist, Walter Freeman. This involved surgical cutting of the frontal lobes of the brain, just behind the eye, and was designed to curb violent behaviour and to relieve clinical depression.

Each of these procedures produced dramatic improvements in some patients whose long-term career as asylum patients otherwise seemed hopeless. But the trigger-happy attitudes of the champions of such 'great and desperate cures', their violent and traumatic nature, and growing evidence of relapses and side-effects, undermined confidence in all of them. Nothing in the literature of madness is so harrowing as the anger expressed by patients subjected to compulsory doses of any of these obnoxious and painful shock procedures.

A paralytic mental patient having his blood sampled at the Vienna Psychiatric Clinic, under the direction of Julius Wagner-Jauregg.

The response of patients themselves to heavy medication ('the liquid cosh') has been more ambiguous, since they can induce lethargy and mental vacancy (the 'zombie' effect). An ex-patient, Jimmie Laing, described the 'Largactil kick': 'You would see a group of men sitting in a room and all of them would be kicking their feet up involuntarily'.[8] The drugs revolution has remained incomplete. A generation ago, the British pyschiatrist William Sargant and other leading members of the profession prophesied that wonder drugs like Largactil would render mental illness a thing of the past by 1990. Such hopes have not been fulfilled.

BACK TO SQUARE ONE?

As we have seen, the asylum movement created its own crises. Patients did not recover as promised. As early as mid-Victorian times, when the asylum-building programme was still in its infancy, even psychiatrists were prepared to admit that a gigantic asylum was a gigantic evil. A full century before the modern antipsychiatry movement, the Victorians had seen the untoward effects of institutionalization. Many psychiatric disorders were recognized to be the products of that very institution claimed to be their cure.

Some of the most bitter critics of the asylum were its patients. There were two standard complaints: one was illegal or improper confinement – the forcible locking up of the sane, usually at family instigation, for underhand purposes, such as to overturn a will or shed an ugly wife; the other, was gross brutality.

Thus mental institutions long suffered a crisis of legitimacy, but little was done. The drugs revolution, the movement for patients' rights, the terminal problems of crumbling asylums – aided by a dose of Treasury parsimony – combined, in

In non-Western nations, mental disorder is treated by a mixture of indigenous and Western methods. Here, a young man in a Chinese asylum in the 1970s is receiving acupuncture on his neck. The Chinese believe that acupuncture works for both what we call somatic and psychological disorders, because they do not recognize the mind/body distinction.

Britain as elsewhere, to launch the 'decarceration' policies popular since the 1960s. Between 1980 and 1989, thirty mental hospitals were closed in Britain and approval was given to the closure of a further thirty-eight by 1995. The ironies of this latest great breakthrough have become all too familiar.

For one thing, the drugs revolution was only half successful. Worse, 'community care' was introduced with little hard cash for care, and little hard thinking about community, and at a time when the British Prime Minister, Margaret Thatcher, went on record as saying 'there is no such thing as society' (a view widely taken as a symptom of a state of delusion on her part). A state of confusion remains. And that is partly because the nature of the beast remains obscure. 'Psychiatry is conventionally defined', wrote Thomas Szasz in the 1970s, 'as a medical speciality concerned with the diagnosis and treatment of mental diseases. I submit that this definition, which is still widely accepted, places psychiatry in the company of alchemy and astrology and commits it to the category of pseudoscience. The reason for this is that there is no such thing as "mental Illness".'[9]

Some find this doctrine liberating, others find it heartless; most think it exaggerated. Nevertheless, it remains true that, even amongst Szasz's critics, there is little agreement as to what mental illness truly is.

From the 1970s, increasing numbers of mental patients were removed from the old hospitals in many European countries and in the USA as part of the policy of 'community care'. Because of failures in medical and welfare provision, they often became homeless street people: violent crimes committed by a few led to growing public concern. What had first seemed a progressive policy came to be regarded as a new form of heartlessness towards a vulnerable population.

CHAPTER 9

John Pickstone

Medicine, Society, and the State

Medicine is not just about knowledge and practice, healing and caring – it is about power: the powers of doctors and of patients, of institutions such as churches, charities, insurance companies, or pharmaceutical manufacturers, and especially governments, in peacetime or in war. This chapter explores the history of these powers in the medicine of Britain, France, Germany, and the USA during the past two centuries (regrettably for space reasons, it excludes most of Asia, Africa, and South America).

This narrative would have been easier to write in 1960, when we were more confident about the progress of medical science, the extension of medical services, and the expanding roles of government. Did anyone then foresee that the containment of costs would become the major focus of health policy, that bioethics would loom so large in public discussion, that market competition would be reintroduced into such advanced welfare bureaucracies as the British National Health Service, or that doctors would be increasingly subjected to lay managements, whether of hospitals or of insurance schemes? The progress-models common up to about 1960 now require more than a little tweaking.

We cannot, however, simply reverse the values, after the manner of some 1960s radicals, so as to present governments as increasingly oppressive and organized

Britain's leading Victorian hospitals were funded largely by subscriptions and donations. This ward of Guy's Hospital in London (*c.* 1900) demonstrates their aspiration to a kind of domesticity.

Some eye hospitals in the former Soviet Union used 'assembly lines'; patients circulated between surgeons, who each did part of the operation. This photograph was taken in 1987.

medicine as progressively enfeebling. That negative version seems no more plausible than its opposite number, even in the affluent West. Whether they run upwards or downwards, linear development models hardly seem adequate. Instead, we must look to the varied workings of medicine in a range of different societies over time.

At one extreme are the societies in which medicine was almost entirely a matter of free markets. For example, in the USA in the 1840s, would-be medical practitioners did not have to be licensed; if they wished to train, they could do so in a variety of competing medical schools, attached to different brands of medicine – herbal medicine and homeopathy as well as the 'heroic' forms of regular medicine. Competition depressed standards. Almost all patients then paid their individual practitioners on a fee-for-service basis. Destitute patients could be treated under a statutory welfare system (or by charity), and some doctors earned part of their salaries in this way; but most were self-employed.

At the other extreme are the societies (or segments of societies) in which most doctors were educated, regulated, and employed by government. Health services of this kind have been developed for the armed forces of many Western countries. Swedish medical services since the eighteenth century have included a substantial component of direct state employment; the former Soviet Union provided health care in this way. From 1948, UK citizens have enjoyed a National Health Service largely funded from taxation.

Between these extremes lie the intermediate institutions that have helped shape medicine in most Western countries: the associations that regulated medical practice, the agencies of 'public health', the poorhouses and hospitals for the destitute, and the friendly societies and other insurance schemes by which workers were protected against unemployment and sickness.

MEDICAL INSTITUTIONS AND POLITICS — AN OVERVIEW

In most of eighteenth-century Europe, medical education and practice were supposed to be regulated by colleges, corporations, or guilds of various kinds. Generally, their powers came to be underwritten by government, or replaced with more direct state control. In some cases, notably in German states, that transition was direct; in others, notably France and the USA, corporate forms weakened or were abolished in favour of free markets, on to which state regulation was later imposed. By about 1900, most Western states were supervising and subsidizing the education of doctors, underwriting the policing of medical conduct, and protecting the regular profession against false claims to qualifications. They did not usually prohibit unlicensed practice, but they required qualifications from the candidates for the increasing number of official medical positions, whether in direct state employment or in agencies supervised by the state.

These national histories of medical regulation corresponded to different patterns of state formation. Where states were relatively strong from the eighteenth century, as in German realms, medicine passed easily from corporate to state regulation, and was later liberalized. Where state powers were initially more restricted, as in Britain and especially the USA in the early nineteenth century, modern forms of medical regulation were developed as governments assumed responsibility for welfare services and public health. In Britain, this happened after about 1830, and the process was greatly complicated by the persistence of older corporations. In the USA, the arguments took place from about 1870, largely unencumbered by earlier institutional forms. Overall, in nineteenth-century nations, one finds a convergence from close state control on the one hand and from free markets on the other, towards the protected, restricted medical markets characteristic of twentieth-century medicine.

Shifting the focus to the politics of public health, we find rather similar cross-national comparisons. German and other strong states tried to improve the health of their populations from the eighteenth century. In France, a concern with the health of the people was central to the Revolution of 1789 and remained an obligation of nineteenth-century governments, advised by elite doctors. In eighteenth-century Britain, public health, like so much else, was a matter of local paternalism and voluntary associations. State responsibility developed in the mid-nineteenth century, as part of the effort to manage the conditions and consequences of an urban industrial economy. That programme was part of the new discipline of political economy and involved a new physiology of the social body. Both of these sciences later proved influential in continental cities and in the USA, as they, too, experienced rapid urbanization (and immigrant poverty). Towards the end of the nineteenth century, the campaigns of the elite doctors, whether for public health or professional powers, were boosted by the researches of Louis Pasteur, Robert Koch, and others; the researchers benefited in turn from the military and imperial expansions that preceded the First World War.

The politics of medical services for the destitute have a rather different history. In Catholic countries around 1750, the bulk of such services was provided by the Church; in Britain, the USA, and most German states, they were the responsibility of local government. Medicine was relatively marginal to the management of the poor, whether this was religious or secular. Doctors were more powerful in the charity hospitals of Britain that served the 'deserving poor' rather than the really destitute, but, even here, control in the eighteenth century rested with lay governors and subscribers. Since then, welfare services for the destitute have mostly come to be provided directly by governments, or at least underwritten by them. The poorhouses of France were 'nationalized' at the Revolution, but many continued to be managed by nursing sisters. In most countries, poorhouses were expanded during the nineteenth century, in line with urbanization. The power of doctors usually increased with state involvement, especially where poorhouses were used for medical teaching. Where they were not so used, medicalization was much slower: British poorhouses were marginal to medicine until the twentieth century.

In Britain and in the USA, charity hospitals rather than poorhouses became the prime site of medicalization and medical education. They were effectively run by doctors from the early nineteenth century, but their political fates diverged in the two countries. In the USA, by 1900, the 'charity' hospitals had begun to compete for patients who could pay their way; they had become part of the medical mar-

Pesthouse in Hamburg, 1746. Throughout the eighteenth century plague remained a major threat in continental Europe, especially to the urban poor. Engraving by Philipp Andreas Kilian after F. S. Heintze.

ket. In Britain, this development was later and more restrained. Between the two world wars, British charity hospitals were subsidized by government, and in 1948 they were 'nationalized' as the key institutions of the National Health Service.

In discussing the increasing powers of organized medicine, the increasing powers of governments, and the ever more complex intertwinings of the two, one must beware simple trajectories or teleologies. The degree of state involvement has varied hugely between countries, and the processes of state involvement can be reversed. The government of Britain is presently trying to reduce its responsibility for medical services, as part of a 'rolling back of the state'. In the USA, the prestige of doctors appears to be declining after a century of steady advance. Western medicine seems to be entering a new political, economic, demographic, and epidemiological era; in Eastern Europe, Asia and the less-developed countries, the future is even more uncertain. As organized medicine changes so, too, will our understanding of its history.

Friendly and other mutual societies

The contrasting political cultures of the UK, continental Europe, and the USA are reflected in their 'friendly societies' – mutual insurance schemes set up in the nineteenth century that protected workers against financial losses from sickness and unemployment, and often came to include arrangements for medical care.

In early-nineteenth-century Germany, employee insurance was encouraged by paternalistic states that controlled most kinds of labour. With the growth of industry and larger employers, German states backed schemes between employer and employee as a kind of neo-feudalism. From the 1880s these schemes were subsidized and supervised in a national programme of health insurance.

British friendly societies, by contrast, were working-class associations, which came to be supervised by government to ensure their financial stability. They were 'nationalized' in 1911, as part of a major extension of state welfare, with the result that British general practitioners gained substantial state incomes, depending on the number of patients they had registered. British insurance schemes had never included specialist or hospital practice, so general medical practice was consolidated much more strongly than in continental Europe or North America.

In France, workers' organizations were restricted by law until 1888; thereafter, mutual societies developed on a voluntary basis, but divisions in the trade-union movement and the resistance of trades people and white-collar workers prevented 'nationalization' until 1930.

In the USA, around the First World War, organized labour and progressive politicians launched a campaign for statutory health insurance that was initially supported by the medical establishment. But support declined with rising medical incomes and the profession threw its growing weight against state schemes, eventually promoting voluntary schemes, to its considerable benefit. American medicine thus remained market-based to an extent unknown in Europe after 1930.

Illustration from the Rules and Orders of a friendly society in the English Midlands, late eighteenth century.

MEDICAL MARKETS IN ENLIGHTENMENT EUROPE

The formal organization of early modern medicine was corporate: colleges of physicians, guilds of surgeons, societies of apothecaries, or combined societies were based in regional or national capitals (see Chapters 4 and 6). One might describe the informal organization of most medicine as 'markets in hierarchical societies'. Physicians were learned men who could elicit the trust of aristocrats and supervise lower grades of doctors. 'Surgeons' were craftsmen, ranging from prestigious attendants on the powerful to local menders of the impoverished sick and wounded. Apothecaries or pharmacists sold remedies and corresponding advice. But hosts of other practitioners – men or women, settled or itinerant, full-time or part-time, trained or untrained – also sold advice, skills, or remedies. And most illnesses, then as now, were treated in the home, usually by women, with no recourse beyond family or neighbours.

All Western countries showed similar patterns of medical work, but they differed in the relative importance of corporate organization and in the links between medicine and the church, which remained strong in southern Europe. The north, and especially Britain, was becoming more secular and

A soup kitchen operated by Quakers in Manchester during the Cotton Famine of 1862.

prosperous; more people could afford 'luxury' purchases, including medicine; communications were improving, and newspapers, which became common in the eighteenth century, carried masses of advertisements for patent medicines, often sold by itinerant vendors.

Cultural leaders were coming to be impressed by natural philosophy and by claims to the ordering of society on scientific principles. Physicians argued that medicine might become as sure as Newtonian physics. They cultivated chemistry and natural history, and tried to classify diseases, often relating them to local conditions (Chapter 5). Surgeons took up anatomy, so establishing their claim to learning. Some apothecaries became chemical manufacturers of, for example, mineral waters; most worried about being undercut by a new breed of retailer, the chemist and druggist. In most Western countries, the growth of markets and the spread of education severely dented the various professional corporations.

In Britain and its North American colonies, medicine changed chiefly by private initiatives – sometimes commercial, sometimes through the 'voluntary' and secular associations that were conspicuous in the increasingly 'polite' society of English county towns (the world of Jane Austen's novels, and of George Eliot's *Middlemarch*). Voluntary associations built most of the hospitals that spread across England from 1720, providing respectable subscribers with a collective means to patronize the deserving poor; doctors, especially surgeons, used them to

'Housewife as family doctor', from a German guide to domestic medicine by Anna Fischer-Dückelmann, 1903.

advertise major operations and to provide clinical experience for their apprentices. In London, such hospitals came to supplement the private anatomy schools newly set up by surgeons, some of whom were also men-midwives or *accoucheurs* (see page 222).

University education, too, could include private enterprise. Oxford and Cambridge universities were stagnant but Edinburgh medical school boosted that city's finances by attracting students from England and North America. In Scottish universities and in the private schools of London, teaching was good business. Indeed, in a sense, education was the most dynamic aspect of the medical economy – knowledge changed much faster than therapies.

In Britain, even public health was often a 'voluntary' matter. Concern with hygiene tended to originate with army and navy doctors, worried by the loss of soldiers and sailors from disease rather than combat, as with scurvy (see page 256). Such concerns were taken up by private 'reformers', who publicized the insanitary conditions in prisons, and indeed in some of the new hospitals. Such reformers were often magistrates, driven by a desire for social discipline, fuelled by notions of scientific improvement. The best known was John Howard, who achieved a national reputation by 'exposing' conditions in prisons. Many physicians also became involved, especially in the newly industrial towns of northern England, where immigrant workers from the countryside suffered the fevers characteristic of army camps, ships, and prisons. In Manchester in 1796, local physicians joined with socially enterprising merchants to set up a fever hospital, and in the hope of supervising lodging-houses and cellar dwellings.

Few of these developments owed much to the Royal College of Physicians, the Company of Surgeons in London, or to the traditional machinery of central and local government. The physicians interested in hospitals, fever, and public welfare were mostly provincial, Scottish-educated and religious dissenters. A campaign to open up the College of Physicians met little success: instead, reformers created new associations for discussion of medical science and philanthropy. One such scheme initiated the 'dispensary movement', through which many cities and smaller towns established charities to provide outpatient care and home-visiting for the sick poor. The new dispensaries came to serve as observatories from which honorary physicians 'discovered' the habitats of the poor. Although some physicians and many surgeons received public monies for the care of paupers in villages or parts of towns, there was little question here of statutory medical policy. British medicine was largely a matter of the free market plus the voluntary associations.

In German states, by contrast, universities and governments were much more prominent in medical matters. Local rulers sought prestige by attracting famous university teachers, who also advised on questions of public health and indeed served as personal physicians. Although some German developments in public medicine and public health were pioneered by religious groupings (as by the Lutherans in the Prussian city of Halle), most were related to 'improvements' in the management of principalities. According to contemporary theories of government, wealth would flow from fertile fields and a healthy population: so infant welfare, breastfeeding, and cleanliness were to be encouraged alongside scientific agriculture. Such German states invented *Medizinpolizei* (medical police, where the meaning of 'police' lies somewhere between 'policy' and 'police force'). Medicine, like many other occupations, was subject to considerable state control, and doctors were employed part-time to supervise public health and attend the local poor. Problems of poverty could also be subjected to scientific management – some paupers were institutionalized and set to work on scientifically minimal diets. Count Rumford (Sir Benjamin Thompson), an American adventurer who devised a scheme for the employment of paupers in Munich, was also the inventor of the soup kitchen; as a physicist he maintained that water became nutritious when boiled with bones.

John Howard (1726–90), the British magistrate turned social reformer, sought to impose order and cleanliness on hospitals, poorhouses, and, especially, prisons.

Written examination for yͤ degree of M.D. Edinͬ University. April, 1855. N.B. yͤ unfortunate undergraduates are in yͤ agonies of composition. × Ane Professor.

Edinburgh medical students writing examinations (in 1855, written exams were still novel); Sir James Young Simpson invigilated.

THE REVOLUTION IN FRENCH MEDICINE

Whilst medical change in Britain tended to occur outside the corporations and the state, and German reforms were often a matter of state policy, France showed both patterns – in rapid succession. Before the Revolution, France had an elaborate hierarchy of medical occupations, from elite physicians in Paris to district surgeons licensed to practise only in the countryside. But most of the physicians who took an interest in public welfare, economic improvement, and the natural history of disease, did so outside the old faculties of medicine, through new societies, sometimes under royal patronage. Elite surgeons also used royal patronage to set up a surgical academy in Paris and to advance their claims to be men of learning. After 1789, the Revolution removed the old faculties and the elaborate systems of corporate regulation of practice, but it also removed the newer institutions under royal patronage. The result was an institutional vacuum, which was indeed the preferred option of the most radical reformers of education and medicine: let patients choose doctors, let students choose teachers, let savants associate together as they wish, with neither state subsidy nor state control.

Such ultra-liberalism could hardly last in a country used to regulation, still less in a country at war. Complaints about unregulated quackery and the urgent need to supply surgeons for the conscript army of the Revolutionary wars meant that new schools of medicine were introduced in 1793. Under Napoleon they were re-ordered, and a national system of medical licensing was established in 1802. Practice was officially restricted to graduate physicians and surgeons, plus a lower order of practitioners – the *officiers de santé*, who received less training and were licensed to practise only on the poor. Thus medical education and licensing became a direct concern of the French state, unmediated by guilds or corporations, although the universities retained some autonomy. Doctors were protected by the state, but they continued to complain of unfair or unlawful competition – from the *officiers de santé*, from the mass of irregular practitioners, and from doctors, who were also pharmacists (pharmacists were subject to state education and licensing as were also midwives and some herbalists). From the Revolution onwards, hygiene was institutionalized as a concern of medicine and of the state. Doctors, especially the Paris professors, served as advisers on public-health matters; indeed, the identification of medicine with public welfare was a recurrent argument against 'ultra-liberal' schemes for the deregulation of medical practice. In nineteenth-century France, voluntary associations of doctors were late and weak compared with those in Britain or the USA.

But the chief international consequence of the French medical revolution stemmed from the re-ordering of the major Paris poorhouses, such as the Hôtel Dieu, just by the cathedral of Notre Dame. Such poorhouses had been managed by the church; they were taken over by the government. The nursing nuns were subordinated to doctors; the paupers, now unprotected by charity or religion, could be sorted out medically, used for teaching, and dissected after death. Surgeons were given parity with physicians and in these 'museums' of medicine, diseases came to be seen primarily as anatomical lesions and explored through a systematic new geography of 'tissues'; peritonitis, for example, was inflammation of the membrane lining the abdominal cavity. Clinical examinations were now applied to find evidence of tissue lesions before death and autopsy: the stethoscope came into use (see page 173) because there was now something to be 'looked' for in the bodies of patients.

This form of practice remained the intellectual frontier of European medicine until after 1850. It came to dominate the big state hospitals of Vienna and Berlin, which boasted of their clinical examinations and autopsies, and to some extent it penetrated the charity hospitals of Britain, where surgeons had already developed their own anatomical approaches to disease. But charity hospitals were sensitive to public opinion, their lay governors feared charges of 'experimentation', and so patients were more or less protected. In Britain, the truly down-and-out – the paupers with no means of support – were mostly in poorhouses rather than charity hospitals. After the Anatomy Act of 1832, paupers without relatives or friends could be dissected after death; in life they were subject to mean and harsh regimes, but were not the subjects of medical teaching.

In many German states, the direct or indirect effects of the French military occupation removed older medical and scientific corporations, and strengthened the links between medicine and government. Medical education and licensing became more directly a matter of government, and cultural nationalism led to a renewal of universities, now dedicated to the advancing knowledge rather than the passing-on of professional information. This assertion of Germanic culture included medicine, usually within idealistic philosophies that were opposed to the 'analytical' knowledge then dominant in Paris. Moreover, many of the German medical schools were in small towns that did not provide the quantities of 'clinical material' essential for the development of the Paris method. For both reasons, professors in these smaller hospitals continued to teach a 'biographical medicine', which included intensive investigations of patients' histories and circumstances. From about 1850, this emphasis on the dynamics of individuals was developed into a more quantitative and physiological 'laboratory' medicine, without the intermediate stage of large-scale, Parisian, 'museum-style' analysis.

MEDICINE, INDUSTRY, AND LIBERALISM

In one sense, Parisian hospital practice was a medicine of the masses – the massed paupers of the teaching hospitals; it was medical practice devised by state-salaried teachers in state institutions attended by students with state bursaries. In Britain, as we have seen, the state was marginal in the eighteenth century, both to the practice of medicine and to the maintenance of public health. But as towns grew rapidly, partly as a result of industrialization, British doctors, too, began to face the 'masses' – not just in hospitals, which became crowded and insalubrious, but in the dense, cheap housing of industrial towns and the poorer quarters of London. In the same towns, doctors experienced intense competition, a loss of traditional rank, and an entrepreneurial culture in which medicine was viewed as merely a trade.

The new industrial towns threatened disease and disorder. Their politicians prescribed remedies: the liberal panaceas of free trade and more individual responsibility. Reformers attacked 'old corruption', including the medicine of the traditional London institutions, but they also argued for new public functions to protect the nascent industrial economy from its social by-products. They campaigned for the reform of poor-relief and for public-health measures. Where possible, they believed, such functions were to be carried out by voluntary associations, or by the new municipal corporations that liberals dominated, with central government perhaps providing legislation or resources.

Questions of medical organization, public health, and poor-relief were integral to political reform as the manufacturing and professional classes exerted themselves against an older England and fought to stabilize a new order. 'Doctors' came to identify with each other. Although a doctor with a prestigious shop might still regard himself as an apothecary, most of the retail end of medicine had been lost to the chemists and druggists. A doctor who held an honorary post at the local hospital would practise as a consultant physician or consultant surgeon, advising other doctors, but he was also the doctor of first resort for richer patients. Such consultants were leaders of the local medical communities, but most doctors now

Meeting of the Royal College of Physicians in London. In the foreground, a candidate undergoes a traditional, informal examination. Etching by Thomas Rowlandson and Augustus Pugin, with aquatint by J. Bluck, from *The Microcosm of London* (1808).

saw themselves as 'general practitioners', even when they still used 'physician' or 'surgeon' as their title. There were far too many graduates in medicine for them all to be confined to the traditional routines of physicians, and most of the surgeons and apothecaries now had some formal training beyond their apprenticeships.

In the search for respectability, and to distance themselves from mere trade, British doctors established local medical societies, especially during the 1830s. There they discussed their economic grievances, but the scientific and clinical content prevented the associations from appearing as mere 'trade unions'. Rather, they resembled the new wave of scientific societies, in which doctors rubbed shoulders with lawyers and the better-educated merchants and gentlemen. Some of the local and regional medical societies attempted to produce journals. They collaborated to form a national association – the Provincial Medical and Surgical Association, which later became the British Medical Association, the voice of general practice.

The world of medicine and its interaction with political reforms was well depicted by George Eliot in *Middlemarch*, especially through the character of the young physician Dr Lydgate:

> [The profession] wanted reform, and gave a man an opportunity for some indignant resolve to reject its venal decorations and other humbug, and to be the possessor of genuine though undemanded qualifications. He went to study in Paris with the determination that when he came home again he would settle in some provincial town as a general practitioner, and resist the irrational severance between medical and surgical knowledge in the interest of his own scientific pursuits, as well as of the general advance: he would keep away from the range of London intrigues, jealousies, and social truckling, and win celebrity, however slowly, as Jenner had done, by the independent value of his work. For it must be remembered that this was a dark period; and in spite of venerable colleges which used great efforts to secure purity of knowledge by making it scarce, and to exclude error by a rigid exclusiveness in relation to fees and appointments, it happened that very ignorant young gentlemen were promoted in town, and many more got a legal right to practise over large areas in the country. Also, the high standard held up to the public mind by the College of Physicians, which gave its peculiar sanction to the expensive and highly-rarified medical instruction obtained by graduates of Oxford and Cambridge, did not hinder quackery from having an excellent time of it; for since professional practice chiefly consisted in giving a great many drugs, the public inferred that it might be better off with more drugs still, if they could only be got cheaply, and hence swallowed large cubic measures of physic prescribed by unscrupulous ignorance which had taken no degrees.[1]

Local and national medical associations worried about irregular competition and conditions of poor-law employment. Many of their members wanted a single

Working-class housing (and cess-pool) in Preston, Lancashire, c. 1840.

national register for all qualified medical men, and a ban on unqualified practice. Some would have liked a national licensing body on which they would have had democratic representation. A few practitioners, but only a few, even in the depressed 1840s, argued for a state medical service, 'endowed' like the Anglican church, affording a decent living even to doctors in poor areas, and with the authority to maintain public health.

For most British doctors, state medicine was a Germanic perversion, but the American example could be equally worrying. There, by the 1840s, anti-elitist politicians had removed the relatively weak forms of medical licensing set up in the decades after Independence. In the resultant free market, medical botanists and homeopaths were on a par with regulars – free to pit their herbs and small-doses against the bleeding and heroic cures of the regular profession. Medical schools in the USA also competed with each other, keeping courses short and cheap so as to attract more students. In Britain, the institutions of regular medicine proved stronger. Pushed by very public criticism – not least the scathing prose of a new medical journal, *The Lancet* – they reformed enough to survive the vitriolic debates of 1825 to 1860, maintaining control over entry to the medical elites and gaining substantial roles in the certification of general practitioners.

Campaigns for radical reform were usually met by the government extending the powers of the old corporations, especially by setting them up as national examining bodies. In 1815, the Tory government had restricted prescribing and dispensing to qualified apothecaries and so provided a framework for a national examination, and thus a major spur to the growth of the private medical schools. This Apothecaries Act increased the power of the Society of Apothecaries while maintaining the subordination of apothecaries to physicians, and excluding from 'apothecary practice' all those general practitioners who had not taken the Society's Licence, even medical graduates. Eight years later the Royal College of Surgeons established a national examination for its Membership diploma, so that LSA and MRCS became the desired dual qualification for general practitioners. The Royal College of Physicians followed, establishing an examination for its Licence, the LRCP, which outranked that of the Apothecaries.

These corporations remained the targets of radical reformers, but the politics were so complex and the interests so confused that legislation was very difficult. Not until 1858 was an Act passed to regularize medical practice in the UK (see page 126). This established a single register for all doctors with recognized qualifications, but it accepted (and so helped secure) all the existing examining bodies, both university and corporate, and did not ban unqualified practitioners. It maintained the principle of 'buyer beware' as regards private practice, but it privileged 'regulars' for the increasing number of 'public' posts. The centralization of the poor law, the inauguration of public-health posts, and concern over military medicine meant that government had a growing interest in regularizing its own medical employees.

German medical reformers meanwhile were pushing simultaneously in the opposite direction. There, liberals wanted a less controlled profession, just as they wanted non-interference in other occupations. They were even ready to forego the ban on unqualified practice that was part of the existing labour laws. In 1869, an Act passed by the Prussian parliament partially deregulated medicine, so approximating the arrangements to those applying in France and developing in Britain. Medical qualifications were protected by the state, though unqualified practice was not illegal.

Interactions between the state and the profession were not limited to medical licensing. For many ordinary doctors, the arrangements for the medical care of paupers were a more pressing, everyday concern, and poor-law reforms were also central to governments' consideration of public health. Population growth had been encouraged throughout Enlightenment Europe, but by the early nineteenth century, especially in urban areas, such policies had given way to worries about the proliferation of the poor. Britain, by the 1820s, seemed to have too many people, half-employed in the countryside or crowded into the new towns. Schemes for the reduction of expenditure on poor-relief included encouragement for the emigration of 1 million paupers (from a population of 12 million). It was hardly surprising that British midwifery charities became less popular, or indeed that the middle classes began to worry about the 'abuse of medical charity', and to formulate schemes for forcing self-reliance. When workers were called 'hands', and hands were plentiful, many workers became fearful of doctors, of their hospitals,

A newspaper cartoon from Rochdale, Lancashire, attacking the local workhouse, 1844.

Removal of 'nuisances' – the reforms of sanitarians

In the early nineteenth century, 'public health' in Britain was a matter for radicals. The epidemic of Asian cholera that attacked Europe in 1831–32, however, scared the nation; sanitary reformers used that fear to underline a core problem – 'the moral and physical decay of the urban poor'.

Degeneracy, it was held, was the precondition for conflagration, whether political or medical: given the degradation, the germs of an epidemic or the words of a demagogue could produce an explosion. Moral and physical cleanliness was therefore to be enforced – through home missionaries, Sunday schools, and better education in basic hygiene. 'Cleanliness was next to Godliness' in this hand-to-hand struggle against barbarism.

The public-health campaign gained momentum through attachment to reform of the poor law, from the extension of civil registration of births and deaths, and by the claim that fever was a major cause of public expenditure. Once the new poor-law system was arranged (1834), expenditures could be easily seen and their causes investigated.

Edwin Chadwick, the Manchester-born social reformer, set himself up to demonstrate that disease was a major cause of poverty (and not the

reverse). In his *Report of the Sanitary Condition of the Labouring Population of Great Britain* (1842) for the British government, he produced evidence to substantiate the message that public dirt caused disease, which caused public expense. With great acumen he narrowed his focus to public expenditure on water supply and drains. Supported by (voluntary) sanitary associations, by some keen medical 'hygienists', and by the recurrence of epidemic cholera, he successfully promoted the Public Health Act of 1848, which encouraged or required the inspection of towns, the removal of 'nuisances', and the provision of piped water.

The effects of these reforms were limited. Industrial demands for clean water, and middle-class demands for cleaner streets and less-noxious rivers, probably outdid 'public health' worries as reasons for municipal expenditure on reservoirs and piping systems. Certainly, Chadwick's economical schemes for piping sewage on to agricultural land came to very little. Coastal towns allowed human waste into the sewers through which water drained from the streets into the sea (or estuaries); the stinking River Thames, flowing by the Houses of Parliament, eventually persuaded the government to invest in major intercepting sewers to divert the nuisance downstream from London.

and of the official precautions against epidemics. The medical profession, not least by encouraging grave-robbing (see page 154), appeared to value the poor more highly as corpses than as patients.

The answer to British worries about excessive expenditure on poor-relief in the first half of the nineteenth century was provided by a group of liberal political economists, headed by Edwin Chadwick, an unemployed lawyer and disciple of the utilitarian philosopher Jeremy Bentham. Traditional British statesmen, more used to war and foreign affairs than to social questions, were all too ready to draw on these new 'experts' and to appoint them to Royal Commissions. The exponents of political economy considered abolishing the poor law, but settled for a massive reform to amalgamate parishes into Poor-Law Unions under Boards of Guardians. Salaried overseers would now be supervised by travelling inspectors; new work-

Inland towns initially developed dry-closet systems, hoping to convert the excremental contents into saleable fertilizers. Manchester, for example, created a huge depot for this conversion; it had railway sidings and a branch canal, but it did not prove profitable. As the city grew, the transport of closet-contents in municipal 'night-soil' carts came to seem an increasing public nuisance. At the end of the century a water-carriage sewerage system was extended into poorer districts; and only then was clean water piped to individual working-class houses.

British 'public health' originated largely in liberal political economy; it also proved influential in continental Europe, where hygiene was more closely tied to regular medicine and to its academic leaders. French specialists had helped provide the data used by Chadwick; they had drawn on the statistical expertise developed by French mathematicians for physics and demography. In the 1820s, Louis-René Villermé and his associates showed that mortality in Paris correlated closely with poverty, and went on to study the textile communities of northern France. Villermé was medically trained, understood hospital statistics, and became active on various governmental hygiene councils; even so, the intellectual basis of his work, like the British and some German studies, lay in the liberal science of political economy.

In Hamburg, English engineers built a sanitary system after the great fire of 1842; but Hamburg was a rather 'British' city because of its North Sea trade. In Munich, the hygiene campaign was led by Max Pettenkoffer, chemist and professor of public health, and in Berlin by Rudolf Virchow, pathologist, anthropologist, and liberal politician, whose report on the textile workers in Silesia owed much to British and French models. Generally, the German sanitary movements were associated with the reformist, oppositional politics of the 1840s and with the tendency of elite German doctors to seek influence through scientific expertise and public opinion rather than through state bureaucracies; their liberal recommendations were part of their hoped-for science of social medicine.

In many Victorian cities, pail-closets were the preferred method of removing 'night-soil' from working-class districts. They were installed and emptied by the municipal authorities, using carts such as these in the Manchester depot.

houses would be built to replace parish poorhouses. No able-bodied paupers would be supported unless they entered the workhouse; and no-one would choose to do so unless they were desperate. The system was designed to deter scroungers. In fact, most workhouse inmates were aged and infirm, or unmarried mothers with no other means of support. They received minimal medical attendance.

Some doctors felt that they, too, were victims of the same hard principles of political economy. Poor-law medical vacancies were advertised, and doctors 'tendered' for the care of a given district's paupers; the lowest tender usually won, provided it also covered the cost of medicines. If local doctors banded together to raise the remuneration, the poor-law Guardians threatened to import a newly qualified doctor, who would work for less. Similar bargaining power was some-

times exerted by the friendly societies, and from the 1820s doctors tried to organize local strikes against them. For early-Victorian doctors, 'professionalization'
was often a desperate response to being treated as tradesmen. Public health would
also come to serve as a 'professional' cause, linking medicine to the protective role
of the state.

In Britain, the association of medicine, materialism, and radical politics is well
known from such novels as *Middlemarch* – George Eliot's common-law husband
was an enthusiast for Positivism, the new religion of science. The politics of most
ordinary doctors, however, are unknown. To the left of the liberals, one can certainly find British doctors who identified more directly with the condition of the
workers; indeed, some felt themselves proletarianized by the development of class
societies and the erosion of the artisan stratum that had provided many of their
own patients. Some of them gave public support to the working-class movement
for political rights (Chartism) or joined the campaigns against the new poor law.
However, the overall voting pattern of British doctors was probably at least as
conservative as the rest of their social class: medicine was still largely a
'carriage-trade'.

SCIENCE AND MORALS

From the mid-nineteenth century, the threat of violent class-conflict declined. In
Britain, as voting rights were extended to some working-class males, the political
parties sought working-class support and consent. They extended primary education, spent money on civic monuments, and softened their attitudes to charities
and poor-relief – at least where these concerned women, children, and the sick.
Higher education was also encouraged (for males), not least to nurture future civil
servants and teachers, whose judgement and cultivation could lend authority to
government and protect against the excesses of democracy. Organized medicine
benefited from these moves towards state authority and the provison of welfare.

After about 1850, the 'condition of England' became a cross-party issue to
which doctors could attach themselves without discomfort. This helped their
struggle for state registration and protection; in turn, the cause of public health
could be projected as 'scientific', involving laboratory experiments as well as
social statistics. John Simon, the first medical officer to Britain's central government, sponsored many investigations in the 1860s; he was also a key supporter of
the Medical Reform Act of 1858. A cultured ex-surgeon with a background in
German idealism, he helped transform 'public health' from a topic of political
campaigns to a matter of incremental, executive advances – scientific, administrative, and legislative. Simon's programme suffered setbacks in the 1870s, however,
when restructuring of the civil service made it subservient to the routines of
poor-relief. At the same time, local sanitary programmes were boosted by smallpox epidemics that helped make the case for isolation hospitals, which local Medical Officers of Health later used for such children's diseases as diphtheria.

From the late 1860s, towns were forced to appoint Medical Officers of Health. With other doctors they preached the science of hygiene and encouraged the public understanding of 'physiology'. But their authority was not uncontested; the laws of health were also crucial to health reformers who were deeply sceptical about regular medicine, especially in its curative aspects. Hygiene in mid-century Britain was still a moral cause – a rationale for better living and a critique of industralism; many of its proponents were women.

The nursing work of Florence Nightingale (see page 226), which became famous from the Crimean war in the 1850s, was in part an attempt to find useful social roles for single ladies, but it was also a campaign for hygiene and moral discipline, especially in hospitals. These were no longer to be crowded depositories for medical and surgical cases, they were to be suburban or rural, with wards designed for ventilation and surveillance – places of restorative regimes and demonstrations of the laws of health. This new view of hospitals appealed to civic authorities, especially when working men also proved ready to contribute to the maintenance of these charities. From the 1860s onwards, local hospitals emerged as key centres of 'community spirit'.

In mid-Victorian Britain, many of the hygienists were homeopaths (see page 114) and other opponents of regular curative practice. Many of them were religious dissenters who opposed medical monopoly as they opposed religious monopoly and state churches. Around 1870, their opposition focused on compulsory vaccination against smallpox and on government measures to force the medical examination – and, if need be, the hospitalization – of prostitutes in towns with army or navy barracks. For these reformers, medicine was a matter for the conscience; those who lived by the laws of nature and of God would have little need for cures, or indeed for the cruel experiments on animals that some doctors seemed to see as integral to scientific advance. Around 1870, vivisection was a major public issue in Britain (see page 183).

Medical men were often involved in disputes about science versus religion. In Britain and Germany, the debate over evolution fuelled longstanding suspicions of 'medical materialism'. In France, especially after 1870, medical republicans, including many prominent parliamentarians, led the fight for secular education and indeed secular medicine. Republicans campaigned to set up lay nursing schools like those of England, and for municipalities to 'laicise' nursing in their local hospitals. But change was slow and uneven, not least because religious sisters were so dependable and cheap to employ. (Britain is historically remarkable for the rarity of 'denominational' hospitals.)

Conflicts between physical and moral paradigms could also be found in discussions of lunacy. Mental diseases were increasingly differentiated and put down to physical causes, either anatomical or merely functional. No-one was cured thereby, and treatment in asylums remained largely 'moral and hygienic'. However, medicalization helped secure the right of doctors to dominate asylums, which had sometimes been questioned earlier in the century. It hid the fact that most of the medical work in asylums was general practice rather than psychiatry; it may have helped the relatives of patients by medicalizing their family's problem and so legitimating incarceration.

The growing authority of medicine and science probably owed much to the claims of experimentalism, especially the physiological experiments on animals made famous by Claude Bernard in Paris and Karl Ludwig and his associates in German universities (see Chapter 5). Their emphasis on the measurement and control of physiological processes in animals and eventually in humans was especially useful to medical educators seeking links between clinical medicine and physical sciences. Governments and large capitalists proved ready to invest in schemes that promised both social welfare and scientific authority.

'Scientific' medicine advanced fastest in Germany, in the new or reformed universities of the USA, and in the university medical schools of England (especially Cambridge and University College London). It was less successful in France and in the British schools dominated by clinicians – the hospital schools in London and the English provinces. In Britain, its progress was called into question by public campaigns against vivisection that were linked to sanitarianism, to feminism, and to other campaigns against cruelty. It could be argued that later nineteenth-century medicine benefited both from (female) sentiment and from (male) science, but not without considerable friction. Much medical rhetoric tried to combine the two appeals: doctors were tender enough to care for their patients as individuals, but tough enough to calculate what was best according to objective statistics and laboratory experiments.

An envelope of 1899 advertising the Anti-Vaccination Campaign.

IMPERIALISM AND SOCIAL WELFARE

By the end of the nineteenth century, technocratic and paternalistic tendencies were becoming dominant in most Western countries. Military reformers argued that improved transport and communications required new forms of large-scale organization under the direction of a highly trained general staff; the German success in the Franco-Prussian war of 1870–71 was persuasive. Industrialists looked increasingly to corporate integration and scientific management rather than to owner-direction and small-scale competition; increasing state regulation of products and of conditions of work operated to the benefit of large companies, who saw state education and welfare as producing and protecting the skilled workforces they now required. National and imperial rivalries, together with worries about the growth of socialism and trade unions, led politicians to cultivate schemes for 'national efficiency', especially those that also secured the loyalty of the working classes. Welfare came back into fashion when fit citizens were required for the armed forces, for empire, or for factories.

In Edwardian Britain, both Conservative and Liberal politicians saw social welfare as the preferred alternative to socialism. The health of infants and school children would be monitored; old age would be cushioned by pensions that workers seemed now to deserve; health insurance, previously limited to workers in friendly societies, would be extended to all working men. In the two decades before the First World War, the foundation of the British welfare state was laid.

Many of the British schemes were borrowed from Germany, where from the 1880s social insurance had been used by Chancellor Bismarck to secure worker loyalty and limit the growth of socialism. Some were borrowed from France, where defeat by Prussia had fed fears of national degeneration and worries about the persistently low birth rate. Such worries helped qualified doctors in their campaign for protection by licensing. State medical insurance was discussed but not introduced, chiefly because organized labour was divided, and the Catholic church and the mass of small employers preferred voluntary schemes.

Some similar patterns can be seen in the USA, where a swing towards professional authority and corporate organization had begun in the 1870s, soon after the Civil War, perhaps to help overcome the sectarianism of religion and the political divides between north and south. Doctors, librarians, plumbers, and many other groups claimed to possess bodies of systematic knowledge that could be taught and used for the public good. Industrial money was laundered into trusts and given to create German-style universities. White America may not have feared industrial or imperial competition, but it did fear the rapid immigration from southern and eastern Europe that funnelled into the cities, threatening disorder and political incoherence.

SCIENTIFIC SOLUTIONS TO SOCIAL PROBLEMS

Scientific solutions for social problems became the mainstay of progressive politicians. Where this meant more demanding and more exclusive medical education, or more rigorous medical licensing, the aims of the progressives coincided with those of organized medicine. In all Western countries, organized medicine benefited considerably both from the extension of welfare and from the increasing acceptance of science as a source of social authority. Investment in medical education and laboratories was particularly successful after 1880, when medical men came to agree that many epidemic diseases were 'caused by' specific microorganisms. This knowledge sharpened many existing developments in sanitary management, in isolation hospitals, clean surgery, and medical diagnostics; it boosted the authority of medical science and so led to further government and charity investment; and it increased the authority of doctors as employees and advisers of the state.

In most countries, it was university medical schools that created the expertise in bacteriology – drawing on existing strengths in microscopy, pathology, and

Satire by George Bellows of
an exercise for business men,
New York, 1916.

chemistry. Some new departments of public health were funded, in part, by undertaking identifications of microbes for local authorities, hospitals, or private doctors. In the USA, Johns Hopkins University in Baltimore pioneered a School of Public Health, as it had also pioneered German-style scientific medicine and the employment of clinical professors on full-time salaries (rather than honorary appointments supplementary to private practice). In Britain, the University of Liverpool developed a major programme in tropical medicine, funded by merchants persuaded that better control of disease would facilitate imperial commerce. In London, the government supported a similar school and research centre. In Germany, the new Reich helped fund Robert Koch and his collaborators (see page 184): their Prussian and Imperial bacteriology was set to replace earlier, more liberal approaches to public health, not least in Hamburg, which suffered badly from cholera in the epidemic of 1892. In France, public subscriptions helped fund a research institute in Paris to honour Louis Pasteur. In the USA, the Rockefeller and Carnegie Foundations channelled industrial money into medical research. The new medical science both shaped and benefited from such major end-of-century concerns as tuberculosis and infant welfare.

Sanatoria for sufferers from tuberculosis had been developed before the recognition of the causative agent, the tubercle bacillus, as extensions of nature-therapy or hygiene; but 'germs' gave them a focus, new regimes, and a link with testing agencies in hospitals and in the community. Germs were used to focus attention in public education campaigns, and governments came to see sanatoria as appropriate for state investment – as ways of restoring working men to health.

In both the voluntary and state-run sectors, sanatoria spread across Europe and North America between 1880 and 1930, and in Britain systematic state support for medical researchers developed out of the concern with tuberculosis and its costs; the Medical Research Committee (later to be renamed the Medical Research Council) was founded in 1913 partly in the hope of finding scientific solutions to tuberculosis (see page 200).

Infant welfare was prominent as a political issue, especially from 1900. Mothers were to be taught about nutrition and cleanliness and health visitors were now to be employed by statutory authorities, thus coming under the control of medical officers. Midwives were to be licensed where (as in Britain) they were previously unregulated; in the USA, midwives came to be replaced by (supposedly) trained medical men. Symptoms such as infant diarrhoea, which had seemed seasonal or even humoral, were now caused by germs and their vectors. Medical officers in factory towns collected statistics on house-fly populations as their colonial colleagues, such as Ronald Ross (see page 188), investigated mosquitoes.

Mental defectives were also topical. Educational developments had made them conspicuous; they were socially recalcitrant and likely to transmit their menace; they came to serve as models of biological degeneracy. What was to be done with children who could not learn? In Britain, as elsewhere, institutions begat institutions: elementary schools led to special schools for the blind, the deaf, for cripples, and for the 'stupid'. Doctors got involved, especially at the turn of the century when 'degeneration of the physical stock' became an issue in all Western countries. From about 1870, doctors had presented themselves as experts on physical constitutions and inheritance; after 1900, they could learn from the new science of genetics that stupidity resulted from a single, recessive Mendelian gene. Although few clinicians were much involved in practice with mental defectives and most public-health officers were suspicious of hereditarian arguments, many doctors took an interest in eugenics – the new science of better breeding. For some it became a great white hope – a way from urban degradation to national strength and order. Eugenic enthusiasm extended across most of the political spectrum, from those who despised the poor to those who wished them free from the burdens of excessive reproduction.

For most of these public medical programmes, support came chiefly from the state, sometimes from charitable associations (which often acted as 'pioneers'), and to a limited extent from the private market (for example, for private sanatoria). But industry, too, came to use the new medicine. Although most pharmaceutical companies (especially in Britain), continued to process traditional

Children being 'disinfected' at a cleansing station in London, 1912.

The eugenics movement

The idea of a science of eugenics was developed by Charles Darwin's cousin, Francis Galton. Building on Darwinian ideas of natural selection, it stressed the role of heredity in many aspects of human life; in the great debate about the competing roles of nature and nurture, it came down heavily on the side of the former. Faced with diseases such as tuberculosis, syphilis, and all manner of psychiatric disorders, eugenicists argued that they were manifestations of inherited defects that degenerated down the generations.

From around 1900, eugenics organizations were created in Britain, Scandinavia, Germany, and the USA – for instance, the UK Eugenics Education Society, founded in 1907. Through education and legislation they promoted 'positive eugenics', encouraging the 'fit' (the upper and middle classes) to have larger families, while (through 'negative eugenics') advocating that the poor and the dregs of society should breed less.

In Britain, the hope was to achieve this essentially by persuasion, but in the USA and Scandinavia the compulsory sterilization of 'defectives' (including psychiatric patients and the mentally deficient) was carried out on an increasing scale. The programme culminated in Hitler's Germany, where the elimination of large numbers of the mentally 'unfit' paved the way for the extermination of Jews and Gypsies.

The scientific basis of eugenics was never well established; brought into ignominy by Hitler and partly overtaken by modern genetics, the eugenics movement had declined by the 1940s.

ONLY HEALTHY SEED MUST BE SOWN!

CHECK THE SEEDS OF HEREDITARY DISEASE AND UNFITNESS BY EUGENICS

A poster published by the Eugenics Society in the 1930s; most of its supporters considered themselves fit to sow.

remedies, or manufacture 'patent remedies' sold by advertisements, a few chemical companies, first in Germany then in the USA, drew on academic chemistry to produce new synthetic drugs allied to dyes (see page 264). Some of them also began to produce 'biologicals', such as vaccines and antisera, sometimes 'taking over' such production from the public laboratories in which it had been pioneered. All these new products involved extensive collaboration between companies, universities, hospitals, and the new research institutes sponsored by states and/or charity. One sees here the beginning of the modern medico-industrial complex, not least in questions of standardization, legislation, and clinical trials.

THE NEW MEDICAL ECONOMY

Market effects were probably clearest for surgery, as the range and number of operative procedures increased rapidly from about 1880. These operations were needed or wanted by self-financing patients as well as by the poor, and they were often performed in patients' homes. The growth of private practice in operative surgery meant that innovative surgeons could become very rich – they thought like inventors and rubbed shoulders with financiers and major industrialists. But as surgeons came to demand elaborate antiseptic or aseptic routines, and as they undertook more and more operations, it became convenient to use private nursing homes or, where possible, public hospitals. In Britain, and especially in the USA, charity hospitals came to admit some private patients; indeed, many charity hospitals and some state hospitals began to employ almoners to ensure that all patients paid what they could towards the cost of their hospital treatment.

A tuberculosis sanitorium built at Paimio, Finland, to a design by Alvar Aalto, 1929–33, exemplifies the interplay of scientific medicine and modernist architecture.

In as much as medical and surgical advances allowed the institutions of medicine to appeal to the self-interest of the better-off, they helped produce a fundamental transformation in the political economy of medicine, visible especially in North America, where many rapidly growing communities lacked established medical institutions. US doctors began their own hospitals, as did religious or racial groups. These hospitals, whether private or charities, competed for paying patients, who by the mid-1890s constituted most of the intake. Outside the hospitals, doctors competed by installing new equipment, such as X-ray machines; in cities, doctors often occupied suites in office buildings dedicated to medicine, where they had access to common facilities.

Public medicine grew, and so did private medicine. Indeed, the distinction between them began to blur as hospitals became more central to both kinds. In most Western countries one sees new 'professional movements' within this new medical economy. While the leading practitioners and educators – the institution men – were negotiating with governments or steering the medical aspects of welfare schemes, many other doctors, especially general practitioners, felt desperately squeezed between the advance of state medicine, the encroachments of charity medicine, and the increasing ability of organized labour to employ doctors.

Friendly societies had employed doctors from the early nineteenth century, especially in the industrial areas of Britain (see page 308). By the end of the century, they were becoming a major element in medical provision for the working classes. More workers could and would pay collectively for medical care, and doctors were worried by this growth of patient-power. The entry of women into medicine – as nurses, midwives, even as women doctors – seemed an additional threat to those average general practitioners whose ideology combined patriarchy with small capitalism. The comments of one doctor sums up attitudes of many of his colleagues at the time:

Elizabeth Blackwell (1821–1910) was the first woman doctor in the US after she graduated at Geneva Medical College, New York State, in 1849. Her pioneering work led to the opening of the Women's Medical College in New York in 1868. Her sister Emily was also a distinguished doctor.

Many of the most estimable members of our profession perceive in the medical education and destination of women a horrible and vicious attempt deliberately to unsex themselves – in the acquisition of anatomical and physiological knowledge the gratification of a prurient and morbid curiosity and thirst after forbidden information – and in the performance of routine medical and surgical duties the assumption of offices which Nature intended entirely for the sterner sex.[2]

To protect their income against all these threats, doctors organized medical guilds – in effect their own trade unions.

Medical syndicalism was much in evidence in Britain, France, and Germany around 1900. In Germany, the medical guilds argued for all doctors to have access to state-regulated insurance practice, and to be paid on a fee-for-service basis, rather than by capitation fees, so improving their bargaining position with the occupational insurance schemes. In Britain in 1911, the doctors reluctantly accepted National Health Insurance for working men, largely because the state scheme incorporated, and so controlled, the medical activities of friendly societies. In fact, most doctors soon found that their new relationship with the state was both more comfortable and more remunerative than their previous condition. They were represented on the local insurance committees, and, because they were paid by capitation, they no longer had to worry about the financial consequences of referring their patients to consultants in the charity hospitals. National Health Insurance thus further differentiated the general practitioner from the hospital doctor, as it also helped establish a stable relationship between the working man and his 'panel doctor'.

MEDICINE FOR CITIZENS, 1920–70

The American Civil War and the Franco-Prussian War had served as models of military and medical organization. The war against the Boers in South Africa at the turn of the nineteenth century had served to worry the British state, not least because of the poor physical health of most of the young men who volunteered to fight. But the First World War of 1914–18 transcended all these in its scale, its horrors, and its duration. For a few years, the major combatant countries were forced to construct medical organizations far larger than their previous (and continuing) civilian systems. Away from the battle-lines, in the cities of Britain, colleges and mansions were taken over as hospitals. Nursing became a major sector of war-work for women, and many doctors learned to work in a large, co-ordinated system – some learned to see the advantages. In the emergencies of war, 'planners', medical specialists, and medical women found opportunities normally denied them.

Much of the system disappeared as the war ended and institutions were returned to their previous medical or non-medical functions, but some new patterns of practice could be carried over, and the expectations of many doctors were permanently changed. For example, British doctors who had specialized in orthopaedic surgery or cardiac medicine under war-time conditions may have returned to more general surgical and medical practices, but they did so with a clearer vision of specialty practice, not least from contact with colleagues from the USA, where a larger private market and more open hospitals had made specialization easier. War-time medicine had aimed to return soldiers to action, so the emphasis of specialists, whether in psychiatry or in cardiology, was on functional disabilities; civilian workers, especially in the armament factories, were the subjects for extensive researches on 'fatigue'. These functionalist attitudes, and the claims of physiologists to a role in scientific management, also carried over into post-war restructuring. For example, at the prestigious Manchester Technical College a physiologist was chosen to head a new department of industrial administration.

Medical teachers and researchers in Britain benefited considerably from war-time projects and from the conviction among higher civil servants that science could render medicine more efficient. In the 1920s, the Medical Research Council was dominated by medical scientists who had the ear of government and who tended to be scornful of mere clinicians, not least the stars of London private practice. Prestigious clinicians reacted by pulling in money for new research char-

A surgical operation (and demonstration) in 1907, in one of the American hospitals run for and by women.

ities, such as the Imperial Cancer Research Fund, but they could not escape from the science/government network. Nor could they counter effectively the claims of medical scientists that disciplined research would eventually provide remedies for disease, and that meanwhile the education of doctors in scientific methods would help create a more efficient health service by eliminating ineffective, if habitual, practices.

Because the British state was now paying much of the cost of general medical care for working men, there was also a financial incentive to study common diseases and to develop a science of 'social medicine'. This broader vision of public health, incorporating social sciences and the new science of nutrition, was developed by medical 'progressives', many of whom were sympathetic to the Labour Party, then replacing the Liberals as the opposition to the Conservatives; some of them were impressed by the organization and scope of 'socialized medicine' in the Soviet Union. The lock-up surgeries run by British general practitioners, and the overcrowded outpatient departments of the charity hospitals, seemed wasteful and haphazard by comparison.

At the end of the First World War, medicine had formed part of national plans for a more collective Britain – a land fit for heroes. A new Ministry of Health was set up and a report (1921) produced by Lord Dawson, an eminent physician based in London, looked to the benefits of state organization, a rationalization of health care based on district hospitals, and primary health centres staffed by general practitioners. But this plan, like so many other hopes, faltered and faded in the economic slump of the 1920s. The decline of the old staple industries severely restricted state spending until the mid-1930s (and rearmament). Little was spent on new hospitals, and there were few major legislative initiatives compared to the 20 years before the First World War. Yet medicine did change significantly.

Partly as a result of the war, and partly as a result of successful campaigns for extension of the vote, women came to play a larger role in politics. Women's political groupings, of both left and centre, campaigned for more maternity hospitals, better midwifery, and better antenatal care. Municipalities and central government obliged, still driven by worries over the quantity and quality of the imperial population. But apart from their 'maternity benefits', most women, as 'non-workers', remained outside the state medical-insurance system, even when this was extended to cover almost all working men. Women and children were comparatively dependent on medical charities, to which working men would now be referred only for specialist or accident care. The only specialized hospital care available from the state was for tuberculosis, which remained a major concern in the interwar years.

By the late 1930s, British medicine had experienced no general reorganization, but in response to specific worries and public demands governments were building up co-ordinated services for tuberculosis, cancer, maternity, and for the care of victims of accidents. Unlike previous government concerns with environment

Allons tous à la consultation

CONSULTATION

Il est plus facile et moins coûteux de **prévenir** la maladie que de la soigner.

A poster used by the American Red Cross in France in 1918 to encourage mothers to bring their babies to infant centres.

and education, these new issues all involved hospitals; specialist hospital consultants were major protagonists and major beneficiaries. At the local level, Medical Officers of Health also became more involved with general hospitals, especially after the abolition of the poor law in 1929, when the former poor-law hospitals were turned over to mainstream local government.

These local authorities were now responsible for a huge range of health services: not just drains and rehousing schemes, but also clinics, health education, special hospitals, and most of the general hospital beds. Only the charity hospitals and general practice remained beyond the reach of local government, and these, as we have seen, were increasingly dependent on central government and subject to some local co-ordination. Hospital services, state or charity, were now for 'citizens' – paupers were no longer segregated and the richer no longer excluded themselves; they tended to use separate blocks in charity hospitals. (George Orwell's *The Road to Wigan Pier* could have featured the private patients' home built in the 1930s beside the charity hospital of that depressed industrial town.)

We might generalize that in most of the 'advanced' countries between the wars, the average man, with his wife and children, became the central focus of organized medicine. The form of the development varied according to the polity and economy concerned. Russia moved in the 1930s from a state-insurance system to a salaried medical and hospitalized service. Germany continued to operate a state-regulated insurance scheme for all the working classes. In Britain, as we have seen, state insurance covered workers for general practice but not for hospital care, for which many working-class families made voluntary contributions to the 'Saturday Funds', once a form of working-class charity, now an informal prepayment scheme. In both Britain and Germany, the insurance schemes were chiefly organized through friendly societies or employer-employee schemes. The middle classes were not covered by state systems, although some paid for private or occupational insurance schemes.

In the USA, the emphasis was on private 'consumers' rather than organized workers or citizens. During the depression of the 1930s, charity hospitals introduced voluntary insurance schemes (the Blue Cross), but commercial companies invaded the hospital-insurance market, partly by offering lower premiums to low-risk households. Doctors' organizations came to accept these insurance schemes as preferable to state intervention; around 1940 they began to organize their own schemes to cover treatment out of hospitals. Many states granted doctors a virtual monopoly for this kind of insurance and medical incomes benefited accordingly. In this way, insurance became part of the market arrangements that dominated most of American medicine. Middle-class families paid for their primary and hospital care through insurance schemes; hospitals competed with each other, and so did doctors. The indigent were covered by the low-grade 'public hospitals' and by the small proportion of 'voluntary hospital beds' that remained assigned to charity cases.

In France, the state-insurance system remunerated patients rather than doctors; there was free choice of doctor and hospital. As in the USA, the public hospitals received little investment and the average citizen now patronized the many private hospitals, often doctor-owned, which benefited from the health insurance system. There was little control on costs.

A Jewish prisoner at Dachau concentration camp is subjected to extreme variations of air pressure in a test for parachute-jumping techniques.

WARTIME MEDICINE

In the First World War, thousands of doctors, nurses, and medical auxiliaries had tended the victims of trench warfare, first in the field then at base hospitals and the crowded, often improvised hospitals back home. Most of the organization was after the fact. In the Second World War, plans were laid in advance; the provision was more scientific, and so were the horrors.

It is easy to demonize the German Nazi party, the Japanese authorities who ran death camps, or the Allied commanders who ended the war by unleashing the atom bomb. But the antisemitism that culminated in the concentration camps had a long history in Germany and was evident enough in other Western countries during the 1930s. German doctors, who had seemed paragons of science, gave disproportionate support to Nazism, and many benefited from the emigration, disqualification, and persecution of their Jewish colleagues. With many honorable exceptions, German medical academics accepted the racial doctrines used to legitimate antisemitism, ranking medical researchers pursued experiments on prisoners, and experts in delousing became experts in mass murder. Medicine was central to this monstrous politics, because it depends on and so helps define the boundaries of humanity. In the case of Nazi medicine, non-Aryan races were formally defined as subhuman and thereby as expendable.

Nazi atrocities came to serve as the major reference point for postwar debates on the ethics of experimentation on humans, but we should also remember the experiments that Japanese doctors and scientists conducted on Chinese victims, not least the fact that the American government kept these atrocities secret and gave amnesty to the perpetrators so as to maintain privileged access to data on germ warfare.

During the Second World War, all the major combatant countries built up unprecedented concentrations of scientific and technical expertise. The key Anglo-American project was the creation of the atom bomb, an enterprise that shaped much military and civilian science into the 1970s. Medical men and women were marginal to this project, although the assessments of the effects of the bomb on its Japanese victims proved foundational for postwar human genetics. The obvious medical counterpart was the development of penicillin, which served as a launch pad for much of the post-war pharmaceutical industry in Britain and the USA (see page 271).

HEALTH SERVICES AFTER THE SECOND WORLD WAR

The success of the antibiotics and the mobilization of new physical techniques further increased popular and governmental faith in medical progress, but in most countries the effects were gradual; only in Britain was there a major postwar reorganization of peacetime medical services.

It was focused on the rationalization of hospital services, which had been funded by the state as part of the war effort and seemed financially too fragile to be returned to the voluntary sector. Liberal and Labour reformers had built on war-time social solidarity to secure promises of major extensions of welfare, including universal medical benefits and free hospital care. Doctors' representatives and most Tory politicians sought secure funding for hospitals, but were unwilling to see the prestigious charity hospitals subordinated in an extension of local authority services. Aneurin Bevan, the imaginative Minister of Health in the postwar Labour administration, nationalized charity as well as municipal hospitals.

Bevan was not an advocate of local government. He wanted the hospitals to be responsible to the Minister and to Parliament; their regional and local organization should then be functional, unimpeded by complexities of ownership. At this level he was content to follow the schemes drawn up by the medical educators and specialists, who, since the 1930s, had been interested in the rationalization of hospital services. Local authorities lost their hospitals and were left with public health services. Because of the resistance of most general practitioners to 'state employment', primary care was extended on much the same basis as had been introduced in 1911, but the whole population was now covered.

Although many reformers came to see the new system as giving too much power to doctors or to local 'philanthropists', the National Health Service proved enormously popular. It allowed considerable levelling-up of services, especially by the appointment of consultants to hospitals outside the main centres of medical teaching. The initial expense proved higher than anticipated, and hopes were soon dashed that proper treatment of the poor would lead to *reductions* in public medical expenditure, yet over the following decades the hospital system proved innovative, efficient, and relatively equitable.

The 1950s saw little investment in new hospital buildings, partly because of shortage of building materials, and partly because the 1950s government gave priority to housing and education. In the early 1960s, the Conservative government produced the first national plan for hospital building, based on the notion of full-service general hospitals in each district. In many towns, it was implemented by adding new ward blocks and technical services on the sites of the old workhouse hospitals. Much of the investment went to teaching hospitals.

In terms of medical professional organization, the NHS strengthened and extended tendencies already evident between the wars. Medical education became more integrated into the hospital regions, each of which was based on a medical school. Grants were provided for undergraduate and postgraduate medical education, and medical careers became more accessible to poor students, although male privilege declined but slowly. All hospital services were now to be supervised by consultants with specialist qualifications, including 'geriatrics', which had scarcely existed in Britain before 1940. In some regions, psychiatric patients also came under the care of consultants in general hospitals rather than in asylums.

All these developments formalized the longstanding, if previously incomplete, division between hospital consultants and general practitioners. Many of the latter had resisted the NHS, and especially the extension of general practice in 'health centres'. They chose to remain in 'small businesses' under contract to the state, and were regarded as inferior to hospital consultants. Not until the 1960s would general practice be renovated, when the threat of health centres run by local government had diminished and GPs could be encouraged to band together in group practices large enough to employ nurses and other auxiliary services.

In the 1930s, local government had loomed large in British health services, but its influence declined when the NHS took over municipal hospitals. By the 1960s it was generally accepted that clinic services would also be transferred to the NHS, leaving only environmental services in the hands of local government. By the late 1970s, after a series of clumsy re-organizations, the future structure of the NHS seemed clear. Hospitals, general practitioners, and public health were to be part of a planned, unified service, based on regions (and their medical schools); central government would decide policy, health-service professionals would manage, local politicians would be involved, and consumers would be represented. Medicine had never seemed so powerful, nor in Britain had services ever been so rationally organized.

Paradoxically, perhaps, the Western countries that were 'occupied' during or after the Second World War did not undertake major re-organization of medical services such as was seen in Britain. France continued to rely on state welfare benefits by which the patient was repaid for most of her/his medical expenditure. Most West Germans continued to use sick-funds that repaid doctors. Most Americans took out private health insurance, often through occupational schemes that were tax-deductible for employers. In the USA and in France, doctors and private

The cancer cause – high investment but meagre returns

From the end of the nineteenth century, doctors in most Western countries became concerned about the growing threat of cancer; they invested hope in X-rays (discovered in 1895), in radium (1898), and in organized scientific research (in Britain, for example, the Imperial Cancer Research Fund was founded in 1902). Cancer hospitals would no longer be homes for the disfigured and dying; they would be centres for inquiry and for the development of therapy.

Between the two world wars, cancer became a major object of governmental health policy, not least in Britain, where the Medical Research Council (MRC) established a nationwide scheme for radium treatment. A few major centres, such as the Christie Hospital in Manchester, came to practise a new kind of medicine based on team-work, set regimes, massive clinical statistics, and technical support from physicists. This kind of medicine was expensive, and it was required by the rich as well as the poor; it tended to break down the habitual distinctions between private and public medicine. By 1939, the British government intended that municipal and county authorities would guarantee their citizens access to diagnostic and therapeutic services for cancer, usually in a specialist cancer-centre.

Cancer was also the object of public, non-governmental campaigns. The American Society for the Control of Cancer (founded 1913) concentrated on public education. The French Anti-Cancer League (1918) promoted public education but also took a leading role in setting up a network of treatment centres. The British Empire Cancer Campaign (1923) focused on finding the cause – it was the clinician's answer to the government's MRC, which they saw as dominated by laboratory scientists. Athough the agencies and forms of medical specializations differed between countries, in all of them, cancer came to be construed as a major public hazard – chronic (like TB) but not infectious, a matter for biomedical research and elaborate physical treatments, rather than for environmental modification.

Research effort and expenditure has increased enormously since the Second World War, but the clinical returns have been meagre, especially for the common cancers. Relatively little has been invested in prevention, even after the uncovering of tobacco as a major cause of lung cancer. As the twentieth century comes to a close, molecular medicine and the promise of genetic therapy have again raised hopes.

A patient receives radioisotope treatment for cancer at the Royal Marsden Hospital, London, in the 1930s.

hospitals competed to offer better medical care; German sick-funds were also competitive to some extent. Such competition drove expenditure upwards.

In the USA, health expenditure increased rapidly, including major capital expenditures on hospitals, often from federal funds. As standards rose, the lack of medical cover for the indigent attracted more attention and in 1965, under President Kennedy, Congress voted to make medical care a social security benefit and to provide grants towards state governments to cover the costs. The result was a massive increase in total medical expenditure.

In post-war France, dependents came to be included in the social-security schemes, which had now been nationalized. Much of the rising expenditure went to private hospitals. They continued to increase in number while 'public hospitals' (old buildings with most of the long-stay patients) languished. But as the French economy recovered, the poverty of the public sector became embarrassing, especially for the supposedly 'elite' hospitals attached to the medical schools. In 1965, the Debré Law invited the affiliation of hospitals with medical schools and offered generous full-time salaries to doctors committed to research and teaching, as well as to patient care. New blocks were added on ancient sites, often housing research laboratories, many of which worked on 'pure science' projects that in other countries would be found in universities or other 'non-clinical' institutions. More generally, the French state took powers to control the development of hospitals – partly to secure better distribution of services, partly to reduce the excess cost arising from the duplication of facilities.

In West Germany, health expenditure had begun to rise rapidly in the 1950s (15 per cent a year); the rises continued during the 1960s, funded by a buoyant economy, and in the 1970s expenditure really took off, increasing much faster than gross national product and giving rise to projections that by the year 2000 half the GNP would be devoted to health. Again, the causes of the rapid increase included hospital policy. Until 1972, the sick-funds had paid towards hospitals established by governments, religious orders, or voluntary associations, but the contributions rarely covered the full cost, so they limited expenditure and building projects. By a Federal Law of 1972, state governments assumed responsibility for hospital building, and sick-funds were required to pay the full daily costs of approved hospitals. These were expensive to run and raised standards for other hospitals. Hence an explosion in costs, so that by the later 1970s Germany, like France and the UK, was looking for ways to restrict expenditure.

In the 30 years since the Second World War, the resources of medicine had grown enormously. Infectious diseases seemed to be conquered (it was commonly, if falsely, believed that viruses as well as bacteria could be killed by antibiotics). Psychotropic drugs were used to control many mental illnesses; there was hope that transplant surgery might provide relief for at least some chronic medical conditions. Doctors, especially in elite hospitals, were oriented towards innovation and so were pharmaceutical companies, which became models of 'research-based' industry, producing a succession of new types of drugs, yet also investing heavily in minor variants within these types. But new medical procedures rarely reduced medical labour or medical costs; they usually involved elaborate tests, the proliferation of paramedical staff, and the provision of drugs – all of which could be very expensive.

Meanwhile, the power and organization of scientific medicine was under attack. From the 1950s, British and American critics of mental asylums had campaigned for 'community care'. From the 1960s, a new wave of feminists queried the increasing hospitalization of normal births: the proportion of institutional deliveries had risen rapidly as confinement times decreased, new hospitals were built, and the birth rate fell. Now feminists called for less interference in birth, and for the right to choose confinement at home. Other consumer groups developed, mobilizing patients and challenging the profession's monopoly of expertise.

The political radicalism of the 1960s tended to present science and technology as aspects of a system of domination that threatened the environment, impoverished less-developed countries, and sapped the ability of Westerners to find fulfilment in community and nature. High-tech medicine came under this criticism. The thalidomide tragedy (see page 276) was a powerful symbol of technical failure. Scientifically educated doctors were portrayed as lacking the human understanding characteristic of interwar GPs. Generally, the left became more critical of the costs (and profits) of high-tech medicine, more ready to argue that professionals tended to pursue private rather than public interests.

Such criticisms were perhaps most prominent in the USA, where the healthcare system was most expensive and least equitable. In Britain, a suspicion of technology and alienation from increasingly bureaucratic hospitals co-existed with public attachment to community services that represented mutual dependence.

It was the cost of high-technology medicine, however, rather than its alienating qualities, that was to determine the next phase of medical politics. From the late 1970s, in most Western countries, the politics of medicine has concentrated on cost-restraint. For 150 years, the political economy of public medicine had focused on death rates in the community; now it is becoming a branch of corporate economics, focused on the costs and benefits of medical services.

HISTORY TOMORROW?

Some economists believe in long-waves – cycles of innovative activity that last a generation or so; they give a pattern to history. Historians of the political have no such resource, unless it be the dialectics of Georg Hegel or of Karl Marx, which are very unfashionable in the 1990s. Can we say anything about the general shape of the analytical narrative in this chapter?

There is more than a suggestion in some histories, including this one, of a kind of oscillation, especially for Britain: late eighteenth-century paternalism gives way to early nineteenth-century liberalism, which gives way to late nineteenth-cen-

Controlling medical expenditure

Throughout the Western world, the oil-price crisis of the mid-1970s heightened concern with the projected costs of welfare and medical systems. The fear then, as now, was that ageing populations were going to impose intolerable burdens on the decreasing body of wage earners, and that advances in medical technology threatened indefinite expense.

Britain was in a good position to control total health expenditure, because almost all of it derived directly from taxation. Except for the cost of prescribed drugs, expenditure in the 1970s was not demand-led; and political decisions controlled the supply side of the system. France sought to limit expenditure by scrutiny of medical expenses, especially in hospitals, and by controlling the provision of hospital services. For expenses beyond those approved by the state, the state remuneration is correspondingly reduced, and because all patients (except those on welfare) make some contribution, there is some small private incentive to keep costs down. Germany, since 1977, has tried to link the sick-fund expenditure to the national average wage, thus setting a global sum within which various kinds of providers must negotiate their provisions and returns.

In the USA, which has led the world in health expenditure, concern about costs have co-existed with problems about access to health services that most European countries regarded as solved. The coverage of the retired and of low-income families under Medicare and Medicaid (1965) was a major step forward, but universal cover remains a much contested project (1995). As in France and Germany, new state initiatives have added to the pressures of reimbursement schemes (commercial or statutory) to produce a major escalation of costs and corresponding worries about cost containment. As in France, the US government introduced powers to limit hospital growth and scrutinize expenditures that were now falling on government. The Reagan governments also tried to shift medical work from hospitals to non-hospital practice. Their preferred instrument was the extension of Health Maintenance Organizations, which undertake the health care of their members on a fixed charge per person and so are supposed to utilize cheaper services wherever possible.

In Britain, too, since 1979, rightist governments have steered medical services towards market arrangements. Frustrated by Britain's economic decline, which they linked to expansion of the state and trade-union power, the neo-liberals led by Margaret Thatcher had their own quarrels with the NHS. To them it was a bastion of trade unionism and producer power, and a huge employer for which a Conservative government preferred not to be responsible. Since it involved neither competition nor costings, it was by definition inefficient. Thatcherites, like the left, were suspicious of service professionals; unlike the left, they also

tury corporatism and professionalism, which develops through the twentieth century until the 1970s, since when it has been increasingly challenged by a resurgence of liberalism, and a return to (early) Victorian values. As a one-sentence summary, this has much to recommend it. The USA shows a similar pattern, displaced towards the liberal pole: the German oscillation takes place nearer the hierarchical, corporatist pole. But patterns are not explanations; what, beyond a dialectic of ideas, would serve to explain such patterns or elucidate the dynamic of our present?

Part of the explanation lies in the interplay of economics, military politics, and population growth. In the late eighteenth century, and again in the early twentieth century, there were strategic and economic reasons for promoting the strength of populations through health care. It seems unlikely that either the economic or the military might of the West will again depend on the aggregate of physical fitness at the level of the nation (or supernation); it is much more likely that Westresented the social-solidarism which the NHS represented.

The neo-liberals preferred markets to service bureaucracies, even when accounting for items of service required much additional administration. In medicine, as in other services, professionals were to be subordinated to managers who were more conscious of costs. Hospitals would be given autonomy as 'trusts'; rather like the old voluntary hospitals but with state funds for work undertaken. General practitioners could also operate as businesses, buying services from the hospitals of their choice. Eventually, on this trajectory, health services will all be provided by independent agencies, funded by the state.

It is as yet unclear whether these huge disruptions of the NHS have produced any increase in efficiency. They have certainly added greatly to the costs of administration and have introduced some new inequities (for example, patients being treated differently depending on whether or not their general practitioner is a 'fund-holder').

It remains to be seen whether health authorities will be able to secure a balance of services that corresponds to public needs rather than the interests of suppliers. Private medicine, which had begun to grow in the 1970s under a Labour government, boomed in the 1980s because employers used private health insurance as a perk for their workforces. Although the private sector remains relatively small in Britain, the risk of American-style inequities will increase substantially if neo-liberal governments allow purchasers of private health insurance to reduce their state contributions, or continue to erode the boundaries between private and public sectors.

Scepticism about medical benefits has grown since the 1960s. Britons now tend to see themselves as 'consumers' of health care rather than citizens who help provide it. However, hospitals in Britain still appear as community institutions, medical charities are popular, and medical education is still prized. The same solidarism restricts the growth of American-style litigiousness; Britons are still reluctant to seek compensation for accidents or even for poor practice, as they are also reluctant to demand extraordinary measures to preserve permanently damaged lives.

Hence it is remarkable that neo-liberals are now pushing medical professionals away from a form of public service that has been demonstrably more efficient and equitable than 'market' alternatives elsewhere, not least because increased costs are given as a reason: if the NHS failed in international comparisons, it was by allowing medicine in Britain to be 'underfunded'.

If costs to the state are held down, it will be less by 'internal competition' than by technical developments, and by shifting costs on to the sick and their families. New forms of surgery promise to reduce hospital stays; psychiatric patients are still being de-institutionalized even when they suffer thereby; the care of the elderly sick has been moved substantially out of hospitals and into nursing and residential homes, for which old people must pay until their capital has almost disappeared. In effect, the benefits of past tax and insurance payments are being reduced as Britain, like most other Western countries, faces an ever larger proportion of 'retired' persons (and the likelihood of unemployment continuing at levels once thought intolerable.

ern businesses (and armed forces) will promote the health and welfare of their own employees, partly for reasons of physical efficiency, partly for the morale and loyalty of highly trained, expensive workforces. There is probably a general confluence, already well established in the USA, between the business as the unit of health-care insurance, and the business as the unit of medical provision. Medicine will probably appear more and more as a service industry, even within taxation-funded systems such as the British NHS. The market version of medicine may come to operate at the level of corporate suppliers and corporate purchasers, with doctors operating as skilled employees rather than as liberal professionals.

Such developments, in the affluent West, will be limited in two ways: by the considerable if diminishing powers of medical professionals, and by the need to provide adequate medicine for the poor. In Britain, the private sector is still small compared with the remaining NHS. (In 1991, 89 per cent of health-care expenditure in the UK came from the public sector compared with 79 per cent in France,

78 per cent in Germany, and 41 per cent in the USA.) Even in the USA, the key medical institutions – the big teaching hospitals – are in some sense producer cooperatives, partly because of their close links with the universities, which are state-owned or public charities and in either case directed chiefly by academics. It is hard to see this system changing rapidly. Yet, throughout the Western world, higher education is being pushed into quasi-market relations and some American firms have claimed to possess sufficient range and depth of expertise in science, teaching, and management to provide the kinds of education and research presently offered by prestige universities. One can perhaps imagine a consortium of medical-technology and medical-care companies setting up a medical school, research institute, and teaching hospital, especially if governments continued to subsidize the students and the patients.

The last point is crucial for, as we have seen, medicine is a very peculiar kind of market. State services developed in all Western countries because much of the population was unable to afford health care of a standard considered adequate by them or by governments. Costs can be spread by commercial or mutual insurance schemes, but these have always left a considerable residual population to be covered by state welfare, and usually to be served by substandard hospitals and clinics. Of course, the incomes of the poor are now much higher, relative to subsistence, than they were in mid-nineteenth-century Britain; but so are the costs of medical services. Governments will continue to support medicine for poor people, partly because of their votes, partly to reduce disaffection and infectious disease, and partly because those in authority can still be embarrassed by 'unneccessary deaths'. Life and death remain ideologically powerful, and health care, even for the poor, is a major issue, not least where the resurgence of infectious diseases, such as tuberculosis, highlights the threat posed by 'lower classes' to the rest of the population.

The key issues for Western health care continue to include equity and community. Should we allow systems that provide the poor with separate, usually inferior services? Can we not maintain equitable services such as were developed by social-democratic governments in Scandinavia and Britain? When measured in terms of health standards against cost, such systems are probably more efficient than more competitive alternatives and they have the considerable political advantage of turning equity into the positive virtue of solidarity. That the economically powerful and politically resourceful share provision with the less fortunate is the best guarantee of efficiency as well as equity.

Such arrangements are now breaking down in eastern Europe as economies decline and can no longer support former standards of service. A small proportion of the population buy Western medicines in hard currencies; the rest suffer, not just from a massive decline in the real resources of the public system but from diversion of expertise to the private sector and the loss of the social and economic co-ordination required to maintain high-technology medicine.

A slum in Jakarta, Indonesia, with the financial district in the background. Western medicines are available for the rich but not for the poor in developing countries.

Some cities in Africa face rather similar problems as their economies are marginalized and the colonial and post-colonial infrastructure fails to be renewed. In addition, of course, many sub-Saharan states also face issues of subsistence and basic sanitation that most European states have considered as solved for at least a century. Old issues are presented in new forms, not least around new pandemics; the prevalence of AIDS in East Africa may have much to do with the patterns of sexual relations, but it also depends on the chronic malnutrition of much of the population, and on the prevalence of other venereal diseases that could be effectively treated.

The West keeps a horrified eye on these sufferings; it intervenes at the margins, from an attenuated conscience and a fear of global consequences. 'Tropical medicine' is no longer required by empires, any more than the former imperial powers require the fitness of their mass citizenry. Internationally, as at home, Western nations have a choice: they can tolerate the increase of inequality and worry later about the consequential threats, or they can seek a broadening of political responsibility. The infrastructure of health – decent food and water, ventilation, and drains (to which we might now add antibiotics and contraceptives) – are, however, not within the control of individuals, or even of the governments of poorer countries.

We often think of medicine as a progress running through recent history. This chapter tells a different story. Medicine is a part of the complex interplay of economic and political history. Its future, like its past, in the 'second' and 'third' worlds as well as in the West, will depend on the shifting patterns of wealth and power.

CHAPTER 10

Geoff Watts

Looking to the future

Modern medicine is powerful and effective, and likely to become more so. Its scientific and technological approach to ill health has yielded unrivalled benefits. Illnesses once unpreventible, symptoms once unmanageable, and conditions once incurable have succumbed to the application of knowledge about the body and its workings. Even the law of diminishing therapeutic returns has so far been offset by the growth in medical research, and the accumulation of still more understanding. For the next decade, and probably beyond, there is every reason to suppose that medicine will continue devising new therapies to combat old enemies.

This hymn of praise is not, however, the complete picture. Medicine is increasingly troubled by doubts and negative developments. While doctors have always had their critics, the past two decades have witnessed a sustained assault on the nature of professional medicine. The social polemicist Ivan Illich opened his book *Limits to Medicine* (1976), by declaring that 'The medical establishment has become a major threat to health. The disabling impact of professional control over medicine has reached the proportions of an epidemic.' Illich's criticisms were more outspoken than most; but his has not been a lone voice.

Some of medicine's most pressing problems are unintended consequences of its success. By way of example, consider a study carried out some years ago at Boston University Medical Center in Massachusetts. A group of doctors followed the progress of more than 800 patients admitted to the medical wards of their hospital. They were looking for iatrogenic complications: for illnesses induced not by nature or circumstance or the patient's own behaviour, but by the drugs and procedures used to diagnose or treat the original condition. Out of the patients admitted during the study, 290 developed one or more iatrogenic disorders – many of them drug-induced. Of these, 76 suffered major complications, and in 15 cases these contributed to their death.

Although as a specialist clinic the Boston Center receives the sickest and most difficult patients, the findings would – to a lesser extent – be true of most hospitals in most places. The discomforting fact is that modern medicine demands a price. And almost as often as it fulfills a promise, it seems to create a moral dilemma or prompt an uncomfortable question – most fundamentally about the purpose of medicine. Despite the wilder ambitions of a few Californians who have had their corpses frozen in the expectation of revival by some omnipotent physician of the future, we may assume that all of us eventually have to die. If medicine succeeded in, for example, eliminating heart disease, many more of us would live slightly longer but then die of cancer. The gain would be, to say the least, questionable. Our ignorance of the ageing process makes it impossible even now to be certain about the long-term effects of our interventions. The ideal health strategy must be to maintain the body in good physical and mental condition until shortly

Opposite: A T lymphocyte, a type of white blood cell, infected with the human immunodeficiency virus (HIV), the causative agent of AIDS. An infected T cell typically appears lumpy and the protuberances coloured green in this electron micrograph are viral particles in the process of budding off from the T-cell membrane. Scientists have made good progress in understanding HIV, building on basic research in cell biology done in the 1960s and 1970s. Because of the fast spread of HIV infection, however, medical science cannot yet stop people contracting the disease or prevent those infected from developing AIDS.

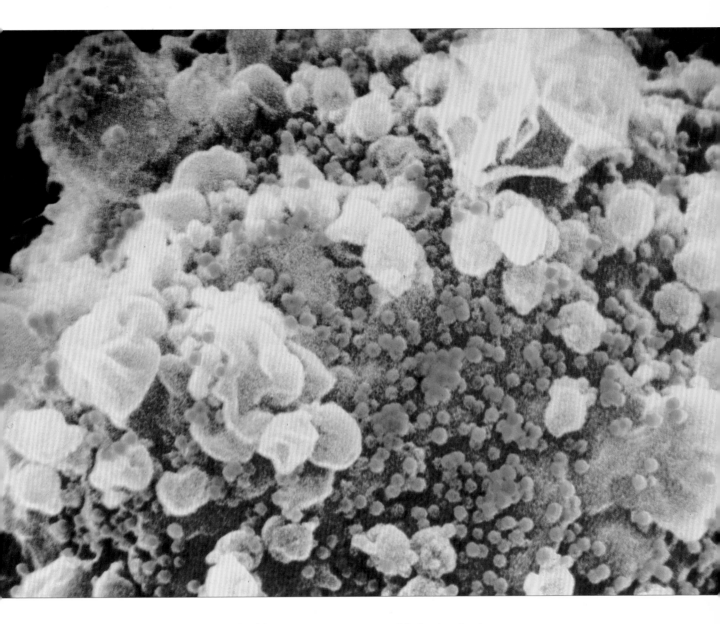

before death: a longer life and a healthy one. But it is just as likely that further increases in longevity will instead offer extra years plagued by degenerative disease and mental impairment. How many people would thank medicine for a gift such as this?

Small wonder, then, that public attitudes to medicine veer so disconcertingly from the laudatory to the censorious. This ambivalence seems set to continue until there is a wider agreement on the purpose of medicine. These conflicts and contradictions will form the substance of much of this chapter. First, though, a caveat.

Predictions about medicine are not new – and many have been wholly wrong. Most are simple extrapolations of present understanding. Once it had become

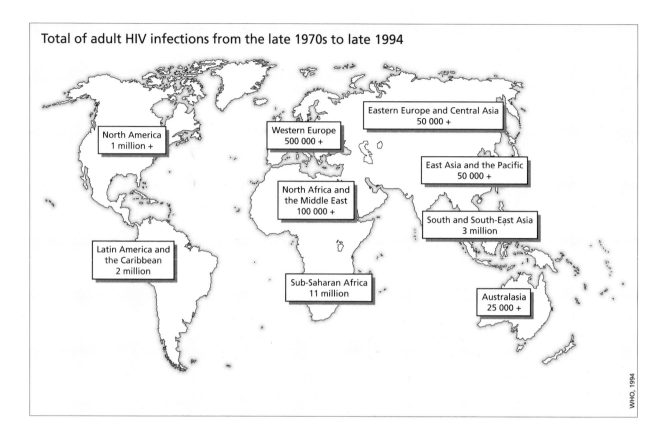

Total of adult HIV infections from the late 1970s to late 1994

North America
1 million +

Western Europe
500 000 +

Eastern Europe and Central Asia
50 000 +

East Asia and the Pacific
50 000 +

North Africa and
the Middle East
100 000 +

South and South-East Asia
3 million

Latin America and
the Caribbean
2 million

Sub-Saharan Africa
11 million

Australasia
25 000 +

WHO, 1994

By the end of 1994, at least 18 million adults had been infected with HIV since the late 1970s/early 1980s, 11 million of them in sub-Saharan Africa. Malaria causes many more deaths than AIDS worldwide, but whereas malaria kills mostly young children, AIDS mainly affects adults in their economically productive years and can devastate not only a family but the economics of a whole community as well. Researchers are working on a vaccine for HIV. But, even if one *is* developed, it may be many years before it is cheap enough for the developing world.

clear that antibiotics could inhibit the growth of bacteria, it required no great insight to predict that new antibiotics would be found or synthesized, and that these would improve the control of bacterial disease. But who predicted the advent of antibiotic resistance, now such a problem? And who can forsee the advent of a new microbe such as the human immunodeficiency virus (HIV)? Likewise, on the credit side, no-one in the 1960s or 1970s could have guessed that surgery for peptic ulcers, then so common, would become a comparative rarity in the late 1980s and 1990s. To have done so would have presumed the existence of a (then undiscovered) drug to stop acid secretion in the stomach. And who could have imagined the burgeoning interest in immunology, its effects on the understanding and treatment of infectious disease, and its use as a tool in almost every branch of medicine?

Neither is expertise a guarantee of exciting, imaginative, and faultless prophesy. The results of a survey of more than twenty 'international medical scientists' organized by the Bristol-Myers pharmaceutical company in 1987 were unremarkable. They suggested, among other things, that the diseases most likely to have been eliminated by the year 2000 are AIDS and measles; that the cure rate for cancer will by that time have risen to about two-thirds (from today's half); and that most coronary bypass surgery will have been replaced by less-invasive techniques, or by drugs able to dissolve the blood clots that otherwise precipitate a heart attack. A first-year medical student would be as capable of this sort of prophesy as any 'international medical scientist'.

For a supreme misjudgement consider the words of the Nobel Prize-winning immunologist Sir Frank Macfarlane Burnet. Research at the level of cells and even molecules has already affected the practice of medicine, and will have an even greater impact in the future. Yet as recently as 1971 MacFarlane Burnet wrote this: 'I believe that biological research can provide gratifying occupation for as many people as have the necessary training, competence and motivation … I do not expect conventional benefits to medicine or technology from biological research to be common in the future. If they should arise they can be accepted as bonuses but need not be sought.'[1] Let this spectacular failure to predict be remembered as I review the direction of medical progress, and identify some of the hurdles and the pitfalls.

THE PROMISE OF MEDICINE

Before the doubts, the promises. The more that is understood of the causes of illness, the greater the potential for prevention. The decline in cigarette smoking in Western countries, for example, will eventually reduce the incidence of cancer in the developed world. Conversly, tobacco consumption in developing countries is increasing by some 2 per cent a year, so they can expect to see a corresponding increase in the disease. Preventive knowledge is effective only if acted on, and there is still little grasp of what makes people act as they do and how they can be persuaded to do otherwise. Any form of prevention that depends on behavioural change will, most likely, continue to be overshadowed by enthusiasm for cures. What follows is an outline of a few of the developments in science and technology that are now shaping the future of medicine. Nowhere is this more evident than in new approaches to inherited disease.

Many illnesses are caused by a defect in a single gene: a single segment of the hereditary material or DNA. Genetic techniques are already used to diagnose such disorders (see later). If undamaged copies of the defective gene could be introduced into the patient's body, the activity controlled by that gene would be restored to normal. This is the basis of gene therapy, itself now on the verge of entering routine practice.

In cystic fibrosis, for example, a defective gene causes patients to produce copious quantities of an abnormal mucus that makes the airways susceptible to various lethal respiratory diseases. In principle, the gene therapist might remove some cells from the lungs and breathing passages, insert normal genes into them, and then return them to the body. Such an approach is feasible for blood or bone-marrow cells; for the airways, it is impracticable. An alternative strategy is to repair the defect *in situ*.

This has already been done by exploiting a virus that colonizes the cells of the airways. Suitably doctored to render it harmless, the virus acts as a carrier for a

Wiping out infections

The successful eradication of smallpox in the late 1970s raised hopes that other infectious diseases would be eliminated. The prospects, however, are not good. Smallpox had a combination of features that set it apart from most other infectious illnesses. It was not especially contagious; it had no animal reservoir; it was easily recognized and diagnosed; there was a very effective vaccine against it; and it was widely feared.

Measles and polio are two of the prime candidates for eradication, especially polio. The World Health Organization has set the year 2000 as the target date for the elimination of polio worldwide, but as long as the polio virus exists it poses a threat. Perhaps the greatest likelihood of success seems at present to lie not with a microbe, but with a parasitic worm. The guinea worm lies beneath the skin and grows up to 60 centimetres in length. It does not kill, but it is a cause of pain and disability to some 10 million people, predominantly in the hot and dry areas of Africa and Asia. A combination of health education and clean drinking water should be enough to defeat it.

Vaccines still have much to offer. Protection against many of the commoner infectious diseases is already possible – although, as with hepatitis B, not always at a price that poor countries can afford. AIDS aside, the most sought-after vaccine is one against malaria. The unicellular blood parasite responsible for this disease has a complex life cycle, each step of which could, in principle, be blocked by a suitable vaccine. One fanciful, but just about plausible suggestion, is

to use suitably treated mosquitoes as a means of immunizing their victims at the same time as they feed on them. More realistic is the vaccine developed by a Colombian physician, Manuel Patarroyo (see page 10). This has the added distinction of being the first vaccine to be chemically synthesized rather than made using a biological process. But trials carried out in Colombia and in Africa have yielded conflicting results. The evidence is still incomplete.

An adult female guinea worm (*Dracunculus medinensis*) emerging from an infected foot. Infection is through drinking water containing a tiny copepod crustacean that harbours the infective larvae of the parasite.

normal version of the abnormal gene. Getting viruses into the lungs presents no problem; an inhaled aerosol will take them where they are needed. The beneficial effects of the new gene should last as long as the viral colonies continue to thrive – and in the handful of patients on whom this experiment has been tried, this is what appears to happen. An alternative way of introducing the genes is to wrap them in fatty envelopes, called liposomes, and blow them in an aerosol into the nose. The long-term benefits of both these strategies remain to be seen.

In some cases gene therapy could turn out to be far simpler, and require nothing more complicated than an injection of the normal or missing gene directly into the tissues in which it is required. This might even apply to Duchenne muscular dystrophy, an incurable disease in which certain muscles become progressively more wasted and so weaker. Muscle cells are able to absorb genetic material. If

DNA containing the gene required to overcome the disease is introduced into the affected muscles, they may take it up and start to manufacture the missing protein.

Other inherited diseases – of which there are several thousand with a familiarity ranging from sickle-cell anaemia (see page 23) and muscular dystrophy to Tay-Sachs and Lesch-Nyan – will demand other strategies. Some are the consequence of single gene defects, whereas others are the result of several such errors. Many hitherto incurable or even untreatable illnesses will soon be candidates for gene therapy. The technique is not limited to inherited disorders. The body makes many natural products able to fight disease: substances such as interferon and interleukin. Gene therapy could be used to increase the output of these substances, or even persuade cells that do not normally make them to do so.

The hereditary material of each human probably comprises some 100,000 genes, only a tiny proportion of which have been identified. But if – or more likely when – the ambitions of a scheme called the Human Genome Project are realized, scientists will have mapped the lot. It will then be possible to identify the defect underlying every inherited disorder and, given sufficient ingenuity and resources, correct it.

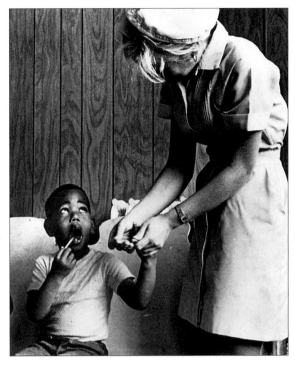

Taking a blood sample to test it for sickle-cell anaemia in 1972. Campaigns in the 1970s to detect carriers of the gene for sickle-cell anaemia among black Americans led to people being stigmatized.

SEQUENCING THE GENOME

The remainder of the 1990s and the beginning of the new millennium will see human biology's first and perhaps only venture into 'big science'. Projects costing tens of millions of pounds and bringing together hundreds of scientists working in international groups have so far been confined to physics. Sequencing the human genome is the biological equivalent of exploring the fine structure of matter. DNA, the hereditary material, is a long, helical, double-stranded molecule built up of pairs of four types of molecular subunits or bases. The order of these base pairs forms a code specifying the structure of all the proteins required to make and run every cell in an organism. The human genome comprises some 3,000 million base pairs, and its full analysis will be an awesome task.

The initial attempts at sequencing were carried out piecemeal, with researchers working on small sections thought to have some special significance – in causing disease, for example. It was in the mid-1980s that scientists conceived the idea of tackling the task more systematically. The Human Genome Project aims to identify the position of every gene on every chromosome, and the order of every one of the millions of base pairs. Japan, Canada, and France are among the countries collaborating in the project; but the leading laboratories are mostly in Britain (for example, at the Sanger Centre in Cambridge and the Institute of Molecular Medicine in Oxford) or in the USA (notably at the National Institutes of Health).

When this aim will be realized and at what cost are still uncertain; but 10 to 15 years, and a price of as many dollars as there are base pairs, would be realistic guesses. By early 1995, only about 5 per cent of the genome had been sequenced, so the project is still in its infancy. In spite of disagreements over patent protection (should the patenting of human genes be permitted?), division of labour, duplication of effort and much else, the project seems certain to progress.

NEW DRUGS — BY DESIGN

The search for new drugs has traditionally relied on trial and error. A chemist might synthesize a new molecule, which a pharmacologist would screen for evidence of useful biological action. Alternatively, a particular molecule might be known to have an action that doctors realize is useful; the chemists could then synthesize variants in the hope of making a more active version. Although this method has yielded large numbers of useful drugs, it is wasteful. Much better would be to design drugs for specific purposes. That is now becoming a reality.

The key to success lies in discovering the processes that control the body's cells, and then manipulating them. For example, much of what cells do is determined by hormones circulating in the bloodstream. These act in a lock-and-key fashion by attaching themselves to hormone-specific sites or receptors located on the membranes of cells. The attachment of the hormone serves to trigger the cell into activity; when the hormone is withdrawn, the cell switches itself off. This offers the pharmacologist several avenues of intervention. By designing a drug molecule that can stick to a receptor of just one particular type, it may be possible to mimic the action of one particular hormone. Or the drug could be made sufficiently like the hormone to attach to its receptor, but not sufficiently similar to activate the cell. Having, as it were, jammed the lock by inserting the wrong key, the cell would be effectively inactivated.

All this, of course, depends on being able to design the right drugs. It is now possible not only to know the atomic make-up of a long-chain molecule but, using a computer, to work out how the molecule will fold on itself. This understanding is vital to drug design because the three-dimensional structure of a molecule is often what determines its properties as a drug. The molecular pharmacologist can view models of drugs and receptors on computer display screens, rotate them, and even find out if one will fit snugly into the other.

The pharmacology of the future will also make greater use of natural chemicals such as interferon, interleukin, and others with less familiar names. By isolating these materials, identifying their roles in the life and control of cells, and then synthesizing them in quantity, it will be possible to manipulate the body's physiology in ways used by the body itself.

MONOCLONAL ANTIBODIES

Antibodies are natural substances – proteins – made by the immune system as part of its defence against invading microbes or other foreign materials that have entered the body. Their value lies in their specificity: usually, one type of antibody molecule will attach itself only to one type of foreign material. When an antigen, as such materials are collectively described, enters the body, the immune system responds by generating large amounts of the corresponding antibody.

The body's output of antibodies is generally adequate for its needs; but to exploit their potential in new ways requires far more pure antibody than can be extracted from an intact, functioning immune system. The monoclonal antibody technique, devised at the Universty of Cambridge in the mid-1970s, is a way of generating a specified antibody in virtually unlimited amounts.

In principle, the technique relies on repeatedly immunizing an animal – originally mice – with the antigen complementary to the required antibody. The cells responsible for manufacturing it are found in the spleen. They can be removed and cultured, but do not survive for long. The key to the Cambridge advance lay in fusing these cells with others able to grow and divide indefinitely, and produced in a type of tumour called a myeloma. The resulting 'hybridoma' cells will grow and proliferate indefinitely, as well as make large quantities of just the one antibody. Suitably adapted, this system can produce any type of human antibody.

Monoclonal antibodies have revived interest in the field of immunotherapy. Moreover, used with ingenuity, they can do things that were previously impossible. Attached to drug molecules, for example, and injected into the bloodstream, antibodies specific for tumour cells will concentrate the drug at the site of the tumour, so minimizing remote side-effects. Alternatively, monoclonal antibodies can be used to inactivate undesirable materials. There is growing evidence that a chemical messenger, misleadingly known as tumour necrosis factor or TNF, plays a part in the sequence of events leading to and maintaining the inflammation in joints afflicted with rheumatoid arthritis. Preliminary attempts at injecting patients with an antibody that binds specifically to TNF – and so neutralizes it – offer the possibility of new biological therapies for this and similar diseases.

The range of applications will be limited only by the imagination of the scientists. For a flavour of the possibilities, consider how one Australian researcher, Warren Jones of Adelaide's Flinders Medical Centre in Australia, is developing a less-invasive method of prenatal testing for fetal abnormalities. A small number of fetal cells cross the placenta and enter the mother's bloodstream – so, in principle, it should be possible to detect abnormalities of the fetus by testing those of its cells present in the mother's blood. Using techniques that increase the amount of genetic material in a cell, it is possible to test for defective genes in a sample containing no more than a dozen or so cells. The trick is first to catch them. As there may be only one fetal cell for every 5 million maternal ones circulating in the mother's blood, this is no easy task.

Right: Surgeons can now operate outside the body using specially designed instruments inserted through small holes in the wall of the abdomen. This 'keyhole' surgical technique is increasingly being used for abdominal operations and is likely to become a standard routine. In the keyhole operation shown here, a surgeon is examining the abdominal organs with a coelioscope. This is a type of endoscope or viewing tube containing optical fibres, a light source, and usually small surgical instruments that can be manipulated by remote control.

Opposite: Promising new drugs are being designed by computer. Researchers first solve the three-dimensional structure of a target molecule involved in a bodily disorder and then build another chemical that fits snugly into the target and blocks its activity. The multicoloured structure at the centre of this picture was developed by a research team in Birmingham, Alabama, to prevent the enzyme purine nucleoside phosphorylase (blue spheres) from interfering with antiviral and anticancer agents.

One solution is to make monocloncal antibodies specific to fetal cells, and then join them to microscopic beads with a metal core. When added to a blood sample, the antibody-coated beads will attach themselves exclusively to the few fetal cells that are present. They can then be separated from the maternal cells using a magnet.

SURGERY – ROBOTS AND KEYHOLES

The notion of robotic surgery is apt to seem not only futuristic but hazardous; the prospect of lying unconscious while an electromechanical device cuts and probes is disconcerting. But until – if ever – computer-controlled machinery can mimic the awareness, adaptability, and knowledge of a human surgeon, such a takeover in the operating theatre is unlikely. A more realistic prospect is of using robots to perform certain tasks requiring great precision.

In replacing a hip, for example, the surgeon has to remove the head of the thigh bone, excavate its interior, and then insert the shaft of the artifical joint. In practice, the area of contact between bone and prosthesis is often less than half; the space is filled out with cement. Increasing the area of contact between bone and metal makes for a more resilient and longer-lasting replacement. And this is precisely what can be achieved by having a robot excavate the interior of the bone. Similar precison is required when operating on structures inside the brain. This organ is ideally suited to robotic surgery because the surrounding skull provides fixed reference points by which to locate any particular part of the brain, and a firm base for mounting instruments.

Details of the anatomy of the bony structures can be supplied to the controlling computer in the form of pictures taken using X-rays or other imaging systems. A double control system requiring the agreement of two computer processors before any action is taken minimizes the risk of mishap – and the whole procedure can be supervised by a human surgeon.

A greater influence on surgery in the near future will be the continuing development of minimally invasive techniques. These allow surgeons to operate from outside the body, so avoiding extensive cuts in its surface. Patients need less anaesthesia, experience less postoperative pain, and can go home sooner – in many cases on the day of the surgery, or the day after.

To see inside the body cavity the surgeon uses a viewing tube or endoscope, often in conjunction with a minature TV camera. The endoscope is pushed through a small hole in the wall of the abdomen, while specially designed instruments are inserted through a further one or two holes. Keyhole procedures already in use include removal of the gallbladder, the appendix, the kidneys, and even quite large sections of bowel, the repair of hernias, the closure of the Fallopian tubes, and removal of the uterus (hysterectomy).

How much surgery will eventually be done in this way is a matter of conjecture, but enthusiasts envisage keyhole techniques becoming standard in at least half of all cases.

TRANSPLANTS OF FETAL TISSUE

Many of the body's tissues can repair themselves; like the skin, they can regenerate if damaged. The nerve cells of the brain are not in this category. Parkinson's disease, for example, is caused by the loss of certain nerves in the part of the brain called the substantia nigra, itself resulting in a fall off of the chemical transmitter dopamine. Attempts to remedy the loss by dosing patients with one of its chemical precursors, called L-dopa, often bring a marked improvement in the symptoms of Parkinson's disease. But the treatment is far from perfect. Hence the attempts to transplant fetal material into the brains of Parkinson's patients.

Whether this will ultimately succeed is still unclear; but if it does, it will be the first of many attempts to use material from fetuses that have been spontaneously or electively aborted. Fetal cells, unlike many of their adult counterparts, can grow and divide, and seem less prone to rejection when placed in another body. Diseases for which this approach might be suitable include Alzheimer's, Huntington's, and diabetes. It might even be possible to use fetal material to repair the damage after a heart attack. The closure of one of the coronary arteries deprives part of the muscular wall of the heart of the oxygen it needs, and so kills it. The muscle cannot repair itself; but if the surgeon could introduce sufficient fetal material, it is possible that the new cells might grow and divide and replace the damaged tissue.

COMPUTERS IN MEDICINE

In medicine as elsewhere, computers will radically alter the way in which medical staff work. The traditional means of storing patient records – a thick wadge of papers bearing semi-legible handwriting, and all too frequently lost – will soon be replaced by a computer memory. Doctors, whether in primary care or in hospitals, will call up the information they require on desktop visual display units. Many case notes are already handled in this way, and it is only a matter of time before X-rays, body scans, and other visual data are similarly stored. All this information would then be instantly available on a display unit in whatever hospital department a patient happened to be visiting.

Diagnosis is also being computerized. Simple tests for blood constituents such as glucose and cholesterol are already available in kits for home use. The development of electronic biosensors will enable many more body fluids to be monitored for the signs of impending ill health.

Some people are prepared to go to any lengths to engage in do-it-yourself diagnosis. Some Japanese researchers forsee the age of the intelligent toilet, equipped to monitor urine and faeces for the presence of blood, sugar, certain proteins, and any other chemicals that might offer clues to an individual's health. Data obtained in this way could be dispatched, down a telephone line, to a central computerized health-monitoring station. On detection of any abnormality, the individual concerned would be contacted and told to visit the doctor.

BENEFITS TO THE POOR

To see medicine's most spectacular achievements you should look to the poor: to the effects of preventive and public health medicine in developing countries. In this century, they have witnessed the dramatic impact of scientific principles on high infant mortality and endemic infections. In due course, patterns of mortality in developing countries will begin to resemble those of the industrial nations, with cancer and cardiovascular disease displacing infections as the main causes of illness and death. Many of these liberated peoples, either through the absence of means or the lack of inclination, have so far failed to limit the growth in their numbers – a catastrophe in the making.

The triumph of death control in the absence of compensating birth control has long been, and remains, socially and ideologically contentious. Countless attempts at planning have been subverted by religious, political, economic, and other vested interests that variously portray population increase as acceptable or even desirable, and all attempts to limit it as conspiratorial or oppressive. Does population increase matter? And in so far as medicine has fuelled it, what role can or should the medicine of the future have in dealing with it?

Only the wildest optimist can believe that population increase represents no conceivable threat. In 1995, there were around 5,700 million of us, and the end of the twenty-first century may see a doubling or even a trebling of this number. More than 90 per cent of the increase will be in developing countries: the have-nots of the planet.

Optimists count on the poor countries of the southern hemisphere undergoing the kind of demographic transition that Europe experienced in the nineteenth century. Before that transition, high birth rates were balanced by high death rates; so the population grew slowly if at all. In the first stage of the transition, health and living standards improved and death rates fell; but because the birth rate remained high, the population began to increase. Only in the third stage did the gains of economic development allow the birth rate to fall; birth and death rates were once more in alignment.

The fact that many countries have already made this transition, however, cannot be taken to indicate that all others can or will. Circumstances in Africa and

A baby being inoculated at a clinic in India. Although smallpox is no longer a threat to the young, measles, diphtheria, cholera, tetanus, influenza, polio, and several other infectious diseases kill millions of children every year, mostly in the poorer countries. Vaccines save lives and prevent disease more effectively than other medications but, for finanicial or logistical reasons, they often fail to reach those whom they would benefit most.

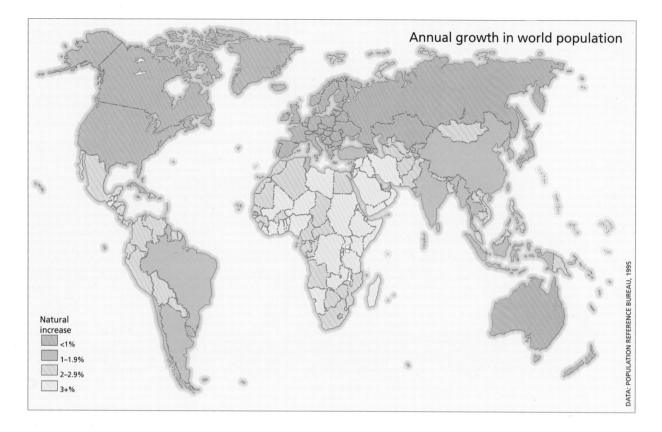

Annual growth in world population

Natural
increase

- <1%
- 1–1.9%
- 2–2.9%
- 3+%

DATA: POPULATION REFERENCE BUREAU, 1995

much of Asia are vastly different from those prevailing in Europe when it went through its demographic transition. Many poor countries are at risk of the negative feedback loop – the 'demographic trap'. It happens when a population entering the first stage of the transition lives in a country with an already overstretched ecosystem – as in the horn of Africa. In these circumstances, a rising population can all too easily precipitate famine. Preventive medicine and public health have tipped many developing countries into the transition before their fragile economies can feed, house, and otherwise sustain the consequent increase in numbers. The next phase of the transition – a lower birth rate – simply isn't happening as rapidly as is needed. In a few cases, it isn't happening at all.

Having contributed so much to the problem, medicine can hardly wash its hands of the matter. It is agreed that there is a vast unmet demand for contraception in developing countries. Although the provision of birth control – depending on the method – is not exclusively or even mainly a medical affair, the cooperation of medicine is vital. Some doctors, notably Maurice King of the Department of Public Health Medicine at the University of Leeds, feel that more radical action may become inevitable.

In 1990, Dr King set out the health problems of the poor, and put them in the context of global ecology.[2] He argued that the celebrated World Health Organization's definition of health as 'a state of complete physical, mental and social

Population growth rates are highest in Africa and the Middle East. By 2010, the world's population of around 5,700 million (mid-1995 figure) is expected to have grown to around 7,000 million and, by 2025, to around 8,000 million.

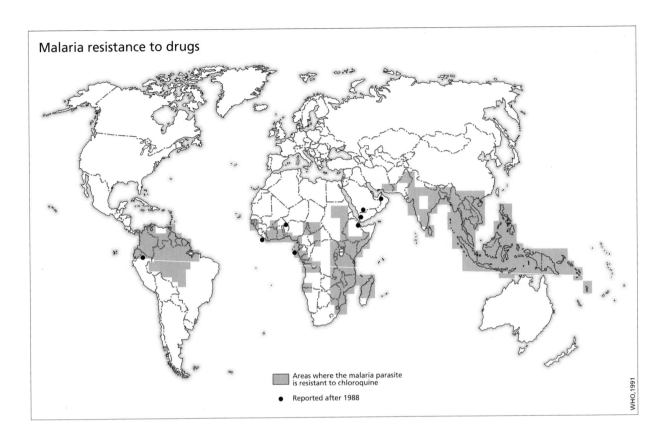

Malaria resistance to drugs

Areas where the malaria parasite is resistant to chloroquine

• Reported after 1988

WHO, 1991

Mosquitoes that carry the malaria parasite have become resistant to insecticides and the parasite itself has developed resistance to anti-malarial drugs. If the insect vector re-establishes itself in areas from which it was once eliminated, and, as a result of global warming, expands into temperate latitudes currently free of the disease, we could see widespread epidemics of malaria in the future. The need for a successful vaccine has never been so acute.

well-being, and not merely the absence of disease' should be amended to include the word 'sustainable' in front of 'state'. He also wrote of the need for the rich countries to modify their lifestyles, of the importance of devising more equal ways of distributing the world's resources, and of the global initiatives that might set these changes in motion. All this, though, was familiar; much less so was the extent to which Maurice King confronted some of the more nightmarish consequences of his dire predictions.

The first hint that he was about to think the unthinkable was an oblique one. 'The reduction of human death rates has always been seen as an absolute good in public health, and unease about population increase has never been an accepted constraint on any public health measure. Will visions of the ultimate effects of population expansion alter this view? Are there some programmes that, although they are technically feasible, should not be initiated because of their long-term population-increasing consequences?'

By way of example Maurice King chose the oral rehydration of children suffering from severe diarrhoea. Although an individual doctor may be duty bound to rehydrate an individual child within his or her care, Dr King questioned whether there is an equal obligation to set up programmes of oral rehydration in the first place. Such measures, he suggested, 'should not be introduced on a public health scale since they increase the man-years of human misery, ultimately from starvation'. In effect, what's the point of denying infants a quick death now when all they face is a lingering and more painful one as adults?

From some authors, these views would have been unacceptable. From Maurice King, a man with a distinguished career in medicine in Africa, they could be repudiated but not dismissed. The article aroused much debate, with critics arguing that Dr King was variously neglecting the unfulfilled desire of many women in poor countries for better (or any) birth control, overstating the strength of the link betwen birth rate and economic development, and generally adopting a defeatist stance. What is significant is that Dr King himself should have felt compelled to voice such an argument; it indicates something of the despair now felt by at least some of those most familiar with the condition and prospects of the poorest of the poor. To make matters worse, there is global warming (see page 358).

FEARS OF THE RICH

The expectations of people living in rich industrial countries are altogether more demanding than those of the poor. The politician Enoch Powell, who served as British minister of health from 1960 to 1963, famously declared that 'there is virtually no limit to the amount of health care an individual is capable of absorbing'. Although this claim is much debated, it is true to say that never before have so many people had their suffering so effectively minimized. Yet far from growing more contented with what they have, many of the citizens of these privileged nations view both present and future with apprehension.

First there is the matter of cost. For decades, developed nations have been accustomed to a rising expenditure on health. At first, this seemed appropriate. But as the proportion of each nation's wealth so deployed has crept steadily upwards, doubts have began to crystallize, especially in the USA where spending on medicine – fuelled by private health insurance and unhindered by the controls operating in state-funded systems – accounts for more than 13 per cent of gross national product (relatively the highest of any Western nation). Although it may be difficult to identify the optimum level of spending on health care, most Americans sense that benefits are not keeping pace with outgoings. Something, they know, will have to be done to limit the flow of dollars. In the absence of a lead from the federal government, some states are trying their own schemes – of which the most draconian and thought-provoking has been devised by Oregon.

The Oregon State Legislature instructed its Health Services Commission to arrange all publically funded (Medicaid) medical services in order of priority, taking account of the views of the public. The commission then worked out the annual cost of providing each of these services. Once the state's annual Medicaid budget had been decided, it would be possible to say how far the money would go. Given x million dollars, items one to n would be paid for; anything below that cut-off point would not.

A warmer planet – impact on health and medicine

The reality of global warming – and, if real, its likely extent – is still debated. But any increase in temperature will have its most immediate impact on health and medicine. Increases in atmospheric temperature would have their most direct effect in the tropics; so once again the poor would find themselves in the firing line. Many infectious and parasitic diseases are spread by intermediate hosts: insects, snails, and small arthropods such as ticks. If temperatures were to increase these carriers of disease would become more widespread, taking with them leishmaniasis, schistosomiasis (bilharziasis), dengue fever, yellow fever, malaria, and much else.

The African form of trypanosomiasis or sleeping sickness is currently confined to the central part of the continent. A warming of about 2°C would allow its insect carrier, the tsetse fly, and with it the geographical boundary of the illness, to shift southwards – perhaps down to South Africa – with potentially severe consequences for humans and for cattle.

Malaria, already re-established in areas from which it had once been eliminated, would also become more widespread. It is worth recalling that malaria was still endemic in parts of southern Europe until the 1950s, and not unusual in Britain during the nineteenth century, especially in wetlands such as the Fens. Any increase in temperature would favour the return of the anopheline mosquito that carries the malaria parasite. And these events would be happening at a time when both the parasite and its insect vector are increasingly resistant to the medicines and insecticides used against them, and when a vaccine is not yet in commercial production.

More generally, lower rainfall would enlarge the areas of the world that face periodic droughts, and so run the risk of malnutrition. This in turn predisposes people to tuberculosis, leprosy, measles, pertussis (whooping cough), and polio. Besides its direct effect on humans, water shortages foster a deterioration in hygiene and public health. Poorer sanitation and contaminated water would encourage the spread of typhoid, cholera, and other such diseases.

Pollution, too, presents a series of uncertain future threats. The worldwide increase in motor traffic has flooded urban atmospheres everywhere with a cocktail of hydrocarbons and oxides of nitrogen. Under the influence of ultraviolet light, certain of the products of motor exhausts react to form ozone. This gas is extremely reactive and damages the delicate membranes lining the airways, causing them to narrow – precisely the problem that troubles people with asthma, who find such a polluted atmosphere difficult to cope with. The number of people consulting a doctor for asthma has doubled in the past decade: powerful, albeit circumstantial, evidence to support those who argue that pollution must be taken more seriously.

Ozone at ground level is a bad thing, but ozone in the upper atmosphere is essential to filter out some of the ultraviolet radiation that would otherwise reach us. The consequences of the much-publicized withering of the ozone layer are already being seen in the rising level of skin cancer in some of the sunnier areas of the globe. How things will develop in the future is difficult to predict – but a 10 per cent decrease in ozone would trigger a 30 per cent increase in rodent ulcer (a slow-growing malignancy of the face) and a 40 to 50 per cent increase in other types of skin cancer. Cataracts of the lens would also become more common. There is also reason to believe that increased exposure to ultraviolet light dampens the immune response generally, so giving a further edge to infectious diseases of all kinds.

None of these things may happen, but, if they do, medicine will find itself having to adapt to new patterns of disease, and facing some almost unimaginable challenges.

Children wear surgical masks to protect themselves from the polluted air in crowded Mexico City.

Public consultation took several forms. Telephone surveys were used to rank twenty-six states of disability. At meetings held throughout Oregon the public was asked to rate the importance of various categories of activity such as 'the treatment of fatal conditions which can't be cured and won't extend life more than five years'. The commission also held public hearings at which special interest groups were able to plead their case. The priority list that finally emerged comprised just over 700 items. In fact, the state's first Medicaid budget under the new system stretched as far as item number 587: treatment for contact dermatitis and other eczema. Item 588, not to be funded, was medical and surgical treatment for acne. Among other items below the cut-off point were infertility services and the treatment of infections in the later stages of HIV disease.

Even its sympathizers recognize the crudity of the Oregon experiment; but it does provide some pointers for anyone contemplating the future of health-care financing. Commentators have pointed out that the Oregon commissioners were simply making explicit a process that happens anyway. All health care is rationed. In a wholly free market it is rationed by the purchaser's capacity to pay for it; in a state-funded system such as Britain's National Health Service it is rationed by the willingness of the government to pay the bills, and by the waiting lists that form when demand for a particular procedure outstrips supply. The Oregon approach defines the choices that have to made, and offers a system for making them. Elsewhere, these decisions are made *ad hoc*, according to political expediency, and in line with professional interests. The means used in Oregon may be deficient; but their end – explicit decisions on what to make available – will surely become a feature of all collectively funded health systems.

A few decades ago, a blocked coronary artery was a death sentence. Then came bypass surgery and, more recently, a technique called coronary angioplasty (shown here). With the help of X-ray imaging, a small balloon on the end of a fine tube is threaded through a vein and into the blocked coronary artery. Pumping up the balloon compresses the obstruction and restores the artery to its normal diameter. The operation is closely monitored in the control room.

Another feature of the Oregon approach was that the commissioners weighted their decisions according to the quality of the patients' lives after treatment. Although this makes the calculations more onerous, it will soon become a regular part of all calculations of medical costs. Finally, there is public consultation. Slavishly following public opinion in making complex technical decisions is foolish; but so is a total neglect of the popular view of what is worth doing. Here, too, Oregon has pointed the way forwards.

The high cost of scientific medicine is not simply a consequence of people seeking and getting more of the same. Many of the diagnostic and treatment innovations devised by medical researchers depend on new and expensive gadgetry. A few decades ago, for example, nothing could be done about blocked coronary arteries. Then came bypass surgery in which small blood vessels taken from the leg are used to fashion a new blood supply to the heart muscle. More recently surgeons have developed a technique called angioplasty, in which, using X-ray guidance, a small balloon on the end of a fine tube is threaded though the blood vessels and into the blocked coronary artery. Pumping up the balloon restores the artery to its normal diameter. Small coiled springs can be placed in the expanded vessel to keep it open. Other researchers are developing lasers with which to unblock the coronary artery from inside. So it has gone on, and so it seems set to continue. With technology, what was once a death sentence can now be repealed. The same is true of most other branches of medicine from kidney transplantation to artificial hips.

New drugs are subject to close scrutiny of their safety and effectiveness, but control over new instruments and procedures is much less rigorous. Although the body scanner – a system for obtaining X-ray pictures of soft as well as bony tissues – was invented in Britain, it was in the USA that the instruments themselves began to proliferate. This rapid spread, however, owed little to good evidence that they improved the outcome of the patients' treatment. They were popular because they were glamorous and they offered physicians another profitable investigation. Proper technology assessment would prevent such excesses. But even when thoroughly applied – which, so far, is seldom – it cannot prevent the extra cost arising through genuinely valuable additions to the doctor's hardware. Short of banning most research and development it is hard to see how the growth of costly advances in medicine can be contained. In this respect, of course, state-financed health systems are in a stronger position; even when a new gadget or procedure is available, they can simply refuse to pay for it. Private expenditure is more difficult to limit.

Optimists see hope in some of the genetic and molecular techniques described earlier. They suggest that costly procedures such as bypass surgery are 'half-way technologies', which will eventually be replaced by cheaper molecular-based approaches for preventing disease or dealing with it at an earlier stage of its development. Their argument is plausible, but not proven. There are, however, some new and improved treatments derived from biomedical research that have already proved to be money savers. For example, the US National Institutes of Health spent 20 million dollars developing a treatment for the chronic skin disease pso-riasis. It relies on giving patients the chemical precursor of a drug that is then acti-vated by exposing diseased areas of skin to ultraviolet light. The annual savings through use of this technique are estimated at almost 60 million dollars. This is a healthy return on research investment; but whether it is typical remains a matter for debate.

Another and deeper disquiet about the future is rooted in the very thing that underpins medicine's success: science. Along with orthodox medicine goes a machine model of the human body. Where kidney disease might once have been considered the consequence of evil spirits, wicked deeds, a malicious deity or some other such influence, it is now viewed as a material problem: a failure of the biological equipment that should be filtering, cleaning, and adjusting the chemi-cal make up of the body's fluids. The renal physician is neither a priest nor a shaman but the physiological equivalent of a domestic plumber. And so it is with most other branches of medicine from gastroenterology to gynaecology; doctors are trained, primarily, as technicians skilled at diagnosing and fixing failed body mechanisms.

To pursue this demanding trade they need sophisticated equipment such as brain scanners, fetal monitors, endoscopes, lasers, radioactive chemicals, artificial hearts, and computers. Learning to handle these things may take months or years; to use them safely often absorbs much of the doctor's attention. It is understand-able that patients may feel alienated, and begin to wonder if the doctor has for-gotten that they are not merely malfunctioning biological mechanisms, but people with problems that go beyond the biological. The doctor as a healer has been replaced, to a varying extent, by the doctor as a body technician. Although grate-ful to receive this form of assistance, most people do not find it sufficient. They need someone prepared to relate to them on a spiritual and human level, and able to appreciate their distress. Sympathy of the kind that a garage mechanic might express when reporting a broken crankshaft is not enough.

One of the first commentators to give clear public expression to these doubts was the London University lawyer Ian Kennedy. In the book based on his 1980 BBC Reith Lectures, he wrote: 'Modern medicine has taken the wrong path … an education which demands high skills in scientific subjects before going to medical school, and involves years of breathing the heady air of one field after another of scientific endeavour once there, produces what it is intended to produce: a doctor who sees himself as a scientist. It may not produce what is so often needed: some-one who can care.'[3]

Medicine thus faces a challenge: to make full use of technology without losing the human contact that has to be part of any satisfactory system of health care. There are many possible remedies. Teaching medical students how to communi-cate with their eventual patients has become a priority. Some medical schools use actors to play the part of patients as students practise their first fumbling attempts

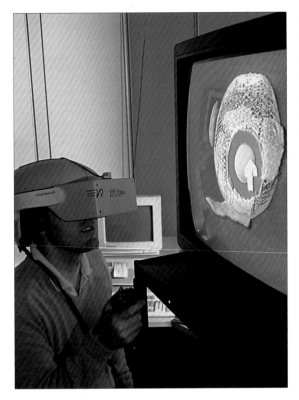

The doctor as a healer has been replaced, to a varying extent, by the doctor as a body technician. Learning to handle sophisticated medical equipment may take months or even years. Here, a researcher wearing a virtual reality (VR) headset practises eye surgery. A surgeon can practise his technique with a VR system or teach students without the need for a live patient. An added advantage of VR is that the procedure can be viewed from all angles, many of which are not visible with a live patient.

to explain difficult ideas or break bad news. The aim is to make the patient rather than the illness the focus of the consultation. Other doctors are turning to complementary medicine, seeking to retain their scientific approach to disease while recognizing that science by itself does not answer all medical needs. There are movements to bring art into hospitals, to reconsider their architecture, to fashion new relationships in which the wishes and feelings of patients are taken into consideration. The success of these and other moves will decide whether the public sees medicine as in broad sympathy with their needs, or as an enterprise from which it feels evermore alienated.

THE FLIGHT FROM SCIENCE

The doctors' dilemma is made no easier by a widespread suspicion of science and technology in general. In spite of their impact on the way we live, ignorance about them are common. Science is thought of as antithetical to human values; technology is associated with pollution, weaponry, and all manner of environmental destruction. Medical science suffers by association and, of course, by its own tragedies and misapplications: thalidomide (see page 276); the overzealous use of life-support systems; the exploitation of unwitting patients as experimental subjects, and so on.

One response has been to seek alternative forms of health care based on other philosophies. To the extent that this is a rejection of what is wrong with orthodox medicine it is sensible and desirable. But in so far as it represents another facet of the flight from science into irrationality, it bodes ill. Some of the bewildering variety of complementary therapies now available – radionics, for example, or the alleged benefits of wearing a crystal or sitting inside any pyramidal structure – can appeal only to the credulous. They discard the exacting framework by which science has so painstakingly attempted to know the world, and replace it with a bogus, back-of-the-envelope mysticism.

The sheer ingenuity of scientific medicine has also created a raft of new ethical dilemmas, which are especially apparent in reproductive medicine.

MORE REPRODUCTIVE DILEMMAS

In vitro fertilization (IVF) has already produced its own crop of ethical issues: the ownership of eggs that have been fertilized and frozen for storage, for example. Still more exotically, surrogate motherhood is now feasible. A couple able to produce healthy sperm and eggs but not to have a child in the normal way can now donate eggs and sperm to be fertilized in the test-tube. The resulting embryo can

Screening for defects

The increasing number of inherited and other congenital disorders that can now be diagnosed before birth offer parents the option of a termination. In amniocentesis, the original method of prenatal diagnosis, a needle pushed through the mother's abdomen is used to extract a sample of the fluid surrounding the unborn child. Fetal cells floating in this fluid can be harvested, cultured, and examined. Their chromosomes reveal abnormalities such as Down's syndrome and, with potentially more sinister consequences, the sex of the child.

In some less-developed countries, for economic and social reasons, male children are the preferred choice of many parents. The effects of unrestricted access to prenatal sex determination are difficult to predict, but some excess of male births would seem likely. At present, many of the countries most likely to use prenatal sex determination are least able to afford it. What might happen to the sex ratio if the scientists devise a cheap method utilizing fetal cells in a maternal blood sample is unnerving to contemplate.

Amniocentesis has now been joined by a technique called chorionic villus sampling or CVS. This involves snipping off a small piece of the placenta, which, as an embryonic tissue, is genetically identical to fetal material. It can be used at an earlier stage of pregnancy: around 10 weeks as opposed to the 16 or so weeks before amniocentesis becomes safe.

The other advance that has brought this field to the fore is the development of techniques of DNA testing by which single gene defects can be identified in fetal cells. There may

be as many as 5,000 of these defects, the best known being cystic fibrosis. This is one of the rapidly growing collection of inherited disorders that can now be identified prenatally. By the early years of next century, we may well be able to test for all of them.

The likelihood that all fetuses will be screened for all defects is remote because most genetic disorders are exceedingly rare. But the question yet to be resolved is the appropriate limit to such testing. There are clear moral arguments in favour of avoiding the birth of a child with cystic fibrosis; but what of a child who is exceptionally short, or less intelligent than average, or who fails in some other way to measure up to a preconceived ideal? There is a pressing need for agreed guidelines.

Genetic screening is not confined to unborn children. As more gene defects are identified, and testing methods developed, it will be possible for would-be parents to confirm or refute any suspicion that they may be carriers of an inherited disease. This, too, will create new ethical dilemmas of the kind that have already been thrown up by the development of a test for Huntington's chorea.

The degeneration of brain cells that underlies Huntington's disease leads to an irreversible dementia and eventually to death. The first signs of the illness do not normally appear until the second half of adult life. The availability of a test for the disease means that adults who are still healthy now have the option of discovering their fate. Some choose to know, some do not. Genetic screening may turn out to offer other disturbing insights into our future well-being.

Amniocentesis – extracting a sample of amniotic fluid from the uterus of a pregnant woman.

Genetic defects can be identified soon after *in vitro* fertilization by sucking one cell out of an eight-cell embryo and analysing its DNA for inherited diseases such as Tay-Sachs, Duchenne's muscular dystrophy, and cystic fibrosis. If the embryo is healthy, it can be transferred, often with several others, back into the woman in the hope that at least one will implant in the uterine wall and continue its development.

then be implanted in the womb of another woman. Genetically speaking, the baby to which she gives birth will be the child of the donor couple. Most societies feel uneasy about the prospect of this 'womb renting', and many countries have made it illegal. But simply because it is technically feasible, attitudes may change; womb renting may one day be no more controversial than adoption or artificial insemination.

IVF has also added another twist to the eugenics story. Prenatal screening for inherited disease requires a willingness to contemplate termination. With IVF, it is possible to fertilize several eggs, allow them to develop to a multicell stage, and then remove from each a single cell for genetic testing. Up to a certain stage of development, all the cells of a dividing egg remain identical, so the loss has no effect on the resulting embryo. In the light of the test results, it is possible to select and implant only defect-free embryos.

The possibility of treating as opposed to merely detecting genetic disorders – gene therapy – has been described already. It continues to provoke public disquiet, some of which actually stem from a misconception. The use of the word 'gene' seems to imply that whatever is done to alter its function – or, in the case of a missing gene, to replace it – will be transmitted to later generations. If this were so, any ill-judged tampering could have adverse consequences for later generations. In fact, this will be the case only if the cells altered are those of the germline that give rise to eggs and sperm. This more ambitious project would indeed rid an individual's progeny of an unwanted gene; but if the potential gains are greater, so, too, are the risks. In the long run, however, it seems likely that this kind of gene therapy will be contemplated.

Moving from the beginning of life to its end, here medical advances are creating additional new dilemmas. When the English poet Arthur Hugh Clough wrote of doctors, 'Thou shalt not kill; but need'st not strive officiously to keep alive', he meant it as a sneer. But he was writing in the nineteenth century, well before the development of life-support systems that can maintain the life of a body whose higher brain centres are no longer functioning: the persistant vegetative state. Strangely, Clough's mocking couplet has become a cherished aphorism used by many doctors to emphasize their awareness of the cruelty of artifically extending the lives of certain seriously ill patients. There is, though, much disagreement about the interpretation of 'officiously'. In 1975, for example, fearful of the power vacuum that would follow the demise of the Spanish dictator Franco, his doctors contrived most horribly to delay his death while the politicians agonized about the succession. Grotesque examples of this kind are, fortunately, rare. But the injudicious use of antibiotics to pull an elderly person through an episode of pneumonia ('old man's friend') when all have agreed that death would be appropriate is not uncommon.

The development of effective life-support systems has opened up another clutch of moral dilemmas related to transplant surgery. Subject to the agreement of relatives, the crucial issue nowadays in timing the withdrawal of life support may be the availability of a would-be recipient of that person's organs. Such arrangements need strict codes of behaviour to ensure that it is the physician supervising the donor patient – as against the doctor in charge of the recipient – who decides that the patient has nothing further to gain from life support.

Reactions to medical practice and innovation vary, as they always have done, from place to place. Religious and social attitudes influence the use of abortion, contraception, artificial insemination, IVF, euthanasia, the use of cadavers to teach anatomy, and much else; and future developments, particularly in reproductive technology and genetic engineering, will continue to startle if not frighten many people.

Some countries are toying with the idea of national bioethics commissions to which these matters could be referred, and from which would come suggestions about legislation and guidelines or codes of professional conduct. A few countries have already set up bodies of this kind; France, for example, has had one for more than decade. There is also something of the kind in Denmark, this organization making particular efforts to inform the public about bioethics, and to seek its views. This approach is less cumbersome than creating a series of *ad hoc* committees to consider individual issues. A standing bioethics commission, already familiar with the territory, should be able to respond without delay. To suggest that developments in medicine merit public scrutiny is not to question the judgement or probity of doctors and medical researchers. Many, already weary of a succession of horror stories and false alarms, would welcome a body in which they, as well as the public, could place confidence. The one certainty is that some branches of medical research have become altogether too ingenious to leave solely in the hands of the researchers.

THE FUTURE OF RESEARCH

The belief that medicine will go on devising new methods of diagnosis and treatment assumes that medical research will continue to flourish. This seems likely; no researcher need lack a project while there are still uncertainties about, for example, the relative importance of environmental as opposed to inherited factors in common diseases from cancer to arthritis. But certain public policy decisions – notably the balance of spending on basic as against targeted or goal-oriented research – could affect the success of attempts to find out. To take cancer as an example, should researchers be given a grant and instructed to find a cure, or should they be funded to carry out whatever studies they think might reveal something about the nature of all cells, malignant and otherwise? This kind of question will increasingly exercise the trustees of charitable research foundations; why should such bodies give their money to scientists who work on cell division in multicellular green algae – organisms not greatly troubled by cancer or any other human disease? In the 1970s, two American doctors made an impressive effort to answer this and similar questions.

Julius Comroe and Robert Dripps of the universities of California and Pennsylvania, respectively, had become troubled by the increasing popularity of targeted research, and the growing doubt that scientists left to their own devices could be counted on to produce useful findings. Anecdotal evidence on this issue is unhelpful. Louis Pasteur was commissioned by the French government to find ways of preventing wine from turning into vinegar, and to stop sheep dying of anthrax. In solving these and other practical problems he effectively created the science of bacteriology: a good advertisement for targeted research. But Wilhelm Röntgen stumbled upon – and saw the medical potential of – X-rays while studying the emissions from a certain type of vacuum tube. His work was basic physics, and had no practical end in view, let alone one to do with medicine.

Comroe and Dripps set themselves the hugely ambitious task of tracking down the sources of the knowledge that underpinned a series of important medical advances. They chose heart, bloodvessel, and lung diseases – these being the branches of medicine in which they themselves worked. With the help of other specialists they compiled a list of significant advances, and then asked forty or fifty experts to vote on their relative importance. For each of the top ten on their lists they identified the bodies of knowledge that had made them possible. In total, they picked out 137 such bodies of knowledge: things such as the development of anticoagulant drugs, the invention of electrocardiography, the identification of blood types, and the management of infection.

Next they identified some 2,500 reports published in the scientific literature that were important in the creation of these bodies of knowledge. With the help of no fewer than 140 consultants they chose 529 key reports for close analysis. In the case of electrocardiography, for example, the chronicle of relevant findings stretches back several hundred years to the first, faultering attempts to understand electricity (see page 167). Key articles in the chain of events leading to the modern electrocardiogram include Luigi Galvani's 1794 report that the discharge of an electric eel could cause heart muscle to contract, and Carlo Matteucci's 1842 observation that a muscle contracts if its nerves are laid across another contracting muscle. When Willem Einthoven first measured a human electrocardiogram in 1901 (see page 141), he was relying on knowledge garnered by people who knew nothing of the existence let alone the significance of electrical rhythms within the heart.

What the stupendous and time-consuming effort of Comroe and Dripps revealed was that 61 per cent of all the knowledge judged to be essential for later

Voluntary euthanasia is, paradoxically, a logical outcome of the success of scientific medicine at fending off death. The low infant mortality and extended lifespans now common in rich countries would have been unimaginable when we lived a hunting and gathering existence. Trauma, infections, and starvation kept the death rate high, and anyone living long enough to develop the chronic and degenerative diseases afflicting twentieth-century people would have counted her- or himself lucky.

Some people, however, are now reluctant to accept this extra life. Alzheimer's and Parkinson's diseases, osteoarthritis, and other such disorders become increasingly likely with age. The gift of a longer life is greatly devalued if, in the end, it has to be paid for in pain, disability, and loss of dignity.

The first step towards voluntary euthanasia, the living will, already has a substantial following. Living wills are documents signed while the signatory is *compos mentis*, and specifying which measures – or none – are to be taken to save or prolong life when, as happens with Alzheimer's, that person is no longer able to make such decisions.

In spite of opposition from many doctors, active euthanasia, too, is finding greater acceptance. The Dutch solution offers the most highly developed model. It effectively decriminalizes the actions of a doctor who administers a lethal injection – provided that the action is in accordance with a series of safeguards. These prevent patients taking the decision quickly or lightly, rule out pressure from relatives, and ensure that euthanasia does not become an automatic panacea.

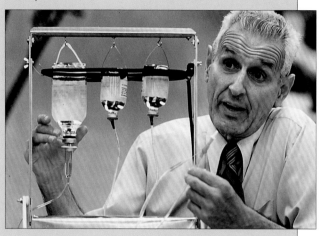

A retired American pathologist, Jack Kevorkian, made headline news in 1990 when he helped Janet Adkins, a woman with Alzheimer's disease, to commit suicide with his 'planned death' machine.

clinical advance were reports of basic research findings. They concluded that clincial research requires different types of research and development, and not one to the exclusion of the other. As far as basic research is concerned, their data revealed a powerful case for the long-term support of 'creative scientists whose main goal is to learn how living organisms function, without regard to the immediate relation of their research to specific human diseases'.[4] In short, basic research pays off.

A contemporary illustration of the extent to which basic research findings can accelerate the understanding of a new malady is HIV disease. AIDS was first recognized as an illness in 1981. In 1983, the American researcher Robert Gallo suggested that it was caused by a retrovirus, a type of virus that carries its genetic information in the form of a molecule of RNA. The following year Luc Montagnier of the Pasteur Institute in Paris succeeded in isolating the virus. By 1986 there was a drug, AZT; preliminary vaccine testing began around the same time. Despite repeated claims that governments have been less than wholehearted in their support for AIDS research, it would be difficult to name any other disease in which understanding has progressed more rapidly. The researchers were able to build on research projects carried out in the late 1960s and 1970s. Much of this went on under the banner of cancer research; but most of it was, in truth, basic cell biology and immunology. The lessons for the future are obvious.

The years since the pioneering work of Julius Comroe and Robert Dripps have seen many attempts at analysing the sources of useful knowledge – and, by extension, the best way of acquiring it. This research has led to the development of technology foresight, an enterprise devoted to the identification and promotion of those areas of strategic research that are likely to yield to the greatest economic and social benefits. Its advocates, arguing that there is not one but many possible futures, seek partly to predict the likely direction of research, and partly also to shape it. The value of technology foresight in medicine, and elsewhere, remains controversial.

CHANGE AND ADAPTATION

Some fear that scientific medicine, driven by its own imperatives and enthusiasms, will continue to plough ahead irrespective of the needs and fears of its recipients. But this is a bleak view, and there are reasons to reject it. While medicine's attachment to scientific models of disease and healing may have created some of the problems, science itself fosters the very scepticism that makes for change and adaptation.

Doctors no longer bow to the authority of long-departed gurus. The idea of relying on the past in the way that physicians for so long viewed the works of Galen as holy writ is now unthinkable. All scientific knowledge is provisional: to be treated not as ultimate truth, but as an understanding that may have to be revised in the light of future discoveries. The very essence of science lies not only in creating hypotheses about the world, but in testing them and, when they fail, replacing them with better ones. It is true that doctors are not scientists as such, and that much supposedly scientific medicine is not as scientific as its practitioners like to suggest. But for all such legitimate carping, medicine does have the kind of mindset in which change is acceptable. So where is the evidence that medicine might be confronting some of the doubts raised earlier, and might even adapt to them?

Of the many hopeful signs that could be offered in evidence, I will pick just three: medicine's renewed interest in the quality of life; its changing attitude towards complementary medicine; and the rise in numbers and importance of patient self-help groups.

QUALITY OF LIFE

Consideration of the quality of patients' lives is not a new phenomenon in medicine. But the doctors' burgeoning interest in curing illness encouraged them to measure their achievements in the most tangible ways. Has the infection been

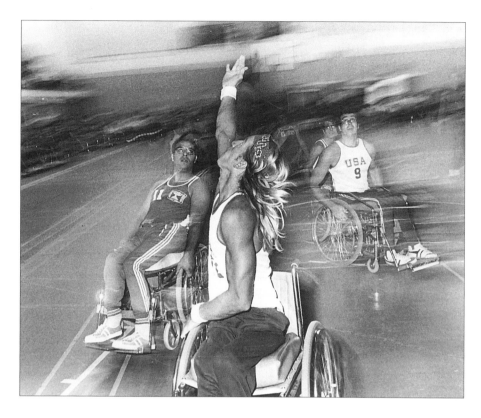

Many disabled people now actively improve the quality of their lives by keeping fit. Basketball players at the 1992 paraplegic games at Stoke Mandeville, England.

eliminated, the disease process halted, and, ultimately, death prevented? These questions can be succinctly and quantifiably answered. That treatments may successfully halt the disease but cause pain and distress, or that a surviving patient would really rather be dead are matters all but eclipsed by the grand imperative to treat and to save life at all costs.

It is hardly surprising that doctors' enthusiasm for using their power to intervene sometimes carries them beyond the wishes of their patients; centuries of medical impotence in the face of illness are still being exorcised. Only when the profession's love affair with its new-found potency had at last begun to cool did it become aware that patients were not always grateful to be kept alive, and were not always convinced that this operation or that course of drugs was really worth having if the price of a longer life was extra years of pain or discomfort.

A concern for quality of life began, formally, to edge its way back on to the agenda. But how to quantify it? Many solutions have been attempted, but most rely on scales of some kind ('On a scale of one to ten, how bad is this pain?') or on comparative rating of various disabilities ('Is it worse to lose an arm or a leg?'). One particularly ingenious attempt at combining quality and quantity of life in a single measurement is the quality-adjusted life year or QALY. This assumes that one year of healthy life is worth as much as two, three, or however many years spent in a state of disease or disability. The value to the patient and to the community of performing a particular medical procedure can then be judged in terms not of the extra years of life it yields, but of the extra number of QALYs. The difficulty, of course, is to establish the appropriate mathematical relationship between a calender year and a QALY.

This has been done by asking people to rate, on a scale from 0 to 100, the extent to which a range of disabilities would reduce their quality of life. Although this sounds disturbingly hit and miss, there are sophisticated methodologies for helping people to establish preferences among dozens or even hundreds of alternatives. The scores that have emerged provide the conversion factors required to translate calendar years into QALYs for a wide range of physical and mental disabilities.

QALYs are most obviously beneficial in evaluating treatment options for an individual: this is what you'll gain from procedure A, this from procedure B. When used by health planners to give priority to treatments they become more controversial. Critics claim, for example, that QALYs discriminate against the elderly. Advocates deny this, and argue that some kind of systematic approach to measuring quality of life is essential if health-care systems are to spend their money wisely.

As the need to curb rising health costs grows more pressing, it seems likely that explicit attempts will be made to take quality of life into account in decision-making. Either way, it is certain that quality of life will become an increasingly important concern in the medicine of the future.

An osteopath examines the back and spine by pressing and manipulating the spinal column and its associated muscles and joints to diagnose dysfunction and to alleviate pain and stiffness. Practitioners of complementary medicine are sometimes better than orthodox doctors at offering comfort in chronic illness and their services are increasingly being sought.

COMPLEMENTARY MEDICINE

Something similar will also be true of complementary medicine. The suspicion of science and of scientific medicine already referred to, and doctors' increasing preoccupation with the technology of their trade, have driven many patients in rich countries to search for methods of healing that they regard as more 'natural'. Doctors, proud of their high-tech gadgetry and their scientific interventions, are now reluctant to see themselves as healers. Yet healers – individuals who offer more than technical solutions to biological problems – are what many people obviously want.

The advent of science offered a new and firmer boundary in the traditional antagonism between approved and non-approved ways of practising medicine. Henceforth, anything scientifically acceptable became 'orthodox', anything not became 'unorthodox'. As the people of many Western countries became more and more enamoured of unorthodox therapies, so the medical establishment mounted periodic offensives designed to fend off the challenge. In great measure they have failed. Indeed, increasing numbers of doctors with an entirely orthodox training have begun to go over to the 'enemy', and to sympathize with the aspirations if not always the methods of the fringe.

Complementary medicine shows no signs of diminishing in public esteem, not least because one of its concerns is for the quality of patients' lives. Looking to the future, how is the rise of unorthodoxy to be regarded? In so far as it relies on unproven methods used by people with little training and less theory, and panders to irrational beliefs, it is to be deplored. And this, of course, is precisely how the medical establishment has chosen to portray it. In fact, this is only part of the truth, and probably a small part.

Some techniques – acupuncture, osteopathy, and chiropractic, for example – have come in from the fringe, and now command the respect of many doctors. Some practitioners of complementary medicine have come to see the logic of trying to establish the efficacy of their methods according to the standards of proof routinely demanded (in theory, at least) by orthodox medicine. The role of healer is one which many unorthodox practitioners are happy to adopt. And in assuming it they sometimes prove better than orthodox medicine at offering comfort in chronic illness, and solace when no treatment is effective. Enlightened doctors know this. And while it would be wrong to suggest that all tensions between the mainstream and the fringe have been or are likely to be overcome, naked antagonism is withering away. So here, too, orthodox medicine, albeit reluctantly, is showing itself able to accept the demands being made by the patients, and adapt accordingly.

SELF-HELP

A third development now helping to shape the future is the advent of patient self-help and support groups. All decisions about health and disease were once regarded by doctors as matters for them alone. Patients had a passive role; having been told what was the matter with them (and sometimes not even that) their only task was to obey whatever instructions the doctor throught fit to issue. But while denied autonomy in strictly medical decisions, they then had to cope alone with the everyday non-medical problems created by their illnesses. Attitudes towards doctors, at least in most developed countries, have changed much in the past few decades. Authoritarianism in medicine has been much eroded; many patients now expect to be advised rather than instructed on their treatment, and given an opportunity to express their own preferences when there is more than one possible course of action.

This climate did much to boost the creation of patient self-help groups. There are now hundreds of these bodies offering practical advice and emotional support to people with all manner of chronic and/or debilitating illnesses from agoraphobia and AIDS to vitiligo and vaccine damage. Often set up with the active assistance of doctors, they provide a forum through which patients can meet and pass on to each other the kind of practical tips that make the difference between coping with an illness, or being defeated by it. These groups will continue to flourish, and become an ever more central part of the response to illness.

UNIVERSAL MEDICINE

Scientific medicine, like the rest of science and technology, has proved itself the most international of all our practical and cultural achievements. The skill, the equipment, and the buildings in which doctors work vary greatly from place to place; but from Bombay to Bloemfontein to Buenos Aires the medicine they practise is recognizably the same. Go to China and you find an elaborate system of traditional medicine; go to India and you find Unani, Ayurveda, and many lesser known brands of healing; go to any developing country and you find systems of herbal medicine. But while all these practices co-exist with scientific medicine, it alone is ubiquitous.

Could there come a time when scientific medicine no longer occupies this dominant position, and some other system commands the global orthodoxy? This seems as improbable as science itself loosing its central role as the way in which we interpret the material world. Once science had emerged, it was soon impossible for medicine to do anything but throw in its lot with this new vision. And as long as science holds its current position, medicine will surely stay with it. Not bounded by it; that is one of its current weaknesses. But rooted, practically and intellectually, within it.

Reference guide to The Cambridge Illustrated History of *Medicine*

Chronology

Selected non-medical events appear in bold

BC

*c.*9000 **Early domestication of plants and animals – rise of new human diseases**

*c.*4000 **First urban centres (Mesopotamia)**

*c.*3000 **Writing invented**

*c.*650 Epilepsy described in Babylonian text

585 Thales of Miletus active; beginnings of Greek philosophy

430 'Plague' of Athens (to 427 BC)

428 **Birth of Plato**

420 Hippocrates of Cos active

399 **Death of Socrates**

384 Birth of Aristotle of Stagira

310 Praxagoras of Cos active

300 Alexandrian Museum and Library founded

*c.*200 Chinese herbal *Pen T'sao*

AD

23 Birth of Pliny the Elder, Roman writer on natural history

40 Celsus's *On Medicine*

60 Dioscorides active

*c.*110 Rufus and Soranus (both of Ephesus) active

129 Birth of Galen of Pergamum

140 Asclepieion of Pergamum rebuilt

165 Antonine 'plague' begins (to 169)

313 **Christianity legalized in Roman Empire**

330 **Constantinople founded as eastern capital of Roman Empire**

350 First hospitals in Eastern Roman Empire

390 Fabiola founds a hospital in Rome

512 Illustrated edition of Dioscorides's *De Materia Medica*

541 First plague pandemic (to 749) and Plague of Justinian (to 544)

610 **Byzantine Empire established**

618 **T'ang dynasty founded in China**

632 **Death of Mohammed**

650 Paul of Aegina active

700 Japan's 'age of plagues' begins

710 **Muslim invasion of Spain**

750 **Abbasid caliphate established in Baghdad**

800 **Charlemagne crowned Holy Roman Emperor**

*c.*850 Hunain ibn Ishaq's *More Questions and Answers*

900 ar-Razi (Rhazes) active

929 **Caliphate established at Córdoba**

979 **Sung dynasty reunites China**

1000 al-Zahrawi (Albucasis) active

1037 Death of Ibn Sina (Avicenna), author of *Canon of Medicine*

1066 **Norman conquest of England**

1080 School of Salerno (to 1200)

1095 **The Crusades (to 1278)**

1123 St Bartholomew's Hospital founded in London

1136 Pantokrator Hospital founded in Constantinople

1187 Death of Gerard of Cremona, translator of Ibn Sina's *Canon*

*c.*1200 Universities of Paris and Oxford founded

1204 **Latin crusaders sack Constantinople**

*c.*1250 First Islamic medical schools in Turkey; anatomy demonstrations at Salerno

1258 **Mongols sack Baghdad; end of Abbasid caliphate**

1275 **Marco Polo arrives in China**

1280 Death of Albertus Magnus ('Doctor universalis')

1284 Mansuri Hospital founded in Cairo

1288 S. Maria Nuova Hospital founded in Florence; death of Ibn an-Nafis, describer of the pulmonary circulation of blood

*c.*1315 First dissection of human corpse by Mondino dei Liuzzi in Bologna

1321 **Death of Dante**

1337 **Hundred Years' War between England and France begins (to 1453)**

1347 Black Death begins (ends 1352)

1363 Guy de Chauliac's *Grande Chirurgie*

1368 **Ming dynasty founded in China**

*c.*1400 Milan institutes a permanent health board

1415 **Portuguese capture Ceuta – beginning of European Expansion**

1424 First recorded regulations for midwives, Brussels

1453 **Ottoman Turks capture Constantinople; end of Byzantine Empire**

*c.*1455 **Gutenberg's Bible printed at Mainz**

1490 Galen's works first printed in Latin

1492 **Fall of Granada; Arabs and Jews expelled from Spain; Christopher Columbus crosses the Atlantic**

1495 Charles VIII's army infected with syphilis during the seige of Naples

1498 **Vasco da Gama sails to India via the Cape of Good Hope**

1500 **Pedro Alvares Cabral claims Brazil for Portugal**

*c.*1510 **African slaves first taken to the New World**

1519 **Magellan begins his circumnavigation of the world (to 1522); death of Leonardo da Vinci;** Thomas Linacre's translation of Galen's *Method of Healing*

1521 **Cortés leads Spanish overthrow of Aztec Empire**

1525 *Hippocratic Corpus* printed in Latin

1526 **Mughal dynasty founded in India**

1534 **Henry VIII of England breaks with Rome**

1540 The companies of Barbers and Surgeons unite in London

1541 Death of Paracelsus

1543 **Nicolaus Copernicus writes of a Sun-centred planetary system;** Andreas Vesalius publishes his great work on human anatomy, *De Humani Corporis Fabrica*

1546 Girolamo Fracastoro's *De Contagione et Contagiosis Morbis* – an early version of the germ theory of disease

1553 Michael Servetus, Spanish physician and theologian, burnt at the stake in Geneva

1559 Realdo Colombo's *De Re Anatomica*

1571 **Portuguese create colony in Angola**

1577 **Francis Drake sets out on his circumnavigation**

1584 **Sir Walter Raleigh sends first of three expeditions to the Americas**

1588 **Spanish Armada defeated**

1590 Death of French surgeon Ambroise Paré

1600 **English Dutch East Indies Company founded**

1601 **English Poor Law system established**

1602 **Japanese dynasty of Tokugawa shoguns begins rule (to 1868)**

1603 **Dutch East Indies Company founded;** Girolamo Fabrizio's study of veins;

1607 **First permanent English settlement in America – at Jamestown, Virginia**

1608 **French colonists found Quebec**

1610 First well-documented Caesarian section (in Germany)

1611 **Authorized 'King James' version of the Bible**

1616 **Death of Shakespeare**

1618 **Pilgrim Fathers leave for the New World in the *Mayflower***

1621 Robert Burton's *The Anatomy of Melancholy*

1628 William Harvey writes on the circulation of the blood

*c.*1630 Obstetrical forceps invented by Peter Chamberlen

1633 French clergyman, Vincent de Paul, founds the Daughters of Charity

1636 **First American university, Harvard College, founded**

1641 René Descartes' *Meditationes de Prima Philosophia*

1642 **Abel Tasman discovers Tasmania and New Zealand; death of Galileo**

1644 **End of Ming Dynasty in China and founding of Qing dynasty by the Manchus**

1647 First New World epidemic of yellow fever begins in Barbados

1648 Johannes Baptiste van Helmont's *Ortus Medicinae*

1653 Francis Glisson describes the liver

1658 **Aurangzeb, Moghul Emperor, begins rule in India**

1660 Robert Boyle's law on the relation between gas pressure and volume; Royal Society of London founded

1663 Marcello Malpighi writes on the lung

1665 Great Plague of London

1666 Thomas Sydenham writes on treating fevers; Acadèmie des Sciences founded in Paris

1672 Regnier de Graaf discovers structures in the ovary, called Graafian follicles after him

1677 Cinchona bark included in the *London Pharmacopoeia* as a fever treatment

1687 **Isaac Newton's *Principia Mathematica***

1690 John Locke's *Essay Concerning Human Understanding*

1701 In Constantinople, Giacomo Pylarini inoculates with smallpox; Yale University founded

1704 **Newton's *Opticks***

1705 Raymond Vieussens describes left ventricle of heart and course of coronary blood vessels

1707 **Death of Aurangzeb and decline of Moghul power in India**; pulse watch introduced by John Floyer

1708 Herman Boerhaave's *Institutiones Medicae*

1709 Great plague in Russia

1714 Gabriel David Fahrenheit constructs the mercury thermometer

1717 Giovanni Maria Lancisi suggests that malaria can be transmitted by mosquitoes; Lady Mary Wortley Montagu brings Turkish practice of smallpox inoculation to England

1721 Obstetrical forceps used by Jean Palfyn

1726 Stephen Hales measures blood pressure of the horse; Edinburgh University Medical School founded

1728 Pierre Fauchard describes how to fill a tooth

1729 **First performance of J. S. Bach's *St Matthew Passion***

1730 First tracheotomy for treatment of diphtheria performed by George Martine

1733 Stephen Hales in *Haemostaticks* describes his measurements of blood pressure; William Cheselden's *Osteographia*

1735 *Systema Naturae* **published by Linnaeus**

1736 First successful appendectomy performed by Claudius Amyand in France; American physician William Douglass describes scarlet fever

1741 Foundling Hospital in London opens

1745 The Company of Surgeons splits from the Barbers in London

1747 First textbook on physiology – Albrecht von Haller's *Primae Lineae Physiologiae*; James Lind discovers that citrus fruits cure scurvy

1748 John Fothergill describes diphtheria in his *Account of the Putrid Sore Throat*

1751 Large public mental institution (St Luke's) opens in London; Robert Whytt demonstrates that pupil contraction in response to light is a reflex motion

1752 William Smellie's *Theory and Practice or Treatise on Midwifery* – first scientific approach to obstetrics; René-Antoine Ferchault de Réaumur discovers that digestion is a chemical process

1753 James Lind's *Treatise of the Scurvy*

1754 First female medical doctor graduates from the University of Halle

1756 First description of casting models for false teeth by Philipp Pfaff

1759 Caspar Friedrich Wolff shows that specialized organs develop out of unspecialized tissue

1761 Leopold Auenbrugger develops percussion technique for diagnosing chest disorders

1763 First American medical society founded in New London, Connecticut

1765 John Morgan founds first American medical school at the College of Pennsylvania, Philadelphia

1766 Albrecht von Haller shows that nervous stimulation controls muscular action

1768 **James Cook charts coast of New Zealand and explores east coast of Australia (returns to England in 1771)**; Robert Whytt's *Observations on the Dropsy of the Brain* – first description of tuberculosis meningitis in children

1771 John Hunter's *The Natural History of the Human Teeth*

1772 **James Cook circumnavigates the southern oceans (to 1775)**; Antonio Scarpa discovers labyrinth of the ear

1773 Lazzaro Spallanzani discovers digestive action of saliva

1774 Joseph Priestley discovers oxygen; William Hunter's *Anatomy of the Human Gravid Uterus*; Franz Mesmer uses hypnosis as a medical treatment

1775 **American Declaration of Independence**; Percivall Pott suggests that environmental factors can cause cancer

1776 **Adam Smith's *The Wealth of Nations***; Matthew Dobson shows that the sweetness of diabetics' urine is caused by sugar; John Fothergill gives first clinical description of trigeminal neuralgia

1780 Luigi Galvani experiments with muscles and electricity

1781 Henry Cavendish determines the composition of water

1784 Goethe, the German poet, discovers human intermaxillary bone

1785 William Withering introduces digitalis

(from the foxglove) to cure dropsy

1789 **George Washington becomes first President of the USA; French Revolution begins**; Antoine-Laurent Lavoisier's *Traité elementaire de Chimie*

1793 Epidemic of yellow fever in Philadelphia; Matthew Baillie describes the appearance of each organ in the first English text on morbid anatomy

1794 Lavoisier guillotined

1795 Thomas Beddoes and Humphry Davy experiment with nitrous oxide, or 'laughing gas'; Sir Gilbert Blane makes use of lime juice mandatory in the British navy

1796 First vaccination against smallpox by Edward Jenner; C. W. Hufeland's *Macrobiotics, or the Art to Prolong One's Life*

1798 Thomas Malthus's *Essay on the Principles of Population*

1800 François Bichat studies postmortem changes in human organs; chlorine used to purify water; Davy makes nitrous oxide in quantity and suggests its use as an anaesthetic; Benjamin Waterhouse is first US physician to use smallpox vaccine

1801 Philippe Pinel advocates a more humane treatment of the insane; Thomas Young discovers the cause of astigmatism

1804 **Napoleon Bonaparte crowned Emperor of France; black republic established in Haiti**

1805 **Battle of Trafalgar**; morphine isolated by Frederick Sertürner

1807 **Slave trade abolished within the British Empire**

1809 First successful ovariotomy (without anaesthetic)

1810 Samuel Hahnemann introduces homeopathy

1811 Charles Bell's *New Anatomy of the Brain*

1812 Benjamin Rush's *Medical Inquiries and Observations upon the Diseases of the Mind*

1815 **Battle of Waterloo; giant eruption of Tambora volcano in Indonesia in April kills thousands of people and causes two cold summers in Europe and N. America**

1816 Stethoscope invented by René Laënnec

1817 First cholera pandemic begins; James Parkinson's *Essay on the shaking palsy*

1818 **Mary Shelley's *Frankenstein***

1821 Charles Bell describes facial paralysis

1822 **Liberia founded as colony for freed slaves**

1823 William Prout discovers hydrochloric acid in stomach secretions; *The Lancet* started

1824 Henry Hickman uses carbon dioxide on animals as a general anaesthetic; second cholera pandemic begins; Justus von Liebig appointed professor of chemistry at Giessen aged 21

1825 **First railway, from Stockton**

to **Darlington**; Pierre Bretonneau performs first tracheotomy

1826   Bretonneau describes symptoms of diphtheria

1827   Richard Bright describes kidney disease

1828   Friedrich Wöhler synthesizes urea

1829   Johann Schönlein describes haemophilia; scandal of William Burke and William Hare, who murdered to supply bodies for dissection

1830   Charles Bell distinguishes different types of nerves

1831   **Charles Darwin joins crew of HMS Beagle**; cholera epidemic starts in Europe; American chemist, Samuel Guthrie, discovers chloroform

1832   **Reform Bill in England**; Pierre-Jean Robiquet isolates codeine; Warburton Anatomy Act legalizes sale of bodies for dissection in England; Thomas Hodgkin describes cancer of the lymph nodes

1834   **New Poor Law in England**; amalgam used for filling teeth; Pierre Louis' *Essay on Clinical Instruction*

1837   **Victoria accedes to British throne**

1838   Registration Act (births, deaths, and marriages) in England

1839   Third cholera pandemic begins; Theodor Schwann defines the cell as the basic unit of animal structure

1840   **First Opium War between China and Britain**; the English quaker Elizabeth Fry founds the Institute of Nursing in London

1841   F. G. J. Henle publishes treatise on microscopic anatomy

1842   Edwin Chadwick's *Report on the Sanitary Conditions of the Labouring Population of Great Britain*

1844   Horace Wells uses nitrous oxide to pull one of his own teeth painlessly

1845   **First failure of Irish potato crop**

1846   **Smithsonian Institution established in Washington DC** (opened in 1855); William Morton uses ether as an anaesthetic at the Massachusetts General Hospital

1847   James Young Simpson uses chloroform to relieve the pain of childbirth; Karl Ludwig invents the kymograph

1848   First Public Health Act sets up General Board of Health in Britain, leading to local medical officers of health; Ignaz Semmelweis introduces antiseptic methods in Vienna

1849   In USA, Elizabeth Blackwell becomes first woman to qualify as a doctor in modern times; Thomas Addison describes anaemia

1851   Hermann von Helmholtz introduces the ophthalmoscope

1853   **David Livingstone's explorations in Africa begin**; smallpox vaccination made compulsory in England; John Snow administers chloroform to Queen Victoria for the birth of Prince Leopold

1854   **Crimean War begins (ends 1856)**; John Snow breaks the Broad Street pump in London

1855   Thomas Addison describes the hormone-deficiency disease that results from malfunctioning adrenal glands

1856   First synthetic dye – mauvine – made by William Perkin

1858   Medical Reform Act sets up Medical Register and General Medical Council in Britain; first edition of *Gray's Anatomy*; Rudolf Virchow's *Cellularpathologie* demonstrates that every cell is a product of another cell

1859   **Charles Darwin's *The Origin of Species***

1860   Nightingale Nursing School founded at St Thomas's Hospital, London

1861   **Outbreak of American Civil War**; Louis Pasteur discovers anaerobic bacteria

1863   Etienne-Jules Marey invents the sphygmograph; fourth cholera pandemic begins

1864   International Red Cross founded

1865   **End of American Civil War and of slavery in USA**; **Gregor Mendel's *Plant Hybridity***; Joseph Lister introduces phenol as a disinfectant in surgery

1866   Thomas Allbutt develops the clinical thermometer

1867   **Russian sells Alaska to USA**; **Dominion of Canada established**; first international medical congress in Paris

1869   **Suez Canal opens**; Jacques Reverdin describes skin-grafting; Sophia Jex-Blake matriculates in medicine at Edinburgh University (but university reverses decision in 1873)

1871   **Darwin's *Descent of Man***

1873   William Osler writes on blood platelets

1874   Louis Pasteur suggests placing instruments in boiling water to sterilize them; London School of Medicine for Women (later the Royal Free Hospital) opened by Sophia Jex-Blake

1875   Public Health Act passed in Britain

1876   **Alexander Graham Bell patents the telephone**; Robert Koch identifies the anthrax bacillus; Cruelty to Animals Act passed in Britain; connection between the pancreas and sugar diabetes discovered

1879   Patrick Manson discovers that mosquitoes transmit filariasis

1880   Charles Laveran isolates blood parasite that causes malaria

1881   Fifth cholera pandemic begins; Institute of Midwives established in London; Louis Pasteur devises a vaccine for anthrax

1882   **Eruption of Krakatoa in the Sunda Straits**; Robert Koch isolates the tubercle bacillus; operation for the removal of the gall bladder introduced

1883   Robert Koch discovers the cholera vibrio

1884   Elie Metchnikoff describes phagocytosis

1885   Louis Pasteur develops a rabies vaccine

1886   **Gold discovered in the Witwatersrand, South Africa**

1889   **Brazil ends Portuguese rule**; Johns Hopkins Hospital opens in Baltimore

1890   Emil von Behring and Shibasabura Kitasato develop vaccines against tetanus and diphtheria; William Halsted introduces surgical gloves

1893   Jean Charcot writes on the use of hypnotism; Daniel Williams performs first open-heart surgery in Chicago; Johns Hopkins Medical School founded

1894   **Nicholas II becomes last Tsar of Russia**; first use of diphtheria antitoxin in Britain, by Charles Sherrington

1895   Wilhelm Röntgen discovers X-rays; Elie Metchnikoff succeeds Louis Pasteur as director of Pasteur Institute in Paris

1896   Antoine Becquerel discovers radiation; Scipione Riva-Rocci invents device for measuring blood pressure

1897   Ronald Ross locates the malaria parasite in the *Anopheles* mosquito; first of seven volumes of Havelock Ellis's *Studies in the Psychology of Sex*

1898   Patrick Manson's *Tropical Diseases*; Pierre and Marie Curie obtain radium from pitchblende

1899   **Boer War begins (ends 1902)**; sixth cholera pandemic; London School of Hygiene and Tropical Medicine founded; aspirin introduced

1900   Sigmund Freud's *The Interpretation of Dreams*; Karl Landsteiner identifies four major human blood groups (A, O, B, and AB); US Army Yellow Fever Commission founded

1901   **Death of Queen Victoria**; first Nobel Prizes

1902   William Bayliss and Ernest Starling discover the hormone secretin; Registration of Midwives Act passed in Britain

1903   **Wright Brothers fly in petrol-powered aircraft**; Willem Einthoven describes the first electrocardiograph

1904   Rockefeller Institute for Medical Research founded in New York

1905   George Washington Crile performs first direct blood transfusion; J. B. Murphy develops first artificial hip joints

1906   Frederick Gowland Hopkins starts experiments on 'accessory food factors' (vitamins); Charles Sherrington's *The Integrative Action of the Nervous System*, a classic of neurology

1907   John Scott Haldane develops method for bringing divers to the surface safely

1908   Sulphanilamide first synthesized

1909   **Industrial production of plastics begins after Bakelite developed**; **Robert Peary and Matthew Hensen reach the North**

Pole; Archbibald Edward Garrod's *Inborn Errors of Metabolism*

1910 Paul Ehrlich announces his discovery of Salvarsan for syphilis – the beginning of modern chemotherapy

1911 **Roald Amundsen reaches the South Pole**; National Insurance Act sets up first state medical insurance scheme in Britain; William Hill develops the first gastroscope

1912 **The *Titanic* sinks on maiden voyage**; Harvey Cushing's *The Pituitary Gland and its Disorders*; Casimir Funk coins the term 'vitamin'

1913 John Jacob Abel develops first artificial kidney; establishment of Medical Research Committee (Council from 1920) in Britain

1914 **Outbreak of First World War; Panama Canal opens**; Alexis Carrel performs first successful heart surgery on a dog; Henry Dale discovers the neurotransmitter acetylcholine in ergot

1916 **Albert Einstein's *General Theory of Relativity***; Walter Gaskell names the involuntary nervous system; Margaret Sanger founds first American birth-control clinic in Brooklyn, New York; Mary Stopes's *Married Love*

1917 Carl Jung's *Psychology of the Unconscious*

1918 **End of First World War**; start of influenza pandemic

1919 **Ernest Rutherford splits the atom; first crossing of the Atlantic by air**

1920 **League of Nations set up**; establishment of Tavistock Clinic, first UK centre for the teaching and deployment of Freud's psychoanalytical ideas

1921 Marie Stopes opens her first birth-control clinic in London; F. G. Banting and C. H. Best isolate insulin

1922 **USSR established**

1923 **Turkish republic formed – end of Ottoman Empire**; Albert Calmette and Camille Guérin develop the BCG vaccine for tuberculosis

1926 First enzyme (urease) crystallized by American biochemist James B. Sumner

1927 Philip Drinker and Louis Shaw develop the 'iron lung'

1928 Alexander Fleming discovers penicillin in a mould; Albert Szent-Györgyi isolates vitamin C

1929 **Wall Street Crash**; Henry Dale and H. W. Dudley demonstrate chemical transmission of nerve impulses; Werner Forssmann develops cardiac catheter

1932 Armand Quick introduces a test to measure the clotting ability of blood; Gerhard Domagk discovers the first sulpha drug, Prontosil

1935 Development of prefrontal lobotomy to treat mental illness; first blood bank set up – in the USA at the Mayo Clinic, Rochester; Hans Zinsser's *Rats, Lice, and History*

1936 Ugo Cerletti describes electroconvulsive therapy

1937 Development of vaccine against yellow fever by Max Theiler and of first antihistamine by Daniel Daniel Bovet; Charles Dodds discovers a synthetic oestrogen (stilboestrol)

1938 New Zealand Social Security Act provides pioneering state medical service; John Wiles develops the first total artificial hip replacement, using stainless steel

1939 **Outbreak of Second World War**

1940 Howard Florey and Ernst Chain develop penicillin as an antibiotic; Karl Landsteiner discovers the Rhesus factor in blood

1941 Norman Gregg links rubella (German measles) in pregnancy and cataract and other abnormalities in children

1942 Report by William Beveridge paves way for the idea of a National Health Service in Britain

1943 Wilhelm Kolff develops first kidney dialysis machine; Selman Waksman discovers the antibiotic streptomycin

1944 Alfred Blalock performs first blue-baby operation

1945 **End of Second World War; beginning of Cold War**; fluoridation of water introduced in the USA to prevent tooth decay

1946 **First meeting of United Nations General Assembly in New York**; start of first randomized clinical trials of strepto-mycin for TB treatment

1948 World Health Organization (WHO) formed within the UN; National Health Service formed in Britain and National Institutes of Health in the USA; Philip Hench discovers that cortisone can be used for rheumatoid arthritis

1951 John Gibbon develops heart–lung machine and operates (1953) successfully using it

1952 Douglas Bevis develops amniocentesis; open-heart surgery begins with implanta-tion of artificial heart valves

1953 E. A. Graham and E. L. Wynder show that tobacco tars cause cancer in mice; James Watson and Francis Crick determine the double-helical structure of DNA

1954 First successful kidney transplant; plastic contact lenses produced

1957 **Treaty of Rome, leading to the establishment (1958) of the European Economic Community**; Albert Sabin develops a live polio vaccine; Clarence Lillehei devises first compact heart pacemaker

1958 Ian Donald uses ultrasound to diagnosis disorders of the foetus

1961 Seventh cholera pandemic begins

1962 **Cuban missile crisis**; lasers first used in eye surgery; thalidomide withdrawn

1963 Measles vaccine licensed for general use in USA; Thomas Starzl's first human liver transplant; the tranquillizer valium introduced

1964 **Outbreak of Vietnam War between N. Vietnam and USA (to 1973)**; home kidney dialysis introduced in the UK and USA

1966 **Cultural Revolution begins in China**

1967 Mammography for detecting breast cancer introduced; Christiaan Barnard performs human heart transplant; Rene Favaloro develops coronary bypass operation; Marburg virus disease recognized

1969 **Neil Armstrong lands on the Moon**; first attempt to use an artificial heart in a human; Patrick Steptoe and Robert Edwards announce the fertilization of human eggs outside the body

1972 Computerized axial tomography (CAT) introduced commercially for medical imaging; first showing of TV hospital drama, *MASH*, based in Korea

1976 Epidemics of Ebola virus disease in Sudan and Zaire

1978 First 'test-tube' baby born in England

1979 World declared free of smallpox

1980 Experimental vaccine against hepatitis B developed

1981 AIDS first recognized by US Centers for Disease Control

1983 First successful human embryo transfers

1986 Human Genome Project set up; gene for duchenne muscular dystrophy discovered

1991 **Collapse of USSR**

1994 The Americas are declared a polio-free zone

1995 WHO given license to develop and distribute Manual Patarroyo's malaria vaccine

Major human diseases

Disease	Cause	Means of transmission
acquired immuno-deficiency syndrome (AIDS)	viruses (HIV-1 and HIV-2)	sexual intercourse; blood products; intraveneous drug use; mother to child in the uterus
amoebic dysentery	amoeba (*Enteramoeba histolytica*)	ingestion in contaminated food and water
Argentine haemorrhagic fever	virus	disease of rodents; probably infects humans through direct contact, or food contaminated with rodent excreta
ascariasis	roundworm (*Ascaris*)	consumption of mature eggs in food or water contaminated with human faeces
beriberi	deficiency of thiamine	historically has affected those with diets centred on rice
Bolivian haemorrhagic fever	virus	disease of rodents that probably infects humans through contaminated food, water, and air
brucellosis	bacterium (*Brucella*)	contact with infected animals
Carrión's disease	bacterium (*Bartonella*)	bloodsucking sandflies
Chagas' disease (American trypanosomiasis)	protozoan (*Trypanosoma cruzi*)	harboured by animals; transmitted to humans by infected bugs
chickenpox (varicella)	virus	human to human
cholera	bacterium (*Vibrio cholerae*)	faecal–oral route, especially in contaminated water
dengue	arbovirus	infected female *Aedes* mosquitoes

Disease	Cause	Means of transmission
diphtheria	bacillus (*Corynebacterium diphtheriae*)	human to human
dracunculiasis (Guineaworm infection)	nematode worm (*Dracunculus medinensis*)	ingested in contaminated water
Ebola virus disease	virus	unsterilized needles and syringes, and other unknown routes
encephalitis lethargica (sleepy sickness)	virus	seems to accompany and follow epidemic influenza
ergotism	ergot fungus (*Claviceps purpurea*)	consumption of ergot-infected grain or grain products
erysipelas (St Anthony's fire)	bacterium (*Streptococcus*)	passed by infected humans through surgical instruments, wounds, and contact
filariasis (includes elephantiasis)	filarial nematode worms	infected mosquitoes
hepatitis A and B	virus	A by ingestion of infected food and water; B through infected blood
hookworm disease (anycylostomiasis)	nematode worms	penetration of the body, typically through the skin of the feet from infected soil
influenza (grippe)	virus	human to human (reservoirs in animals)
Lassa fever	virus	urine from rodents, then human to human
leishmaniasis	protozoan (*Leishmania*)	bloodsucking sandflies
leprosy	bacillus (*Mycobacterium leprae*)	human to human after prolonged contact

Disease	Cause	Means of transmission
leptospirosis (Weil's disease)	spirochaete bacteria (*Leptospira*)	contact with infected animals, especially their urine
malaria	protozoans (*Plasmodium*)	bite of infected female mosquitoes, especially *Anopheles*
Marburg virus disease	virus	apparently through the blood of infected monkeys or humans
measles (rubeola)	virus	human to human
mumps	virus	human to human
onchocerciasis (river blindness)	filarial nematode worms (*Onchocerca*)	blood-feeding flies
pellagra	deficiency of niacin (vitamin B_3)	historically has affected those with diets centred on maize
pinta	spirochaete bacteria (*Treponema*)	skin-to-skin contact
plague	bacterium (*Yersinia pestis*)	bite of a flea from an infected host, usually a rat
poliomyelitis (polio)	virus	faecal–oral route
protein-energy malnutrition	usually weaning to low-protein diet	mostly affects children in the developing world; worsened by infection
relapsing fever	spirochaete bacteria (*Borrelia*)	lice and ticks
Rift Valley fever	viruses	bloodsucking sandflies
Rocky Mountain spotted fever	rickettsia	ticks
rubella (German measles)	virus	human to human
scarlet fever	bacteria (*Streptococcus*)	close human contact

Disease	Cause	Means of transmission
schistosomiasis (bilharziasis)	trematode worm (*Schistosoma*)	penetration of the skin in contaminated water
scurvy	deficiency of ascorbic acid (vitamin C)	affects those on diets lacking fresh fruits and vegetables, such as sailors
sleeping sickness (African trypanosomiasis)	protozoan (*Trypanosoma brucei*)	bite of a tsetse fly
smallpox (variola)	poxvirus	airborne droplets, human to human
syphilis (venereal)	spirochaete bacteria (*Treponema*)	sexual intercourse or from mother to child in the uterus
syphilis (non-venereal)	(same as above)	human (usually children) to human through mucous membranes
tetanus (lockjaw)	bacterium (*Clostridum*)	through wounds
trachoma	bacterium (*Chlamydia trachomatis*)	from eye to eye via the fingers; by eye-seeking flies; from mother to baby
trichinosis	nematode worm (*Trichinella spiralis*)	consumption of under-cooked meat, usually pork
tuberculosis	bacillus (*Mycobacterium*)	human to human
tularaemia (rabbit fever)	bacterium (*Francisella tularensis*)	contact with infected animals
typhoid and paratyphoid	bacteria (*Salmonella*)	faecal–oral route
typhus (ship fever, prison fever)	rickettsia	bite of fleas, lice, and mites
whooping cough	bacterium (*Bordetella pertussis*)	mainly airborne
yellow fever	virus	bite of infected mosquitoes, especially *Aedes*

Notes

Introduction (pp. 6–15)

1 Lord Horder, 'Whither medicine', *British Medical Journal* vol. i (1949), pp. 557–60 (quote p. 58).

2 Lewis Thomas, 'Biomedical science and human health – the long-range prospects'. Paper presented at a Festschrift in honour of Dr Otto Westphal, Freiberg, 1 February 1978.

Chapter 2 (pp. 52–81)

1 Quoted in J. V. Kinnier Wilson and E. H. Reynolds, 'A Babylonian treatise on epilepsy, *Medical History* vol. 34 (1990), p. 192.

2 Quoted in H. E. Sigerist, *A History of Medicine I: Primitive and Archaic Medicine* (New York, Oxford University Press, 1951), p. 324.

3 Ibid., p. 334.

4 The Hippocratic Corpus, *Epidemics* vol. I, ch. 11 (*c.* 410 BC).

5 J. Chadwick and N. Mann (transl.), *The Medical Works of Hippocrates* (Oxford, Blackwell, 1950), p. 67.

6 Galen, *On Diseases Hard to Cure* (*c.* AD 180); extract transl. from M. Meyerhof, 'Arabische Bruchstücke Galens', *Südhoffs Archiv* vol. 22 (1929), p. 83.

7 Galen, *On Examining a Physician* (*c.* AD 177), ed. A. Z. Iskandar (Berlin, Akademie Verlag, 1988), p. 65.

8 Lapo Mazzei, *Advice in Time of Plague* (1401); extract in I. Origo (ed.), *The Merchant of Prato* (London, Penguin Books, 1963), p. 309.

9 Margery Kempe, *The Book of Margery Kempe* (Penguin Books, 1985); quoted by R. Porter, *A Social History of Medicine* (London, Weidenfeld & Nicolson, 1987), p. 108.

Chapter 3 (pp. 82–117)

1 Quoted in Timothy P. Weber, 'The Baptist tradition', in Ronald L. Numbers and D. W. Amundsen (eds), *Caring and Curing: Health and Medicine in the Western Religious Tradition* (New York, Macmillan, 1986), p. 291.

2 Quoted in Richard Palmer, 'The Church, leprosy and the plague in Medieval and Early Modern Europe', in W. J. Sheils (ed.), *The Church and Healing* (Oxford, Basil Blackwell, for the Ecclesiastical History Society, 1982), pp. 79–100 (quote p. 97).

3 W. H. S. Jones (transl.), 'The sacred disease', in *Hippocrates* (London, Heinemann, 1923), vol. 2, p. 141.

4 N. D. Jewson, 'The disappearance of the sick man from medical cosmology, 1770–1870', *Sociology* vol. 10 (1976), pp. 225–44.

5 Michaela Reid, *Ask Sir James* (London,

Hodder & Stoughton, 1987), p. 201.

6 R. Latham and W. Matthews (eds), *The Diary of Samuel Pepys*, 11 vols (London, Bell & Hyman, 1970–83), vol. 3, p. 237.

7 Ibid., vol. 5, p. 359.

8 Barbara Duden, *The Woman Beneath the Skin: A Doctor's Patients in Eighteenth-Century Germany*, transl. Thomas Dunlop (Cambridge, MA, Harvard University Press, 1991), pp. 89–90.

9 E. L. Griggs (ed.), *Collected Papers of Samuel Taylor Coleridge*, vol. I (Oxford, Clarendon Press, 1965), p. 256: Coleridge to Charles Lloyd, Sr., 14 November 1796.

10 Gustav Broun, 'The amputation of the clitoris and labia minora: a contribution to the treatment of vaginismus'; transl. from the German by Jeffrey Moussaieff Masson in *A Dark Science: Women, Sexuality, and Pyschiatry in the Nineteenth Century* (New York, The Noonday Press, 1988), pp. 128–38.

11 Thomas Beddoes, *Essay on the Causes, Early Signs, and Prevention of Pulmonary Consumption for the Use of Parents and Preceptors* (Bristol, 1799), p. 6.

12 Quoted in Susan Sontag, *Illness as Metaphor* (London, Allen Lane, 1979), p. 29.

13 Quoted in W. S. Lewis (ed.), *The Yale Edition of Horace Walpole's Correspondence*, 48 vols (New Haven, Yale University Press, 1937–83), vol. 25, p. 402.

14 Quoted in R. W. Chapman (ed.), *The Letters of Samuel Johnson*, 3 vols (Oxford, Clarendon Press, 1952), letter 891, vol. 3, p. 81.

15 Quoted in J. W. Warter (ed.), *Southey's Common-Place Book* (London, Longman, 1831), p. 551.

16 'Bec's birthday', in Harold Williams (ed.), *The Poems of Jonathan Swift*, 3 vols (Oxford, Clarendon Press, 1937), vol. 2, p. 761.

17 Edward Shorter, *From Paralysis to Fatigue: A History of Psychosomatic Illness in the Modern Era* (New York, Free Press, 1992).

18 W. H. Helfand, 'James Morison and his pills', *Transactions of the British Society of the History of Pharmacy* vol. 1 (1974), pp. 101–35.

19 Charles E. Rosenberg and Janet Golden (eds), *Framing Disease: Studies in Cultural History* (New Brunswick, NJ, Rutgers University Press, 1992).

Chapter 4 (pp. 118–53)

1 [George] Bernard Shaw, Preface (1911) to *The Doctor's Dilemma: A Tragedy* (Harmondsworth, Penguin, 1946), p. 76.

2 William Buchan, *Domestic Medicine: Or, A*

Treatise on the Prevention and Cure of Disease, 10th edn (London, 1788; first published 1769), pp. 162–3.

3 Adolf Kussmaul, *Jugenderinnerungen* (Stuttgart, 1922), pp. 222–3.

4 W. Brockbank and F. Kenworthy (eds), *The Diary of Richard Kay, 1716–51, of Baldingstone, near Bury: A Lancashire Doctor* (Manchester, Chetham Society, 1968), pp. 162–4.

5 Arthur E. Hertzler, *The Horse and Buggy Doctor* (New York, 1938), p. 117.

6 Isabella Beeton, *The Book of Household Management* (London, 1861), p. 1065.

7 Samuel Gross, *Then and Now: A Discourse Introductory to the Forty-Third Course of Lectures in the Jefferson Medical College of Philadelphia* (Philadelphia, 1867), p. 30.

8 Richard H. Shryock, 'Selections from the Letters of Richard D. Arnold, M. D., *Johns Hopkins Hospital Bulletin* no. 42 (1928), pp. 156–71 (quote p. 164).

9 James B. Herrick, *Memoirs of Eighty Years* (Chicago, University of Chicago Press, 1949), pp. 100–1.

10 Edward Sutleffe, *Medical and Surgical Cases: Selected During a Practice of Thirty-eight Years* (London, 1824), pp. 409–10.

11 Benjamin Rush, 'Observations and reasoning in medicine' (1791), in Dagobert D. Runes (ed.), *The Selected Writings of Benjamin Rush* (New York, Philosophical Library, 1947), p. 249.

12 William Douglass, *A Summary, Historical and Political, of the . . . Present State of the British Settlements in North America*, 2 vols (Boston, 1755), vol. 2, pp. 351–2.

13 John Burns, *Dissertation on Inflammation*, 2 vols (Glasgow, 1800), vol. 1, pp. 117–20.

14 *The Spectator in Four Volumes* (London, Dent, 1945), vol. 1, (24 March 1711), pp. 64–5 .

15 D[aniel] W. Cathell, *The Physician Himself and What He Should Add to the Strictly Scientific* (Baltimore, 1882), p. 139.

16 Q. J. C. Yeatman, quoted in I. S. L. Loudon, 'The origin of the general practitioner', *Journal of the Royal College of General Practitioners* vol. 33 (1933), pp. 13–18.

17 Karl Stern, *The Pillar of Fire* (New York, Harcourt, 1951), pp. 102–3.

18 Hertzler, *Horse and Buggy Doctor* (1938), op. cit. (note 5), pp. 101-10.

19 D[aniel] W. Cathell, *Book on the Physician Himself from Graduation to Old Age*, Crowning edn (Philadelphia, 1924), p. 132.

20 A. Conan Doyle, 'A false start', in *Round the*

Red Lamp, Being Facts and Fancies of Medical Life (1894), 14th edn (London, 1912), pp. 61–2.

21 Hertzler, *Horse and Buggy Doctor* (1938), op. cit. (note 5), p. 9.

22 William Victor Johnston, *Before the Age of Miracles: Memoirs of a Country Doctor* (Toronto, Fitzhenry and Whiteside, 1972), p. 58.

23 Quoted in Walter Rivington, *The Medical Profession* (London, 1879), pp. 338–9.

24 Anon, 'St Bartholomew's Hospital: Casualty Department', *The Lancet* vol. i (11 January 1879), pp. 59–60 (quote p. 60).

25 Joseph McDowell Mathews, *How to Succeed in the Practice of Medicine* (Philadelphia, 1905), p. 133.

26 George T. Welch, 'Therapeutical superstition', *Medical Record* vol. 44 (8 July 1893), pp. 33–8 (quote p. 35).

27 Thomas Hall Shastid, *My Second Life* (Ann Arbor, 1944), pp. 40-1.

28 Alfred T. Schofield, *Behind the Brass Plate: Life's Little Stories* (London, 1928), p. 111.

29 A. Conan Doyle, *The Stark Munro Letters* (London, 1895), p. 208.

30 Robert I. Lee and Lewis Webster Jones, *The Fundamentals of Good Medical Care* (Chicago, 1922; Publications of the Committee on the Costs of Medical Care, no. 22), p. 244.

31 James Mackenzie, *The Future of Medicine* (London, 1919), p. 171.

32 Quoted in Erna Lesky, *Die Wiener Medizinische Schule im 19. Jahrhundert* (Graz: Böhlau, 1978), pp. 146–7.

33 Cathell, *The Physician Himself* (1882), op. cit. (note 15), p. 18.

34 William N. Macartney, *Fifty Years a Country Doctor* (New York, 1938), p. 56.

35 Herrick, *Memoirs of Eighty Years* (1949), op. cit.(note 9), p. 105.

36 W. Burton Wood, 'Pulmonary tuberculosis in general practice', *The Lancet* vol. ii (4 October 1930), pp. 726–30.

37 Cathell, *Book on the Physician Himself* (1924), op. cit. (note 19), pp. 187–8.

38 Bernhard Naunyn, *Erinnerungen, Gedanken und Meinungen* (Munich, 1925), p. 516.

39 Jacob Bigelow, 'On the medical profession and quackery' (1844), in Bigelow, *Modern Inquiries: Classical, Professional, and Miscellaneous* (Boston, 1867), pp. 199–215 (quote p. 214).

40 Oliver Wendell Holmes, 'Currents and counter-currents in medical science' (1860), in Holmes, *Medical Essays, 1842–1882* (Boston, 1911), pp. 173–208 (quotes pp. 184, 203–4).

41 William Osler, *The Principles and Practice of Medicine* (New York, 1892), p. 75.

42 Hertzler, *Horse and Buggy Doctor* (1938), op. cit. (note 5), pp. 99–100.

43 Max Neuburger, *Hermann Nothnagel: Leben und Wirken eines deutschen Klinikers* (Vienna, 1922), pp. 146, 159, 162, 406, n. 20.

44 [Autobiography] *Barney Sachs, 1854–1944* (New York: privately printed, 1949), p. 48.

45 Quoted in C[larence] B. Farrar, 'The four doctors', in *Proceedings of the Seventh Annual Psychiatric Institute, September 16, 1959* (Princeton: New Jersey, 1959), pp. 105–16 (quote p. 110).

46 C.B.F. [Clarence B. Farrar], 'I remember Osler, Psychotherapist', *American Journal of Psychiatry* vol. 121 (1965), pp. 761–2 (quote p. 762).

47 Lewellys F. Barker, *Time and the Physician* (New York, 1942), p. 270.

48 G[eorge] Canby Robinson, *The Patient as a Person: A Study of the Social Aspects of Illness* (New York, 1939), pp. 9–10, 410–14.

49 Francis Weld Peabody, *The Care of the Patient* (Cambridge, 1927), p. 34.

50 William R. Houston, *The Art of Treatment* (New York, 1936), pp. 72, 74.

51 Cathell, *Book on the Physician Himself* (1924), op. cit. (note 19), pp. 63–4.

52 Guy de Maupassant, *Mont-Oriol* (Paris: Gallimard, 1976; first publ. 1887), p. 238.

53 Joseph S. Collings, 'General practice in England today: a reconnaisaance', *The Lancet* vol. i (25 March 1950), pp. 555–85 (quote p. 577).

54 Rivington, *The Medical Profession* (1879), op. cit. (note 23), p. 54.

55 Wilmot Herringham, 'The consultant', *British Medical Journal* vol. 2 (10 July 1920), pp. 36–8 (quote p. 36).

56 John Brotherston, 'Evolution of medical practice', in Gordon McLachlan and Thomas McKeown (eds), *Medical History and Medical Care* (London, Oxford University Press, 1971), pp. 87–125 (quote p. 108).

57 Cathell, *Book on the Physician Himself* (1924), op. cit.(note 19), p. 33.

58 Naunyn, *Erinnerungen* (1925), op. cit. (note 38), pp. 164–5.

59 Macartney, *Fifty Years a Country Doctor* (1938), op. cit. (note 34), pp. 75–8.

60 Ralph W. Tuttle, 'The other side of country practice', *New England Journal of Medicine* vol. 199 (1 November 1928), pp. 874–7 (quote p. 876).

61 W. Stanley Sykes, *A Manual of General Medical Practice* (London, 1927), pp. 54–5.

62 Keith Hodgkin, *Towards Earlier Diagnosis in Primary Care* (1963), 4th edn (Edinburgh, Churchill Livingstone, 1978), p. ix.

63 J. M. Last, 'The iceberg: "Completing the clinical picture" in general practice', *The Lancet* vol. ii (6 July 1963), pp. 28–31 (quote p. 30).

64 Sykes, *A Manual of General Medical Practice* (1927), op. cit. (note 61), p. 2.

65 John H. Budd, 'Art vs. science in medicine: a look at public perception of physicians', *Postgraduate Medicine*, vol. 69 (1981), pp. 13–19 (quote p. 15).

66 Herrick, *Memoirs of Eighty Years* (1949), op. cit. (note 9), p. 103. Herrick was present at the scene, involving an unnamed family physician.

Chapter 5 (pp. 154–201)

1 Roger French, *William Harvey's Natural Philosophy* (Cambridge, Cambridge University Press, 1994), p. 78.

2 Andrew Wear (ed.), *William Harvey: The Circulation of the Blood* (London, Dent, 1990), p. 3.

3 Friedrich Hoffmann, *Fundamenta Medicinae*, transl. and introduced by Lester S. King (London, MacDonald, 1971; first published 1695), p. 5.

4 Quoted in A. C. Corcoran, *A Mirror up to Medicine* (Philadelphia, J.B. Lippincott, 1961), p. 60.

5 Quoted in W. F. Bynum, *Science and the Practice of Medicine in the Nineteenth Century* (New York, Cambridge University Press, 1994), p. 98.

6 Ross Ronald, *Memoirs, with a Full Account of the Great Malaria Problem and its Solution* (London, John Murray, 1923), pp.223–4.

7 Quoted in Corcoran, *A Mirror up to Medicine* (1961), op. cit. (note 4), p. 261.

8 Thomas Lewis, 'The Huxley Lecture on clinical science within the university', *British Medical Journal* vol. 1 (1935), pp. 631–6.

Chapter 6 (pp. 202–45)

1 Jerome, *The Principal Works of Jerome*, transl. by the Hon. W. H. Freemantle (Oxford, James Parker; New York, The Christian Literature Co., 1893), p. 190.

2 Quoted in W. B. Howie, 'Medical education in eighteenth-century hospitals', *Scottish Society for the History of Medicine, Report Proceedings* (1969–70), pp. 27–46 (quote pp. 41–2).

3 Quoted in Toby Gelfand, '"Invite the philosopher, as well as the charitable"; hospital teaching as private enterprise in Hunterian London', in W. F. Bynum and R. Porter (eds), *William Hunter and the Eighteenth-Century Medical World* (Cambridge, Cambridge University Press, 1985), pp. 129–52 (quote p. 146).

4 Quoted in R. Porter, *Doctor of Society: Thomas Beddoes and the Sick Trade in Late Enlightenment England* (London, Routledge, 1991), p. 77.

5 J. Hemlow (ed.). *The Journals and Letters of Fanny Burney (Madame D'Arblay)*, 12 vols (Oxford, Clarendon Press, 1972–84), vol. 6, p. 598f.

6 Sir William Osler, 'The nurse and the patient', in *Aequanimitas and Other Addresses*, 2nd edn (London, H. K. Lewis, 1906), p. 163.

Chapter 7 (pp. 246–77)

1   Quoted in Wilfrid Blunt and Sandra Raphael, *The Illustrated Herbal* (London, Frances Lincoln, n.d.), p. 20.

2   Charles Singer, 'The herbal in antiquity', *Journal of Hellenic Studies* vol. 47 (1927), pp. 1–52 (quote p.22).

3   E. Stone, 'An account of the success of the bark of the willow in the cure of Agues', *Philosophical Transactions of the Royal Society* vol. 53 (1763), pp. 195–200.

4   Anonymous, 'Yo-Ho-Ho. Pulv. Ipecac. Co. (Dover's Powder', in *Round the Fountain* (London, St Bartholomew's Hospital Medical Journal, 1923).

5   *The Journal of Joseph Banks in the* Endeavour, with a commentary by A. M. Lysaght (Guildford, Genesis Publications, 1980), pp. 213–14.

6   Ibid., between pp. 214 and 215.

7   Victoria Glendinning, *Trollope* (London, Pimlico, 1993), p. 63.

8   Sir William Osler, 'Teaching and thinking'; address given at McGill Medical School in 1894, reprinted in *Aequanimatas,* 3rd edn (London, H. K. Lewis, 1941), pp. 119–29 (quote p. 121).

9   *The Lancet* vol. i (1853), p. 453.

10 Quoted by H. H. Dale, in 'Acetylcholine as a chemical transmitter of the effects of nerve impulses', *Journal of the Mount Sinai Hospital* vol. 4 (1937–8), pp. 401–29.

11 James Lind, Preface to *A Treatise on the Scurvy* (London, 1753).

Chapter 8 (pp. 278–303)

1   Aretaeus the Cappadocian, *The Extant Works,* ed. and transl. by Francis Adams (London, The Sydenham Society, 1856).

2   William Pargeter, *Observations on Maniacal Disorders* (Reading, for the author, 1792), p. 31.

3   William Perfect, *Select Cases in the Different Species of Humanity* (Rochester, 1787), pp. 1–4.

4   John Locke, *An Essay Concerning Human Understanding,* ed. by P. H. Nidditch (Oxford, Clarendon Press, 1975), pp. 160–1.

5   Samuel Tuke, *Description of the Retreat, an Institution Near York for Insane Persons of the Society of Friends,* facsimile of the 1813 edn, ed. by R. Hunter and I. Macalpine (London, Dawsons, 1964), pp. 146–7.

6   C. Dickens and W. H. Wills, *A Curious Dance Around a Curious Tree* (1852); reprinted in *Charles Dickens' Uncollected Writings from Household Words* (Bloomington, Indiana University Press, 1968), vol. 2, pp. 281–91.

7   U. Cerletti, 'Electroshock therapy', in F.

Marti-Ibanez, A. M. Sackler, M. Sackler, and R. Sackler (eds), *The Great Physiodynamic Therapies in Psychiatry: An Historic Appraisal* (New York, Hoeber-Harper, 1956), pp. 93–4.

8   Jimmie Laing and Dermot McQuarrie, *Fifty Years in the System* (Edinburgh, Mainstream, 1989), p. 89.

9   Thomas S. Szasz, *The Myth of Mental Illness: Foundations of a Theory of Personal Conduct,* rev. edn (New York, Harper and Row, 1974), p. 1.

Chapter 9 (pp. 304–41)

1   George Eliot, *Middlemarch: A Study of Provincial Life* (London, Dent in Everyman's Library; first published 1871–2), pp. 149-50.

2   W. Rivington, *The Medical Profession* (Dublin and London, 1879), pp. 135–6.

Chapter 10 (pp. 342–72)

1   Frank Macfarlane Burnet, *Genes, Dreams and Realities* (Aylesbury, Medical & Technical Publishing, 1971).

2   Maurice King, 'Health is a sustainable state', *The Lancet* vol. 336, pp. 664–7 (1990).

3   Ian Kennedy, *The Unmasking of Medicine* (London: Allen & Unwin, 1981), p. 26.

4   Julius Comroe and Robert Dripps, 'Scientific basis for the support of biomedical science', *Science* vol. 192, pp. 105–11 (1976).

Further Reading

General and reference works

Ackerknecht, E. H., *A Short History of Medicine* (Baltimore, Johns Hopkins University Press, 1968). Probably the best brief history.

Ackerknecht, E. H., *Therapeutics from the Primitives to the Twentieth Century* (New York, Hafner, 1973).

Brieger, Gert H., 'History of medicine', in Paul T. Durbin (ed.), *A Guide to the Culture of Science, Technology and Medicine* (New York, Free Press, 1980), pp. 121–96.

Bynum, W. F., 'Health, disease and medical care', in G. S. Rousseau and R. Porter (eds), *The Ferment of Knowledge* (Cambridge, Cambridge University Press, 1980), pp. 211–54.

Bynum, W. F. and Porter, Roy (eds), *Companion Encyclopedia of the History of Medicine*, 2 vols (London, Routledge, 1993). The most up-to-date work of reference.

Castiglioni, Arturo, *A History of Medicine*, transl. and edited by E. B. Krumbhaar (New York, Alfred A. Knopf, 1941).

Clarke, Edwin, *Modern Methods in the History of Medicine* (London, Athlone Press, 1971).

Conrad, Lawrence et al., *The Western Medical Tradition: 800 BC to AD 1800* (Cambridge, Cambridge University Press, 1995).

Garrison, Fielding H., *An Introduction to the History of Medicine* (Philadelphia, Saunders, 1960; first published 1917).

Howells, John G. and Osborn, M. Livia, *A Reference Companion to the History of Abnormal Psychology*, 2 vols (London, Greenwood Press, 1984).

Illich, I., *Limits to Medicine: The Expropriation of Health* (London, Marion Boyars, 1976; paperback edition, Penguin, 1977).

Jordanova, L. J. 'The social sciences and history of science and medicine', in P. Corsi and P. Weindling (eds), *Information Sources in the History of Science and Medicine* (London, Butterworth Scientific, 1983), pp. 81–98.

Kiple, Kenneth F. (ed.) *The Cambridge World History of Human Diseases* (Cambridge, Cambridge University Press, 1993).

Magner, Lois N., *A History of Medicine* (New York, Marcel Dekker, 1992).

McGrew, Roderick E., *Encyclopedia of Medical History* (New York, McGraw-Hill, 1985). An extremely useful work of reference.

McKeown, T., *The Role of Medicine: Dream, Mirage or Nemesis?* (London, Nuffield Provincial Hospitals Trust, 1976; Princeton, Princeton University Press, 1979; Oxford, Blackwell, 1979).

Morton, L. T., *A Medical Bibliography (Garrison and Morton): An Annotated Checklist of Texts Illustrating the History of Medicine,* 4th edn (Aldershot, Hants, Gower, 1983).

Neuburger, Max, *History of Medicine*, transl. by Ernest Playfair, 2 vols (London, H. Frowde, 1910–25).

Olby, R. C., Cantor, G. N., Christie, J. R. R., and Hodge, M. J. S. (eds), *Companion to the History of Modern Science* (London, Routledge, 1989).

Payer, Lynn, *Disease-Mongers: How Doctors, Drug Companies, and Insurers are Making You Feel Sick* (New York, Wiley, 1992).

Pelling, Margaret, 'Medicine since 1500', in P. Corsi and Paul Weindling (eds), *Information Sources in the History of Science and Medicine* (London, Butterworth Scientific, 1983), pp. 379–407.

Shryock, Richard H., *The Development of Modern Medicine: An Interpretation of the Social and Scientific Factors*, 2nd edn (New York, Alfred A. Knopf, 1947; reprinted Madison, University of Wisconsin Press, 1980). A dated but highly stimulating work.

Sigerist, Henry E., *Civilization and Disease* (Ithaca, Cornell University Press, 1943; reprinted Chicago, University of Chicago Press, 1962).

Sigerist, Henry E., *A History of Medicine I: Primitive and Archaic Medicine* (New York, Oxford University Press, 1951).

Sigerist, Henry E., *A History of Medicine II: Early Greek, Hindu and Persian Medicine* (New York, Oxford University Press, 1961).

Singer, Charles and Underwood, E. Ashworth, *A Short History of Medicine* (Oxford, Clarendon Press, 1928; 2nd edn, New York, Oxford University Press, 1962).

Sournia, Jean-Charles, *The Illustrated History of Medicine* (London, Harold Starke, 1992). Very finely illustrated.

Temkin, O., *The Double Face of Janus and Other Essays in the History of Medicine* (Baltimore, Johns Hopkins University Press, 1977).

Walton, John, Beeson, Paul B. and Bodley Scott, Ronald (eds), *The Oxford Companion to Medicine*, 2 vols (Oxford, Oxford University Press, 1986).

Webster, Charles, 'The historiography of medicine', in P. Corsi and P. Weindling (eds), *Information Sources in the History of Science and Medicine* (London, Butterworth Scientific, 1983), pp. 29–43.

Contemporary research in the history of medicine is comprehensively listed in two ongoing publications: *Bibliography of the History of Medicine*, no. 1– (Bethesda, National Library of Medicine, 1965–), an annual with quinquennial cumulations; and *Current Work in the History of Medicine. An International Bibliography* (Wellcome Institute for the History of Medicine, London, 1954–). A cumulation of *Current Work*, and most secondary literature of the twentieth century until 1977, is listed in the Wellcome Institute for the History of Medicine's, *Subject Catalogue of the History of Medicine*, 18 vols (subject section, 9 vols, biographical section, 5 vols, topographical section, 4 vols (Munich, Krays International, 1980). Material since 1977 is listed on card files and on computer in the Wellcome Library.

The history of disease (Chapter 1)

Ackerknecht, Erwin H., *History and Geography of the Most Important Diseases* (New York, Hafner, 1965).

Akroyd, W. R., *Conquest of Deficiency Diseases* (Geneva, World Health Organization, 1970).

Anderson, Roy M. and May, Robert M., *Infectious Diseases of Humans: Dynamics and Control* (Oxford, Oxford University Press, 1991).

Ashburn, P. M., *The Ranks of Death: A Medical History of Conquest of America* (New York, Coward-McCann, 1947).

Burnet, Sir Macfarlane, *Natural History of Infectious Disease*, 3rd edn (Cambridge, Cambridge University Press, 1962).

Cartwright, Frederick F., *Disease and History* (New York, Thomas Y. Crowell, 1972).

Cohen, Mark Nathan, *The Food Crisis in Prehistory: Overpopulation and the Origins of Agriculture* (New Haven and London, Yale University Press, 1977).

Crosby, Alfred W., *Ecological Imperialism: The Biological Expansion of Europe, 900–1900* (Cambridge and New York, Cambridge University Press, 1986).

Crosby, Alfred W., *The Columbian Exchange: Biological and Cultural Consequences of 1492* (Westport, CT, Greenwood Press, 1972).

Dobyns, Henery F., *Their Numbers Become Thinned* (Knoxville, University of Tennessee Press, 1983).

Dubos, René and Dubos, Jean, *The White Plague: Tuberculosis, Man, and Society* (Boston, Little Brown, 1952).

Fiennes, Richard, *Zoonoses of Primates: The Epidemiology and Ecology of Simian Diseases in Relation to Man* (Ithaca, Cornell University Press, 1979).

Harrison, Gordon A., *Mosquitoes, Malaria, and Man* (New York, Dutton, 1978).

Henschen, Folke, *The History and Geography of Diseases*, transl. by Joan Tate (New York, Delacorte Press, 1962).

Hoeppli, Reinhard, *Parasitic Diseases in Africa and the Western Hemisphere: Early Documentation and Transmission by the Slave Trade* (Basel, Verlag für Recht und Gesellschaft, 1969).

Hopkins, Donald R., *Princes and Peasants:*

Smallpox in History (Chicago, University of Chicago Press, 1983).

Kiple, Kenneth F., *The Caribbean Slave: A Biological History* (Cambridge, Cambridge University Press, 1984).

Kiple, Kenneth F. (ed.), *The Cambridge World History of Human Diseases* (Cambridge, Cambridge University Press, 1993).

Livingstone, Frank B., *Abnormal Hemoglobins in Human Populations* (Chicago, Aldine, 1967).

McGrew, Roderick E., *Encyclopedia of Medical History* (New York, McGraw-Hill, 1985).

McKeown, Thomas, *The Origins of Human Disease* (Oxford and New York, Basil Blackwell, 1988).

McKeown, Thomas, *The Modern Rise of Population* (London, Edward Arnold, 1976).

McNeill, William H., *Plagues and Peoples* (Garden City, NY, Anchor Press/Doubleday, 1976).

Ramenofsky, Ann, *Vectors of Death: The Archaeology of European Contact* (Albuquerque, University of New Mexico Press, 1987).

Roe, Daphne A., *A Plague of Corn: The Social History of Pellagra* (Ithaca, Cornell University Press, 1973).

Scrimshaw, Nevin S., Taylor, Carl E. and Gordon, Jack E., *Interactions of Nutrition and Infection* (Geneva, World Health Organization, 1968).

Stannard, David E., *Before the Horror: The Population of Hawaii on the Eve of Western Contact* (Honolulu, University of Hawaii Press, 1989).

Wrigley, Anthony and Scofield, Roger S., *The Population History of England, 1541–1871* (Cambridge, MA, Harvard University Press, 1981).

Zinsser, Hans, *Rats, Lice, and History*, 4th edn (London, Routledge, 1942).

The rise of medicine (Chapter 2)

Edelstein, L., *Ancient Medicine* (Baltimore, Johns Hopkins University Press, 1987).

Estes, J. Worth, *The Medical Skills of Ancient Egypt* (Canton, MA, Science History Publications, 1989).

Jackson, R., *Doctors and Diseases in the Roman Empire* (London, British Museum Publications, 1988).

Jones, Peter Murray, *Medieval Medical Miniatures* (London, British Library, 1984).

Lloyd, G. E. R., *The Revolutions of Wisdom* (Berkeley, University of California Press, 1987).

Longrigg, J. N., *Greek Rational Medicine* (London, Routledge, 1993).

Nutton, V., *From Democedes to Harvey* (London, Variorum, 1988).

Siraisi, N. G., *Medieval and Early Renaissance Medicine* (Chicago, University of Chicago Press, 1990).

Temkin, O., *Hippocrates in a World of Pagans and Christians* (Baltimore, Johns Hopkins University Press, 1991).

Ullmann, Manfred, *Islamic Medicine* (Edinburgh University Press, 1978).

What is disease? (Chapter 3)

Balint, M., *The Doctor, His Patient, and the Illness* (London, Pitman, 1957).

Black, Nick *et al.* (eds), *Health and Disease: A Reader* (Milton Keynes, Open University Press, 1984).

Bynum, W.F. and Porter, Roy (eds), *Companion Encyclopaedia of the History of Medicine*, 2 vols (London, Routledge, 1993).

Caplan, A.L., Engelhardt, H.T., and MacCartney, J.J. (eds), *Concepts of Health and Disease* (Reading, MA, Addison-Wesley, 1981).

Currer, Caroline and Stacey, Meg, *Concepts of Health, Illness and Disease: A Comparative Perspective* (Leamington Spa, Berg, 1986).

Douglas, Mary, *Purity and Danger: An Analysis of Concepts of Pollution and Taboo* (Harmondsworth, Penguin, 1966).

Dubos, René, *The Mirage of Health* (New York, Harper, 1959).

Engelhardt, Jr, H. Tristram, 'The concepts of health and disease', in Tristram Engelhardt and Stuart F. Spicker (eds), *Evaluation and Explanation in the Biomedical Sciences* (Dordrecht, Reidel, 1975), pp. 125–141.

Fee, Elizabeth and Fox, Daniel M. (eds), *AIDS, The Burdens of History* (Berkeley, Los Angeles and London, University of California Press, 1988).

Fee, Elizabeth and Fox, Daniel M. (eds), *AIDS: The Making of a Chronic Disease* (Berkeley, Los Angeles and London, University of California Press, 1992).

Flew, Anthony, *Crime or Disease?* (London, Macmillan, 1973).

Foucault, M., *Naissance de la Clinique: Une Archéologie du Regard Médical* (Paris, Presses Universitaires de France, 1963); transl. by A. M. Sheridan Smith as *The Birth of the Clinic* (London, Tavistock, 1973).

Gilman, Sander L., *Seeing the Insane* (New York, Brunner, Mazel, 1982).

Gilman, Sander, *Disease and Representation: From Madness to AIDS* (Ithaca, Cornell University Press, 1988).

Gilman, Sander L., *Difference and Pathology* (Ithaca, Cornell University Press, 1985).

Helman, C., *Culture, Health and Illness* (Bristol, Wright, 1984).

Illich, I., *Limits to Medicine: The Expropriation of Health* (London, Marion Boyars, 1976; paperback edition, Harmondsworth, Penguin, 1977).

Keele, K., *Anatomies of Pain* (Oxford, Blackwell Scientific Publications, 1957).

King, Lester S., *The Philosophy of Medicine: The Early Eighteenth Century* (Cambridge, MA, Harvard University Press, 1978).

King, Lester S., *The Growth of Medical Thought* (Chicago, University of Chicago Press, 1963).

Kleinman, A., *Social Origins of Distress and Disease: Depression, Neurasthenia, and Pain in Modern China* (New Haven, Yale University Press, 1986).

Parsons, Talcott, *The Social System* (Glencoe, IL, Free Press, 1951).

Riese, Walther, *The Conception of Disease, its History, its Versions and its Nature* (New York, Philosophical Library, 1953).

Risse, G., 'Health and disease: history of the concepts', in W. T. Reich (ed.), *Encyclopedia of Bioethics*, vol. 2 (New York, Free Press, 1978), pp. 579–85.

Rosenberg, Charles E. and Golden, Janet (eds), *Framing Disease: Studies in Cultural History* (New Brunswick, Rutgers University Press, 1992).

Sacks, Oliver, *A Leg to Stand On* (London, Duckworth, 1984).

Sontag, S., *AIDS as Metaphor* (Harmondsworth, Allen Lane, 1989).

Taylor, F. Kräupl, *The Concepts of Illness, Disease and Morbus* (Cambridge, Cambridge University Press, 1979).

Turner, Bryan S., *Medical Power and Social Knowledge* (London and Beverly Hills, Sage Publications, 1987).

Watts, Geoff, *Pleasing the Patient* (London, Faber, 1992).

Primary care (Chapter 4)

Beeson, Paul B. and Maulitz, Russell C., 'The inner history of internal medicine', in C. Maulitz and Diana E. Long (eds), *Grand Rounds: One Hundred Years of Internal Medicine* (Philadelphia, University of Pennsylvania Press, 1988), pp. 15–54.

Bliss, Michael, *The Discovery of Insulin* (Toronto, McClelland and Stewart, 1982).

Brotherston, John, 'Evolution of Medical Practice', in Gordon McLachlan and Thomas McKeown (eds), *Medical History and Medical Care* (London, Oxford University Press, 1971), pp. 84–125.

Cartwright, Ann and Anderson, Robert, *General Practice Revisited: A Second Study of Patients and Their Doctors* (London, Tavistock, 1981).

Foster, W. D., *A Short History of Clinical Pathology* (Edinburgh, Livingstone, 1961).

Hodgkin, Keith, *Towards Earlier Diagnosis in Primary Care*, 4th edn (Edinburgh, Churchill Livingstone, 1978; first published 1963).

Johnston, William Victor, *Before the Age of Miracles: Memoirs of a Country Doctor* (Toronto, Fitzhenry and Whiteside, 1972).

King, Lester S., *The Medical World of the Eighteenth Century* (Chicago, University of Chicago Press, 1958).

Koos, Earl Lomon, *The Health of Regionville: What the People Thought and Did about It* (New York, Columbia University Press, 1954).

Loudon, I. S. L., *Medical Care and the General Practitioner, 1750–1850* (Oxford, Clarendon Press, 1986).

Parssinen, Terry M., *Secret Passions, Secret Remedies: Narcotic Drugs in British Society, 1820–1930* (Philadelphia, Institute for the Study of Human Issues, 1983).

Peterson, M. Jeanne, *The Medical Profession in Mid-Victorian London* (Berkeley, University of California Press, 1978).

Porter, Roy (ed.), *Patients and Practitioners: Lay Perceptions Of Medicine in Pre-industrial Society* (Cambridge, Cambridge University Press, 1985).

Reiser, Stanley Joel, *Medicine and the Reign of Technology* (Cambridge, Cambridge University Press, 1978).

Rosenberg, Charles, 'The practice of medicine in New York a century ago', *Bulletin of the History of Medicine*, vol. 41 (1967), pp. 223–53.

Rothstein, William G., *American Physicians in the Nineteenth Century: From Sects to Science* (Baltimore, Johns Hopkins University Press, 1972).

Shorter, Edward, *Bedside Manners: The Troubled History of Doctors and Patients* (New York, Simon and Schuster, 1985); republished with a new preface as *Doctors and Their Patients: A Social History* (New Brunswick, NJ, Transaction Publishers, 1991).

Shorter, Edward, *From Paralysis to Fatigue: A History of Psychosomatic Illness in the Modern Era* (New York, Free Press, 1992).

Sneader, Walter, *Drug Discovery: The Evolution of Modern Medicines* (Chicester, Wiley, 1985).

Starr, Paul, *The Social Transformation of American Medicine* (New York, Basic Books, 1982).

Stevens, Rosemary, *Medical Practice in Modern England: The Impact of Specialization and State Medicine* (New Haven, Yale University Press, 1966).

Stevens, Rosemary, *American Medicine and the Public Interest* (New Haven, Yale University Press, 1971).

Taylor, Stephen, *Good General Practice* (London, Oxford University Press, 1954).

Warner, John Harley, *The Therapeutic Perspective: Medical Practice, Knowledge, and Identity in America, 1820–1885* (Cambridge, MA, Harvard University Press, 1986).

Medical science (Chapter 5)

Booth, Christopher, *Doctors in Science and Society: Essays of a Clinical Scientist* (London, British Medical Journal, 1987).

Brock, Thomas D., *Robert Koch: A Life in Medicine and Bacteriology* (Madison, WI, Science Tech Publishers, 1988).

Bulloch, William, *The History of Bacteriology: University of London, Heath Clark Lectures, 1936* (London, Oxford University Press, 1938); reprinted in 1960 (New York, Dover, 1979).

Bynum, W. F., *Science and the Practice of Medicine in the Nineteenth Century* (Cambridge, Cambridge University Press, 1994).

Bynum, W. F. and Porter, Roy (eds), *Companion Encyclopedia of the History of Medicine* (London, Routledge, 1993). Various chapters offer the best up-to-date short summaries of particular dimensions of medical science.

Coleman, William and Holmes, Frederic L. (eds), *The Investigative Enterprise: Experimental Physiology in Nineteenth-Century Medicine* (Berkeley, Los Angeles, and London, University of California Press, 1988).

Cunningham, George J., *The History of British Pathology* (Bristol, White Tree Books, 1992).

Foster, W. D., *A Short History of Clinical Pathology* (Edinburgh, Livingstone, 1961).

Foster, W. D., *A History of Medical Bacteriology and Immunology* (London, Heinemann, 1970).

Frank, Robert G., *Harvey and the Oxford Physiologists: Scientific Ideas and Social Interaction* (Berkeley, University of California Press, 1980).

Fye, W. Bruce, *The Development of American Physiology: Scientific Medicine in the Nineteenth Century* (Baltimore, Johns Hopkins University Press, 1987).

Goodfield, June G., *The Growth of Scientific Physiology* (London, Hutchinson, 1960).

Hall, Thomas S., *Ideas of Life and Matter: Studies in the History of General Physiology 600 B.C. to 1900 A.D.*, 2 vols (Chicago, University of Chicago Press, 1969).

Harvey, William, *An Anatomical Disputation Concerning the Movement of the Heart and Blood in Living Creatures*, transl. by G. Whitteridge (Oxford, Blackwell Scientific, 1976).

Long, E. R., *A History of Pathology* (New York, Dover Publications, 1965).

Maulitz, Russell C., *Morbid Appearances: the Anatomy of Pathology in the Early Nineteenth Century* (Cambridge and New York, Cambridge University Press, 1987).

Roberts, K. B., *The Fabric of the Body: European Traditions of Anatomical Illustration* (Oxford and New York, Clarendon Press, 1992).

Rothschuh, Karl E., *History of Physiology* (original German edn, 1953); edited and transl. by G. B. Risse (Huntington, NY, Robert E. Krieger, 1973).

Singer, C. and Underwood, E. Ashworth, *A Short History of Medicine* (New York and Oxford, Oxford University Press, 1962).

Hospitals and surgery (Chapter 6)

Abel-Smith, B., *The Hospitals 1500–1848: A Study in Social Administration in England and Wales* (London, Heinemann, l964).

Ackerknecht, Erwin H., *Medicine at the Paris Hospital, 1794–1848* (Baltimore, Johns Hopkins University Press, 1967).

Cartwright, F. F., *The Development of Modern Surgery* (London, Arthur Barker; New York, Thomas Y. Crowell, 1967).

Dally, Ann, *Women Under the Knife; A History of Surgery* (London:,Hutchinson Radius, 1991; New York, Routledge, 1992).

Freidson, Eliot (ed.), *The Hospital in Modern Society* (London, Collier and MacMillan, 1963).

Gelfand, Toby, *Professionalizing Modern Medicine: Paris Surgeons and Medical Science and Institutions in the 18th Century* (Westport, CT, Greenwood Press, 1980).

Granshaw, Lindsay, *St. Mark's Hospital, London: A Social History of a Specialist Hospital* (London, King's Fund, 1985).

Granshaw, Lindsay and Porter, Roy (eds), *The Hospital in History* (London, Routledge, 1989; paperback edition, 1990).

Granshaw, Lindsay, 'The hospital', in W. F. Bynum and Roy Porter (eds), *Companion Encyclopedia of the History of Medicine* (London, Routledge, 1993), pp. 1173–95.

Haeger, Knut, *The Illustrated History of Surgery* (New York, Bell, 1988).

Hunt, Tony, *The Medieval Surgery* (Woodbridge, Sussex, Boydell Press, 1992).

Hurwitz, Alfred and Degenshein, George A., *Milestones in Modern Surgery* (New York, Hoeber-Harper, 1958).

Jones, Colin, *The Charitable Imperative: Hospitals and Nursing in Ancien Régime and Revolutionary France*, Wellcome Institute Series in the History of Medicine (London and New York, Routledge, 1989).

Lawrence, Christopher (ed.), *Medical Theory, Surgical Practice: Studies in the History of Surgery* (London and New York, Routledge, 1992).

Lawrence, Ghislaine, 'Surgery (traditional)', in W. F. Bynum and Roy Porter (eds), *Companion Encyclopedia of the History of Medicine* (London, Routledge, 1993), pp. 957–79.

Nightingale, Florence, *Notes on Hospitals* (London, John W. Parker & Son, 1859).

Pickstone, John, *Medicine and Industrial Society: A History of Hospital Development in Manchester and its Region 1752–1946* (Manchester, Manchester University Press, 1985).

Pouchelle, Marie-Christine, *The Body and Surgery in the Middle Ages*, transl. by Rosemary Morris (New Brunswick, Rutgers University Press, 1990).

Poynter, F. N. L. (ed.), *The Evolution of Hospitals in Britain* (London, Pitman, 1964).

Ravitch, Mark M., *A Century of Surgery: 1880–1980*, 2 vols (Philadelphia, J. B. Lipincott, 1982).

Risse, Guenter, *Hospital Life in Enlightenment Scotland: Care and Teaching at the Royal Infirmary of Edinburgh* (Cambridge, Cambridge University Press, 1986).

Rosenberg, Charles E., *The Care of Strangers: The Rise of America's Hospital System* (New York, Basic Books, 1987).

Stevens, Rosemary, *In Sickness and in Wealth: American Hospitals in the Twentieth Century* (New York, Basic Books, 1989).

Taylor, Jeremy R. B., *Hospital and Asylum Architecture in England 1840–1914: Building for Health Care* (London/New York, Mansell, 1991).

Thompson, J. D. and Goldin, G., *The Hospital: A Social and Architectural History* (New Haven and London, Yale University Press, 1975).

Tröhler, Ulrich, 'Surgery (modern)', in W. F. Bynum and Roy Porter (eds), *Companion*

Encyclopedia of the History of Medicine
(London, Routledge, 1993), pp. 980–1023.
Wallace, Anthony F., *The Progress of Plastic
Surgery: An Introductory History* (Oxford,
William A. Meeuws, 1982).
Wangensteen, Owen H. and Wangensteen, Sarah
D., *The Rise of Surgery: From Empiric Craft to
Scientific Discipline* (Minneapolis, University of
Minnesota Press, 1978; Folkestone, Kent,
Dawson, 1978).
Woodward, J., *To Do The Sick No Harm: A Study
of the British Voluntary Hospital System to 1875*
(London and Boston, Routledge & Kegan
Paul, 1974).

Drug treatment and the rise of pharmacology (Chapter 7)
Binden, J. S. & Ledniger, D. (eds), *Chronicles of
Drug Discovery* (New York, Wiley, 1982).
Bliss, M., *The Discovery of Insulin* (Toronto,
McClelland & Stewart, 1982).
Blunt, Wilfrid and Raphael, Sandra, *The
Illustrated Herbal* (London, Francis
Lincoln/Weidenfeld & Nicolson, n.d.).
Holmstedt, B. & Liljestrand, G., *Readings in
Pharmacology* (Oxford, Pergamon Press,
1963).
Pagel, W., *Paracelsus: An Introduction to
Philosophical Medicine in the Era of the
Renaissance*, 2nd rev. edn (Basel, Karger,
1982).
Parascandola, J., *The Development of American
Pharmacology: John J. Abel and the Shaping of a
Discipline* (Baltimore amd London, Johns
Hopkins University Press, 1992).
Ross, W. S., *The Life/Death Ratio: Benefits and
Risks in Modern Medicines* (New York, Reader's
Digest Press, 1977).
Sneader, W., *Drug Discovery: The Evaluation of
Modern Medicines* (Chichester, Wiley, 1985).
Weatherall, M., *In Search of a Cure: A History of
Pharmaceutical Discovery* (Oxford, Oxford
University Press, Oxford, 1990).

Mental illness (Chapter 8)
Alexander, Franz G. and Selesnick, Sheldon T.,
*The History of Psychiatry: An Evaluation of
Psychiatric Thought and Practice from
Prehistoric Times to the Present* (London, Allen
& Unwin, 1967).
Barham, Peter, *Closing the Asylum: The Mental
Patient in Modern Society* (Harmondsworth,
Penguin, 1992).
Feder, L., *Madness in Literature* (Princeton,
Princeton University Press, 1980).

Foucault, Michel, *La Folie et la Déraison: Histoire
de la Folie à l'Age Classique* (Paris, Librairie
Plon, 1961); abridged as *Madness and
Civilization: A History of Insanity in the Age of
Reason*, transl. by Richard Howard (New York,
Random House, 1965).
Howells, John (ed.), *World History of Psychiatry*
(New York, Bruner/Mazel, 1968).
Howells, John G. and Osborn, M. Livia, *A
Reference Companion to the History of Abnormal
Psychology* (Westport, CT, Greenwood Press,
1984).
Hunter, Richard and Macalpine, Ida, *Three
Hundred Years of Psychiatry: 1535–1860*
(London, Oxford University Press, 1963).
Ingleby, David (ed.), *Critical Psychiatry: The
Politics of Mental Health* (Harmondsworth,
Penguin, 1981).
Laing, R. D., *The Divided Self* (New York, Random
House, 1969).
Peterson, D. (ed.), *A Mad People's History of
Madness* (Pittsburgh, University of Pittsburgh
Press, 1982).
Porter, Roy, *Mind Forg'd Manacles: Madness and
Psychiatry in England from Restoration to
Regency* (London, Athlone Press, 1987; paper-
back edition, Penguin, 1990).
Porter,Roy, *A Social History of Madness* (London,
Weidenfeld & Nicolson, 1987; paperback edi-
tion, 1989).
Porter, Roy, *The Faber Book of Madness* (London,
Faber, 1991).
Scheff, Thomas, *Being Mentally Ill: A Sociological
Theory* (Chicago, Aldine Press, 1966).
Scull, Andrew, *The Most Solitary of Afflictions:
Madness and Society in Britain, 1700–1900*
(New Haven and London, Yale University
Press, 1993).
Scull, Andrew, *Decarceration: Community
Treatment and the Deviant – A Radical View*,
2nd edn (Oxford, Polity Press; New
Brunswick, Rutgers University Press, 1984).
Sedgwick, Peter, *Psychopolitics* (London, Pluto
Press; New York, Harper and Row, 1982).
Simon, Bennett, *Mind and Madness in Ancient
Greece* (Ithaca, Cornell University Press, 1978).
Skultans, V., *Madness and Morals: Ideas on
Insanity in the Nineteenth Century* (London and
Boston, Routledge & Kegan Paul, 1975).
Szasz, Thomas S., *The Manufacture of Madness*
(New York, Dell, 1970; London, Paladin, 1972).
Szasz, Thomas S., *The Myth of Mental Illness:
Foundations of a Theory of Personal Conduct*
(London, Granada, 1972; revised edn, New
York, Harper and Row, 1974).

Szasz, Thomas S., *The Age of Madness: The History
of Involuntary Mental Hospitalization Presented
in Selected Texts* (London, Routledge and
Kegan Paul, 1975).

Medicine, society, and the state (Chapter 9)
Fox, Daniel, *Health Policies, Health Economics:
The British and American Experiences,
1911–1965* (Princeton, Princeton University
Press, 1986).
Hollingsworth, J. Rogers, *A Political Economy of
Medicine: Great Britain and the United States*
(Baltimore, Johns Hopkins University Press,
1986).
Hollingsworth, J. Rogers, Haget, Jerald, and
Hanneman, Robert A., *State Intervention in
Medical Care: Consequences for Britain, France,
Sweden and the United States, 1890–1970*
(Ithaca, Cornell University Press, 1986).
Klein, Rudolf, *The Politics of the NHS* (London,
Longman, 1983).
Rosen, George, *A History of Public Health* (New
York, MD Publications, 1986).
Rosenberg, Charles E., *The Care of Strangers: The
Rise of America's Hospital System* (New York,
Basic Books, 1987).
Starr, Paul, *The Social Transformation of American
Medicine: The Rise of a Sovereign Profession and
the Making of a Vast Industry* (New York, Basic
Books, 1982).
Stevens, Rosemary, *Medical Practice in Modern
England: The Impact of Specialization and State
Medicine* (New Haven, Yale University Press,
1966).
Stevens, Rosemary, *In Sickness and in Wealth:
American Hospitals in the Twentieth Century*
(New York, Basic Books, 1989).

Looking to the future (Chapter 10)
Austyn, J. M. (ed.), *New Prospects for Medicine*
(Oxford, Oxford University Press, 1988).
Helman, C., *Culture, Health and Illness* (Bristol,
Wright, 1984).
Illich, I., *Limits to Medicine: The Exploration of
Health* (London, Marion Boyars, 1976; paper-
back edn, Penguin, 1977).
Kennedy, I., *The Unmasking of Medicine* (London,
Allen & Unwin, 1981).
McKeown, T., *The Role of Medicine* (Oxford,
Blackwell, 1979).
Pietroni, P., *The Greening of Medicine* (London,
Gollancz, 1990).
Wilkie, T., *Perilous Knowledge* (London, Faber,
1993).

Index of Medical Personalities

General Index

Acknowledgements

Every effort has been made to obtain permission to use the copyright material listed below; the publishers apologize for any errors or omissions and would welcome these being brought to their attention.

PHOTOGRAPHS

Gemeente Musea Delft, Delft *cover*; **Wellcome Institute Library**, London *half-title*, 24, 25, 35, 39, 43, 46, 47, 48, 55, 57, 68, 70, 79, 81, 82, 84, 89, 92, 93, 94, 98, 100, 102, 108, 110, 111, 112, 115 (© Little, Brown and Company, 1980), 116, 121, 125, 126, 127, 129, 140, 141, 146, 147, 155, 156, 159, 160, 161, 163, 164, 166, 172, 173, 174, 177, 187, 188, 191, 194, 200, 203, 209, 210, 218*t,b*, 219, 220, 222*l,r*, 227, 231*l*, 236, 243, 247, 252, 253, 254, 256, 258, 262, 274, 275, 278, 282, 284, 285, 289, 290, 292, 293 (Royal Medico-Psychological Association Library), 296, 297 (© H. Kimpton, London), 304, 308, 309, 311*t,b*, 314, 326, 331; **Memling Museum**, Bruges *title-page*; **Science Photo Library** (J. C. Revy) 7, (Moredun Animal Health Ltd) 23, (BSIP, LECA) 239, 350, (NIBSC) 343, (CDC) 346, (Hank Morgan) 359, 362, (Will & Deni McIntyre) 363, (BSIP, Roux) 370; **The Alan Mason Chesney Medical Archives of The Johns Hopkins Medical Institutions**, Baltimore 8, 182, 197, 237; **British Library**, London 9, 58, 204; **Frank Spooner/Gamma-Liaison** 10 (R. Gaillarde), 367; **Network** (Bilderberg/R. Drexel) 11, (Barry Lewis) 369; **Panos Pictures** (Penny Tweedie) 12, 303, (Ron Giling) 17, (unnamed photographer) 50, (C. Paul Harrison) 267, (Sean Sprague) 341; *Nature*, **Macmillan Magazines Ltd** 16 (Professor Alan Walker), 19 (courtesy of Dr Simon Davis); **Manchester University Museum** 20 (courtesy of Joann Fletcher); **The Natural History Museum**, London 21; **Fratelli Alinari** 28, 52, 205, 212; **Hulton Deutsch Collection** 29, 41, 44, 124, 149, 185, 238, 242, 325, 329; **AKG, London** 33, 110, 119, 122*r*, 137, 143, 167, 170 (Kunsthistorisches Museum, Vienna), 190 (Wyeth Laboratories, Philadelphia), 211, 230 (Boston Medical Library, Francis A. Countway Library of Medicine, Boston), 261, 263, 266, 278, 307, 310; **Trinity College/University Library, Cambridge** 37, 64, 75; **Clark Spencer Larsen**, University of North Carolina 45; **Iowa State University Library/University Archives** 49; **British Museum** (courtesy of the Trustees) 53; **Vatican, Biblioteca Apostolicana**, Rome 59; **Ancient Art & Architecture Collection** 61; **Bibliothèque Nationale**, Paris 63, 250; **Sonia Halliday Photographs** (André Held) 66, (Hassia) 248; **Victoria & Albert Museum** (by permission of The Board and Trustees) 72; **Sächsische Landesbibliothek/Deutsche Fotothek** (A. Rous) 76; **Bodleian Library**, Oxford 77, 80; **Museum of London** 78*t*, 288; **Scala** 78*b* (Archivio di Stato, Lucca), 91 (Vatican), 206 (Museum voor Schone Kunsten, Gent); **Museum für Volkerkunde, Berlin/Werner Forman Archive** 83; **Arxiu MAS** 84 (Academia S. Fernando), 131 (Museo de Bellas Artes, Seville), 139 (collection of Doña Carmen Marañon Vinda de Fernández de Araoz, Madrid); **St Bartholomew's Hospital Archives/Prudence Cumming Associates** 87; **York City Art Gallery** 97; **US National Library of Medicine**, Bethesda 103; **Tate Gallery**, London 107, 135; **Hahnemann University Archives**, Medical College of Pennsylvania and Hahnemann University, Philadelphia 114; **Bridgeman Art Library** 118 (Tate Gallery, London); **New York Historical Society**, Olds Collection no. 96 22*l*; **Bildarchiv Preussischer Kulturbesitz**,

Berlin 130, 178; **E.T. Archive** 134, 181, 183, 246, 259, 265*l,r*, 271*t*, 322; **Topham** 148, 332; *The Spectator*, London 152; **J.-L. Charmet** 169, 175, 223 (Musée Carnavalet), 295 (Académie Nationale de Médicine); **Institut für Geschichte der Medizin der Universität**, Vienna 180, 301; **Brown Brothers** 186; **MacQuitty International Collection** 202, 241, 302; **Fotomas/Barnaby's Picture Library** 208, 231*r*; **Museum der Stadt/Fotostudio Otto** 214; **Royal College of Surgeons of England** 217, 225; **Jefferson Medical College, Thomas Jefferson University**, Philadelphia 230; **Österreichische Galerie**, Belvedere, Vienna 235; **Dr Simon Fishel**, NURTURE (Nottingham University Research and Treatment Unit in Reproduction) 240; **Powell Moya Archive** (Colin Westwood) 245; **Österreichisches Nationalbibliothek**, Vienna 249, 251; **Popperfoto** 271*b*, 276, (AFP) 358; **Studio Basset** 279 (Musée des Beaux-Arts de Lyon); **Visual Arts Library** 287 (Courtauld Institute, London); **Mary Evans Picture Library** 299 (Freud Family Archive); **Novosti**, London 305; **Manchester Central Library**, Local Studies Unit 316, 318, 319; **Rochdale Community Services Department** 317; **Philadelphia Museum of Art**, reproduced from *Medicine and the Artist* (*Ars Medica*) by permission, 324; **Range/Bettmann** 327, 347; **Museum of Finnish Architecture**, Helsinki 328; **Royal Marsden Hospital Archive/Pictorial Press** 335; **Dr William M. Larson**, Center for Macromolecular Crystallography, University of Alabama, Birmingham 351; **Ann & Bury Peerless** 354; **Jones Institute for Reproductive Medicine**, Eastern Virginia Medical School 364.

MAPS AND DIAGRAMS

26, adapted from 'The bubonic plague' by C. McEvedy, Copyright (1988) *Scientific American* Inc., all rights reserved; 31, from 'North America' by Frank C. Innes, in *The Cambridge World History of Human Disease* (Cambridge University Press, 1993); 34, from Paul F. Russell, Luther S. West, and Reginald D. Manwell, *Practical Malariology* (W. B. Saunders, 1946), fig. 128; 42, from George K. Strode (ed.), *Yellow Fever* (McGraw-Hill, 1951), fig. 67; 74, adapted from Edward P. Cheyney, *The Dawn of a New Era, 1250–1453* (Harper & Row, 1962); 158, from Charles Singer and C. Rabin, *A Prelude to Modern Science* (Cambridge University Press, 1946), fig. 21/ Wellcome Institute Library, London; 344, reproduced, by permission of WHO, from 'The current global situation of the HIV/AIDS pandemic', *Weekly Epidemiological Record* vol. 70 (2), 8 (1995), map 2; 355, data from Population Reference Bureau, *World Population Data Sheet, 1995*; 356, reproduced, by permission of WHO, from 'World malaria situation, 1989, Parts I and II', *Weekly Epidemiological Record* vol. 66 (22–23), 157–63, 167–70 (1991), Map 91363.

For their help with the preparation of this book, Sarah Bunney thanks the staff of the Wellcome Centre Photographic Library, Dr Peggy Jefferies of the University of Reading, and Nigel Wright of European Map Graphics; John Pickstone acknowledges the helpful comments of Toby Gelfand, Ron Numbers, Patrice Pinell, Roy Porter, Paul Weindling, and Paul Wilding; and Roy Porter records his immense gratitude to Frieda Houser and Caroline Overy of the Wellcome Institute.